Endoscopic
Surgery

MOSBY'S PERIOPERATIVE NURSING SERIES

Endoscopic Surgery

Kay A. Ball, RN, BSN, MSA, CNOR

Nurse Educator/Consultant
Lewis Center, Ohio

with 445 illustrations

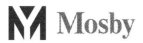 Mosby

St. Louis Baltimore Boston Carlsbad Chicago Naples New York Philadelphia Portland
London Madrid Mexico City Singapore Sydney Tokyo Toronto Wiesbaden

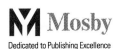

Dedicated to Publishing Excellence

A Times Mirror
Company

Publisher: Nanci L. Coon
Editor: Michael S. Ledbetter
Developmental Editor: Nancy L. O'Brien
Project Manager: Mark Spann
Production Editor: Anne Salmo
Designer: Judi Lang

A NOTE TO THE READER:

The author and publisher have made every attempt to check dosages and nursing content for accuracy. Because the science of pharmacology is continually advancing, our knowledge base continues to expand. Therefore we recommend that the reader always check product information for changes in dosage or administration before administering any medication. This is particularly important with new or rarely used drugs.

Printed in the United States of America
Composition by Arthur Morgan Company, Inc.

Mosby–Year Book, Inc.
11830 Westline Industrial Drive
St. Louis, Missouri 63146

Library of Congress Cataloging-in-Publication Data

Ball, Kay, RN.
     Endoscopic surgery / Kay A. Ball.
    p.   cm. — (Mosby's perioperative nursing series)
Includes bibliographical references.
ISBN 0-8151-0600-9
1. Endoscopic surgery. 2. Surgical nursing. I. Title.
  II. Series.
    [DNLM: 1. Surgery, Endoscopic—nurses' instruction.
  2. Perioperative Nursing—methods.   WO 500 B187e 1997]
  RD33.53.B35   1997
  617'.05–dc20
  DNLM/DLC
  for Library of Congress   96–44663
                                      CIP

97 98 99 00 01 / 9 8 7 6 5 4 3 2 1

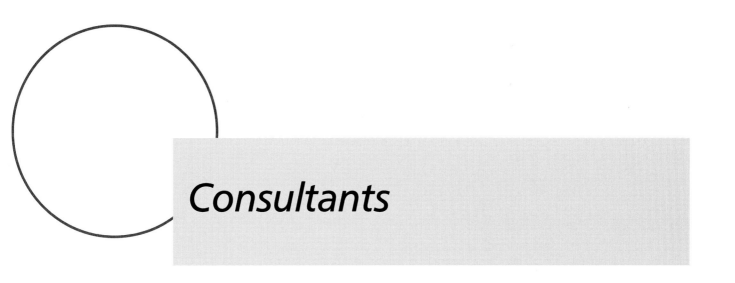

Consultants

Sandra L. Dunn, RN, CNOR, BSEd
Clinical Educator
St. Lukes Hospital Medical Center
Phoenix, Arizona

Sherrie Holliman, RN, CNOR
Director, Surgical Technology
Thomas Technical Institute
Thomasville, Georgia

Marilyn A. Hunter, RN, PhD, CNOR
Program Director Surgical Technologies
Daytona Beach Community College
Daytona Beach, Florida

To Cassidy Disco Ball

*My first grandchild,
my link to the future*

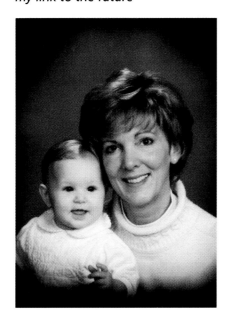

8/27/97

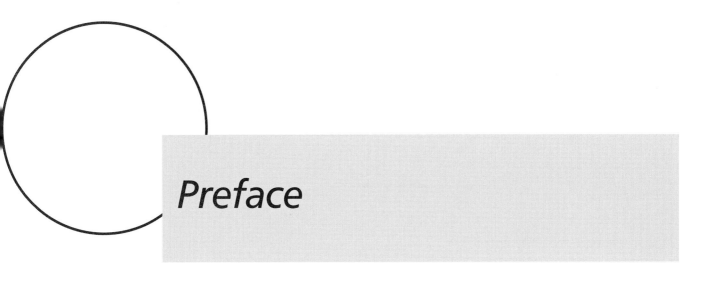

Preface

Endoscopy has evolved and matured so quickly over recent years that significant effects have been felt by perioperative nurses. The rapidity of endoscopic advancements has challenged perioperative nurses to master this technology quickly and adapt their practices to provide safe and appropriate patient care during the various endoscopic procedures.

I remember the first time I observed an endoscopic procedure as a student nurse years ago. Laparoscopic surgery was being performed on a woman for endometriosis. I watched in eager anticipation as the surgeon manipulated the laparoscope inside her abdomen to identify and ablate the endometrial implants. Several times he showed me what he was doing through the laparoscope since cameras and monitors were not used very often during laparoscopic procedures at that time. I was very impressed with the technical equipment and instrumentation that enabled this procedure to be performed with great ease. The perioperative nurses had modified their nursing skills to this new, evolving endoscopic technique. Even though the nurses made their work look very easy, the instruments and equipment were very confusing to a novice like me who wasn't used to this type of minimally invasive surgery. I needed a nursing book explaining endoscopic procedures to help me understand and develop my endoscopic skills, but none was available at that time.

This incident happened more than 20 years ago, but the need for knowledge of and skills for endoscopic surgery remain today. Endoscopic procedures continue to evolve as techniques, equipment, instrumentation, and patient care become more sophisticated and exact. The perioperative nurse must stay current with these changes and new developments. *Endoscopic Surgery* provides an easy-to-understand educational guide to help simplify the complex aspects of endoscopic surgery.

This book was written to help nurses master the art and technology of endoscopic surgery with the following two goals in mind:
1. To examine the evolution and impact of endoscopy and the nursing practices that have been adapted to accommodate these technological advancements.
2. To highlight the technology of endoscopy, including instrumentation, equipment, video systems, and energies used through an endoscope. The hundreds of photographs and drawings found throughout the book help illustrate and simplify the complexity of this technology.

Chapters 1 and 2 describe the history of endoscopy and its impact on perioperative nurses. Chapters 3 and 4 detail the various roles and responsibilities of the members of the endoscopic team, as well as the requisite education and training. Chapters 5 and 6 discuss how nursing care and considerations for the patient undergoing endoscopy have been incorporated into the organized and practical steps of the nursing process.

The next five chapters discuss the technical aspects of endoscopy that the perioperative nurse must understand to provide a safe surgical environment. Chapter 7 describes endoscopic instruments and their uses in detail, while Chapter 8 discusses the care needed to reprocess and maintain instrumentation. Chapter 9 focuses on devices ranging from light sources to insufflators that are used during endoscopic procedures. Chapter 10 discusses video technologies, and Chapter 11 describes the various energies used through an endoscope.

I want to acknowledge the great number of endoscopy-related surgical companies who helped supply me with information, illustrations, and graphics of various endoscopic devices or techniques. The illustrations used throughout the book were contributed not to promote a product or company but rather to characterize and enhance the text. My gratitude also is extended to my nursing colleagues and physicians who provided experience and knowledge to foster a greater understanding of endoscopic surgery.

Special recognition goes to my husband, Dan, who patiently supported me through the adventure of writing this book. His wisdom and experience helped me create the words needed to communicate my message.

Lastly I would like to acknowledge a new breath in my life, my first grandchild. Cassidy Disco Ball represents the future to me As I look at her tiny face, feel her soft skin, and cuddle her warm, little body, I embrace tomorrow. By the time she is an adult, endoscopy will be so common that open procedures will be a thing of the past. Dedicating this book to her represents the capture of today's foundation of endoscopic skills and knowledge that will continuously grow and evolve to be applied in tomorrow's surgical arena.

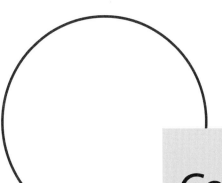

Contents

11   *ENDOSCOPIC ENERGIES AND DIAGNOSTIC TOOLS* 165

APPENDIX

Endoscopic
Surgery

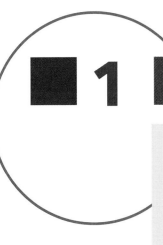

The Evolution of Endoscopy

ENDOSCOPY DEFINED

In recent years health care has experienced an amazing reformation that has completely changed the way in which many surgical procedures are now performed. Physicians no longer need to make large incisions to access body organs or cavities. Instead, surgical entry is achieved through small incisions (Fig. 1-1) or natural body openings (Fig. 1-2) that provide a passage for surgical instruments. The internal structures are viewed directly through a lens or on a video monitor while the surgical procedure is performed using endoscopic instrumentation (Fig. 1-3).

Endoscopy is the inspection of body organs or cavities by means of an endoscope, which is a device consisting of a tube and optical system. Because it provides the means to perform minimally invasive procedures, patients usually experience less postoperative discomfort and recover more quickly than patients who undergo more invasive procedures. Endoscopy has begun to be widely used as advancements in endoscopes, cameras, endoscopic instrumentation, and surgical techniques have evolved.

THE BEGINNING OF ENDOSCOPY

Endoscopy may have had its start with the curiosity to look inside body cavities or canals. During the time of Hippocrates II (460 to 375 B.C.), physicians were able to examine the rectum with a rectal speculum to determine where problems were located (White and Klein, 1991). Other speculums were used to examine other areas of the body, such as the vaginal canal. The first

time that light was used for better visualization was when an Arab named Abulkasim in A.D. 1012 used a mirror to reflect light into the vagina (White and Klein, 1991). Tulio Caesare Aranzi (1585) designed the first endoscopic light, which was a crude instrument that he used to look into the nasal cavity. As the light source, it used solar rays passing through a small hole that were brought to a focus with a spherical glass flask filled with water (White and Klein, 1991).

THE 1800s

As time went on, physicians and researchers wanted to look into other internal body organs and structures. In 1805 in Frankfurt, Germany, Bozzani, an obstetrician, visualized the inside of the urethra using an unwieldy tube as an endoscope and candles as the light source (White and Klein, 1991). However, he was soon censured by the medical community of Vienna for being too inquisitive. Segalas of France in 1826 refined this instrumentation by adding a cannula to the endoscope that would act as an obturator to allow easier insertion. He also added a series of mirrors that reflected the light into the urethra, aiding in the visualization (White and Klein, 1991).

Desormeaux is credited as being the father of endoscopy. In 1835 he developed the first true cystoscope and urethroscope; as the light source kerosene lamp light was reflected through a mirror system (White and Klein, 1991). In 1869 Commander Pantaleoni of England refined the Desormeaux endoscope and used the resulting instrument to look inside the uterus and cauterize a hemorrhagic growth with silver nitrate (White and Klein, 1991). This marked the birth of hysteroscopy.

1

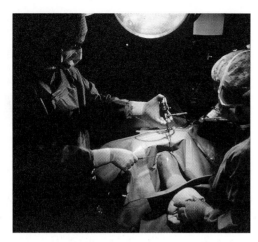

Fig. 1-1   A small incision is made to access the knee joint during an arthroscopic procedure. (Courtesy Kimberly-Clark Corp, Roswell, Ga.)

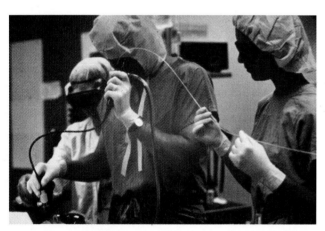

Fig. 1-2   A flexible endoscope is inserted through a natural body orifice to access the respiratory system during bronchoscopy.

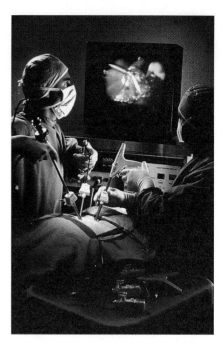

Fig. 1-3   A laparoscopic procedure is performed as internal structures are observed on the monitor. (Courtesy Ethicon Endo-Surgery, Inc., Cincinnati, Ohio.)

The first crude optical system within an endoscope made its debut in 1877, when a German physician by the name of Nitze added a lens system to the endoscopic tube (White and Klein, 1991). Following Edison's invention of the incandescent lightbulb in 1880, Dittel in 1887 added a small incandescent lightbulb at the end of the cystoscope to provide more direct illumination (White and Klein, 1991). By the end of the nineteenth century, endoscopic procedures, such as cystoscopy, proctoscopy, laryngoscopy, and esophagoscopy, had become widely accepted and used in almost all major health care centers.

THE EARLY 1900s

The first person to perform an endoscopic procedure of the abdomen was a gynecologist by the name of Ott from Petrograd who called his procedure "ventroscopy." An article describing this procedure was published in 1901. The procedure involved the creation of a small anterior abdominal incision, through which a speculum was passed; a head mirror was used to reflect light into the area (White and Klein, 1991). Also in 1901 Kelling, a surgeon from Dresden, performed an experiment in which he inserted a cystoscope into a dog to demonstrate a new procedure he called "coelioscopy" for the examination of the abdominal viscera. Pneumoperitoneum was established through the passage of filtered air through a separate needle inserted into the abdominal cavity, thus marking the performance of the first closed-cavity endoscopic procedure (White and Klein, 1991). In 1910 Jacobaues, of Stockholm, was the first to try this new technique on human subjects; not only was he able to view the abdominal (peritoneal) area, but also he was able to view the thoracic (pleural and pericardial) region (White and Klein, 1991).

The ability to look into the abdomen has been advanced by many physicians over the years. In 1912 Nordentoft and his brother, of Copenhagen, were the first to place the patient in the Trendelenburg position to enhance visualization of the abdominal organs and structures (White and Klein, 1991). In 1924, Zollikofer, of Switzerland, described the use of carbon dioxide for insufflation, identifying it as the gas of choice for this purpose because of its quick absorption (White and Klein, 1991). A German named Kalk, known as the father of modern laparoscopy, in 1929 developed a foreoblique (135-degree) viewing system that enabled enhanced visibility and made it possible to more accurately diagnose abdominal pathologic conditions. He put the system to much use in the many procedures he performed. He also introduced the second-hole puncture that allowed for a more controlled technique for biopsying the liver (White and Klein, 1991).

During this same era, Takagi, at Tokyo University in Japan, studied the principles of endoscopy and in 1918 performed the first successful endoscopy of the knee joint, carrying out this procedure on a cadaver (Gruendemann and Fernsebner, 1995). In 1921 Bircher used the Jacobaues laparoscope to perform "arthroendoscopy" of the knee (Gruendemann and Fernsebner, 1995).

The first gastroscopes, called "electroscopes," were introduced by Bruening in 1907, but it was not until 1932 that the first semiflexible gastroscope was developed by a man named Schindler (Gruendemann and Fernsebner, 1995). Part of the scope was flexible to facilitate insertion, but the shaft of the portion of the scope located in the stomach had to be straight so that the 50 or more lenses could function. At that time, specialists noted that gastroscopy done using this crude endoscope required great skill and training on the part of the physician. They also remarked that the patient had to have the anatomy of a sword swallower to tolerate the procedure.

The applications of laparoscopy expanded from diagnostic uses to actual operative treatments when in 1933 Fervers lysed abdominal adhesions and biopsied different tissues under direct visualization (White and Klein, 1991). In 1941 Powers and Barnes, of the University of Michigan, first described their experience fulgurating fallopian tubes with an electrical current transmitted through the endoscope to effect sterilization (White and Klein, 1991).

THE LATER 1900s

In 1952 a revolutionary endoscopic technique made its debut when Fourestier, Gladu, and Valmiere developed a method to transmit light along a quartz rod from the proximal to the distal end of the endoscope (White and Klein, 1991). With more intense light to illuminate the abdominal structures, pictures could now be taken. Even with these advancements, however, many surgeons in America were not impressed. In 1967 British physicist Harold Hopkins designed a superior ocular system that used a series of large, rod-shaped quartz lenses that provided brighter, clearer images (Gruendemann and Fernsebner, 1995).

In 1968 interest in laparoscopy was renewed in the United States with the advent of fiberoptics, which greatly improved lighting and visualization. Since then the growth of laparoscopy has been astonishing. Because of the overwhelming interest in laparoscopy and the phenomenal growth in the use of the techniques, a new organization, the American Association of Gyneco-

logical Laparoscopists was formed and held their first meeting in 1972, with more than 600 people in attendance (White and Klein, 1991).

Some of the common open gynecologic surgical procedures began to be converted into procedures involving laparoscopic entry. Steptoe and Edwards in 1970 described the laparoscopic retrieval of oocytes, which advanced in vitro fertilization techniques (White and Klein, 1991). In 1973 Shapiro and Adler removed an ectopic pregnancy through the laparoscope (White and Klein, 1991). As endoscopic instrumentation was developed and refined, other laparoscopic gynecologic procedures, such as laparoscopic adhesiolysis, adnexectomy, ovariectomy, myomectomy, and treatment of endometriosis, quickly became the standard of care. In 1977 Kurt Semm introduced the first carbon dioxide pneumoautomatic insufflator to facilitate the induction of a pneumoperitoneum and to replace the manual technique of introducing carbon dioxide through a needle (Gruendemann and Fernsebner, 1995).

Different kinds of energy began to be transmitted through the endoscope and alternate techniques of doing so were initiated, allowing for advanced gynecologic operative techniques to be performed. For example, in 1985, Lomano described photocoagulation of pelvic endometriosis using the neodymium:yttrium-aluminum-garnet laser (Nd:YAG) (Fig. 1-4) (Lomano, 1985). In 1987 Perez performed the first successful presacral neurectomy through the laparoscope (Figs. 1-5 and

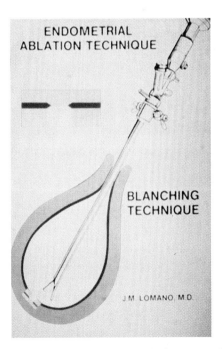

Fig. 1-4 Dr. Jack Lomano described photocoagulation of the endometrium using the Nd:YAG laser to treat menorrhagia. (Courtesy Jack Lomano, M.D., Sanibel, Fla.)

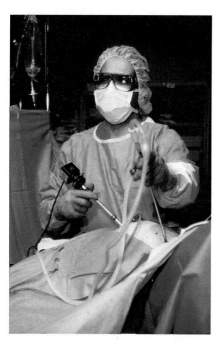

Fig. 1-5 Dr. Jim Perez performed the first successful presacral neurectomy through the laparoscope. (Courtesy Jim Perez, D.O., Columbus, Ohio.)

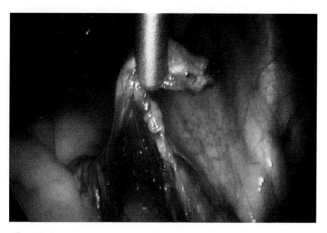

Fig. 1-6 Laparoscopic view of a presacral neurectomy being performed. (Courtesy Jim Perez, D.O., Columbus, Ohio.)

1-6) (Perez, 1990). Also in 1987 Reich described the first laparoscopic use of bipolar electrosurgery for the management of large-vessel hemostasis (Reich, 1987); in 1989 he and his colleagues also reported on the first laparoscopic hysterectomy (Reich, 1989).

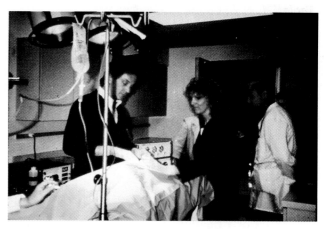

Fig. 1-7 Dr. Leonard Schultz successfully performed a laparoscopic cholecystectomy on a dog in 1985.

THE LAPAROSCOPIC REVOLUTION

Laparoscopy has become increasingly accepted for the treatment of many traditional open procedures. After gynecologist Kurt Semm performed the first laparoscopic appendectomy in 1983, general surgeons began to show interest in learning more about these less intrusive techniques (White and Klein, 1991).

One of the first laparoscopic cholecystectomies attempted on a dog was performed by Leonard Schultz in 1985, with help from gynecologist Jack Lomano and (author) Kay Ball (Fig. 1-7). Soon general surgeons realized that many traditional procedures could be performed through the laparoscope. The first laparoscopic cholecystectomy performed on a human subject in the United States was described in 1988 by McKernan and Saye (Gruendemann and Fernsebner, 1995). Since then many other endoscopic techniques have been refined so that they could be performed through the laparoscope; these include hernia repair, bowel resection, and fundoplications. (A history of endoscopy is outlined in Table 1-1.)

With the evolution of endoscopy, especially laparoscopy, it has been possible to convert many major surgical procedures once performed using open techniques into less invasive procedures. The benefits accruing to the patient include less postoperative discomfort, shortened hospitalizations, and quicker return to normal activities. Surgical professionals, researchers, and industry representatives have combined their respective wisdom, experience, resources, and creativity to rapidly advance the art of endoscopy. Given the continual and substantial advancements predicted for the future, the enthusiasm for the technique will likely endure.

Table 1-1 ▪ *Milestones of endoscopy*

Year	Physician/Researcher	Contribution
460–375 B.C.	Hippocrates II	Examined rectum with a speculum
1012–1013	Abulkasim	Light reflected into vagina with a mirror
1585	Tulio Caesare Aranzi	Looked into nasal cavity, with sun rays focused by flask filled with water
1805	Bozzani	Looked into urethra with tube, using candles as light source
1826	Segalas	Developed scope obturator for easy insertion into urethra; also developed a series of mirrors to reflect light
1835	Desormeaux	Developed first effective endoscope
1869	Pantaleoni	Designed first hysteroscope; used to cauterize growth inside uterus
1877	Nitze	Developed crude optical system, with lenses within scope
1880	Edison	Invented incandescent lightbulb
1887	Dittel	Placed incandescent lightbulb at end of cytoscope
1901	Ott	Performed first abdominal endoscopic inspection ("ventroscopy")
1901	Kelling	Demonstrated "coelioscopy" for the examination of the abdominal viscera on a living dog with pneumoperitoneum; first closed-cavity endoscopy
1907	Bruening	Developed first gastroscope
1910	Jacobaues	Performed first closed-cavity endoscopy on humans (abdominal and thoracic)
1911	Bernheim	First in the United States to view the peritoneal cavity using a proctoscope
1912	Nordentoft	First to describe use of Trendelenburg position during endoscopy
1918	Takagi	Performed knee joint endoscopy
1918	Getze	Developed an automatic spring needle
1921	Bircher	Used Jacobaues scope for arthroendoscopy
1924	Zollikofer	Described carbon dioxide as gas of choice for endoscopy of abdomen
1929	Kalk	Father of Modern Laparoscopy; developed fore oblique viewing system and second-hole puncture
1932	Schindler	Developed first semiflexible gastroscope
1933	Fervers	Performed first operative laparoscopy
1938	Verres	Developed a modified spring needle to induce pneumothorax
1941	Powers and Barnes	Used fulgurated tubes with electrical current for sterilization through endoscope
1952	Fourestier, Gladu, and Valmiere	Developed method to transmit light along a quartz rod as an external light source
1953	Thomsen	Took color photographs of cul-de-sac
1967	Hopkins	Designed lens system with large quartz rods
1968		Fiberoptics introduced
1970	Steptoe and Edwards	Performed first laparoscopic retrieval of oocytes
1972		Formation of the American Association of Gynecological Laparoscopists
1973	Shapiro and Adler	Performed first removal of ectopic pregnancy through a laparoscope
1977	Semm	Developed the first carbon dioxide pneumoautomatic insufflator
1985	Lomano	Performed first laparoscopic photocoagulation of endometriosis with Nd:YAG laser
1985	Schultz, Lomano, and Ball	Performed one of the first laparoscopic cholecystectomies on a dog
1987	Perez	Performed first laparoscopic presacral neurectomy
1987	Reich	First to perform laparoscopic bipolar electrosurgery for large-vessel hemostasis
1988	McKernan and Saye	Performed first laparoscopic cholecystectomy on a human subject
1989	Reich	Performed first laparoscopic hysterectomy

REFERENCES

Gruendemann BJ, Fernsebner B: *Comprehensive perioperative nursing, Vol 2, Practice*, Boston, 1995, Jones and Bartlett Publishers, p 449.

Lomano JM: Photocoagulation of early pelvic endometriosis with the Nd:YAG laser through the laparoscope, *J Reprod Med* 30(2):77, 1985.

Perez JJ: Laparoscopic presacral neurectomy, *J Reprod Med* 35(6):625, 1990.

Reich H: Laparoscopic oophorectomy and salpingo-oophorectomy in the treatment of benign tubo-ovarian disease, *Int J Fertil* 32(3):233, 1987.

Reich H, DeCaprio J, McGlynn F: Laparoscopic hysterectomy, *J Gynecol Surg* 5:213, 1989.

White RA, Klein SR: *Endoscopic surgery*, St. Louis, 1991, Mosby, p 3.

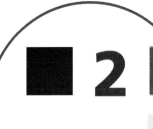

The Impact and Future of Endoscopy

THE IMPACT OF ENDOSCOPY

The evolution of endoscopy has had a profound impact on health care and spawned some interesting trends. Health care providers and patients have both eagerly watched this technology unfold.

Impact of Media Attention

The expansion of endoscopy has been fostered indirectly by the media. The frequency with which the media has introduced and promoted new endoscopic applications has escalated as celebrities have been the beneficiaries of the most current technology that health care can offer. When former Vice President Dan Quayle underwent a laparoscopic appendectomy, the media was eager to describe this relatively new surgical approach to the public. Prior to this, most people had not even known of the existence of this procedure.

Publicity has significantly affected the public's interest in and acceptance of endoscopy. The media is always eager to promote new advanced endoscopic techniques, especially if there is a patient who agrees to be interviewed about the procedure. The testimonial and endorsement of such a patient heightens the public's awareness and acceptance of the procedure. Through the resulting public pressure, many physicians who may not have wanted to learn new endoscopic techniques have been forced to assimilate this technology into their practices.

Compelling media stories about endoscopy are sometimes misunderstood by the public, however. The media may describe a new technique using an unwarranted sensationalism that distorts the reality of the surgery. The endoscopic approach may be publicized as the best method of surgery, but in reality some patients may not even qualify for this type of procedure. Patients may then request the endoscopic technique, whether they fulfill the selection criteria or not. This has caused great frustration on the part of health care professionals but, on the other hand, has also brought a lot of attention to endoscopy in recent years. It therefore falls to nurses and physicians to educate patients on the true facts about an endoscopic procedure—the indications for it and its advantages and disadvantages versus those of the open technique.

Impact of Endoscopic Research

As with any new developments in health care, research is vital to facilitating acceptance and change. In this regard, more research is needed to demonstrate the many different benefits of various endoscopic procedures, and definitive objective results are vital to prove the value of endoscopy versus that of open procedures. However, such research requires that there be dedicated people who are willing to take the time to advance the art and science of endoscopy. Today many health care facilities, universities, manufacturers of surgical devices, and foundations are eager to assist physicians and nurses with such research projects by providing the necessary funding. Findings from outcome analyses of endoscopy results must then be published so that they can be shared with other health care professionals.

It is vital, however, as endoscopic findings are published that members of the health care community be able to interpret research results. Following are some basic guidelines for reviewing the endoscopic research literature (*Laparosc Surg Update,* 1994a):

- What is the publication? Is it reputable? For example, a laparoscopy article that explains the technique of hernia repair published in an infection control journal may not have as much merit and be as believable as one published in a recognized laparoscopy journal. Consistency with the focus of the journal is preferred.
- Is the journal peer reviewed? This ensures the validity of the research and the appropriateness of the article.
- Who is writing the paper? Is the author reputable?
- Is there a connection between the author and the industry? What is this connection? Is the author on the payroll of the industry mentioned in the research?
- Are endoscopic products being compared? This may send up a red flag if the article is trying to promote one product over others.
- Is the research method sound and repeatable?
- Is the study being funded by industry? This may cause a bias within the study. Always check the acknowledgments to find out if industry was involved.
- What references have been made? If a profound statement that could be challenged has been made, check the reference that is listed. Is the reference really valid?
- Are there many references listed or only a few? If there appears to be a consensus among many different sources, then the statement or information is probably legitimate.
- Is the reference significant and reliable? Did the reference come from a peer-reviewed publication? Articles usually are peer reviewed, but poster displays of research studies are usually not.

Acceptance of endoscopic techniques will increase as long as comprehensive research findings and objective results are presented. To encourage this acceptance, follow-up studies must be more complete and comprehensive. Currently, some physicians cite tremendous postoperative results from a particular endoscopic procedure but fail to report the response rate with regard to patient follow-up. For example, a surgeon might cite a 100% "no recurrence" rate for patients who have undergone laparoscopic hernia repairs, but perhaps 45% of the patients have not been contacted for follow-up. There must be at least an 80% patient follow-up rate for there to be confidence in the success data reported (*Laparosc Surg Update*, 1994c).

Economic Impact of Endoscopy

The economic impact of endoscopy must be carefully examined to ensure that financial decisions about the technology are valid. Financial experts within the health care facility should be consulted whenever an economic analysis is being performed to ensure accuracy and to ensure that the factors being analyzed are appropriate.

The procurement process, financial considerations, and cost containment all influence whether an endoscopic procedure can be economically justified.

Technology procurement

The popularity of endoscopy has made it necessary for health professionals to acquire comprehensive technology assessment and management skills. Detailed plans for procurement regarding purchasing, maintaining, and storing endoscopic equipment and instrumentation are vital. The entire surgical team, including physicians, nurses, and technologists, must be involved in every phase of the procurement process to ensure success and economic viability.

The team approach to purchasing endoscopic equipment and instrumentation is vital and must consist of a systematic process of procurement. By involving different health care professionals in this procedure, a sense of ownership is fostered that helps make the system work. The procurement team could involve the operating room director, physicians, the financial administrator, the purchasing agent, and others who can offer expertise during this process. Staff nurses and technologists also must be involved, because they are often the ones responsible for the operation, maintenance, and acceptance of the device.

As with any advanced technology purchases, the procurement process for endoscopic equipment and instrumentation should consist of the following steps (Ball, 1995):

1. Justification—to ensure that the device is needed and that there is interest in using the device.
2. Evaluation—to actually try using the device to determine its acceptability and ease of use.
3. Acquisition—to procure the device. There are a variety of financial options that can be employed, depending on the economic status of the health care facility.
4. Incorporation into the endoscopic armamentarium. Staff nurses and technologists are critical to the success of this phase.

Input from physicians is needed during the evaluation phase to make sure the product is appropriate and useful. During the procurement process the team must assess and compare product quality, warranties, acquisition costs, hidden costs, and alternative products. The standardization of devices also necessitates systematic evaluation of the various products on the market. Being able to standardize surgical instruments and supplies saves money and decreases confusion among the surgical team members.

Financial considerations in endoscopy

The trend toward managed care (managing the cost of care) compels health care professionals to focus on the expense of endoscopic procedures. When determining the economic impact of a procedure, the actual cost of the procedure is the most valuable piece of information to compare with the estimated income from the procedure, instead of merely the patient charge. Often the patient charge includes hospital markups that may be inconsistent; therefore the actual cost to perform the procedure represents a more realistic cost analysis or comparison.

When determining the true economic impact of an endoscopic procedure, the time it takes for the patient to become completely healed and resume normal living activities also should be included. If only the actual cost of the procedure is considered without a consideration of the patient's recovery time, this does not reflect an accurate economic appraisal of the total surgical experience and the benefits of endoscopy.

Many health insurance organizations today are not totally happy with the popularity of some endoscopic procedures. Even though an endoscopic experience may cost less than that of an open procedure, more money is ultimately being spent because the less invasive procedure can be performed on more patients. For example, laparoscopic cholecystectomy is now being performed on more patients than the open procedure because it is less invasive and the recovery time is shortened. People who in the past opted not to have the open procedures are now agreeing to have the endoscopic technique. Those patients who could not tolerate an open procedure also are opting for the endoscopic procedure. In addition, many surgeons are lowering the threshold of the patient selection criteria so that more patients can qualify to have the endoscopic procedure. It is for reasons such as these that the total volume of patients undergoing endoscopic procedures, and hence the amount of health care monies spent, has increased. This has had a significant financial impact on managed care organizations and insurance carriers. A leading health maintenance organization determined that between 1988 and 1992 the cost per procedure for cholecystectomy declined 25.1% but the frequency with which cholecystectomy procedures were performed increased nearly 60% (*Laparosc Surg Update*, 1994b).

Another consideration in reviewing the financial impact of endoscopy is the physician's level of skill. When a physician is learning the skills required to perform a specific endoscopic procedure, the cost of the procedure can be greater because more operative time may be required. The cost to perform a procedure will naturally decrease as physicians become more skilled, thus decreasing the surgical time needed. If the physician continues to take more surgical time or requests specific endoscopic instruments or supplies that are more expensive, the managed care organization or the third-party insurance carrier may eliminate him or her from the list of physician choices.

The cost of endoscopic procedures may also be increased at teaching facilities that provide resident and intern training. This is a result of extra time needed to provide education and training during the procedure. The cost for repair services also may be greater at a teaching institution, because less experienced professionals are more prone to breaking instruments and equipment.

Another financial consideration pertaining to endoscopic procedures is the decision to use single-use versus reusable products. (This topic is discussed in greater detail in Chapter 8.) When deciding whether to purchase single use or reusables, some of the variables to review include the following:

- The actual cost of the product
- The number of uses of the product
- Reprocessing costs
  - Supplies and equipment
  - Sterilizing and disinfecting devices
  - Staffing time
  - Staff education
  - Risk of transmission of disease during reprocessing
- Availability of product
- Disposal costs
- Inventory costs
- Storage costs
- Purchasing costs
- Product quality and reliability

Cost containment

Surgical managers are learning ways to creatively cut endoscopic procedure expenses while controlling their operating and capital budgets. During a cost-cutting campaign to curtail spending, a surgical department found that physicians were very willing to cooperate in cost-saving efforts if objective instead of subjective information was provided. Physicians were shown their own costs for specific endoscopic procedures in comparison with those of their colleagues, who were not identified. This motivated physicians to compete with one another to try to minimize the costs of their procedures. The surgery department successfully and significantly curbed expenses in a short time. Now the physicians expect to see how their costs compare with those of their colleagues each quarter (*Laparosc Surg Update*, 1994d).

Many other measures have been initiated by nurses, physicians, and other health care professionals to curtail costs. For example, one hospital surgery suite in Michigan switched to using trocar kits instead of individually packaged trocars with sheaths. The staff found that they were using two 5-mm trocars in most laparoscopy cases. So, in an attempt to control costs, trocar kits containing one trocar with two sheaths were purchased instead. Even though disposable trocars are usually preferred because of their sharpness, the physicians had no problems with reusing the same trocar to make another port during the procedure. This project saved $14,000 in 1 year (*Laparosc Surg Update*, 1995a).

In another cost-containment project, the expense of performing laparoscopic appendectomies was noted. The cost of the laparoscopic procedure was found to be $1962.13 whereas that of the open procedure was $1744.26, a difference of $217.87. During the laparoscopic procedure, a linear cutter costing $338 was used. A suggestion was made to use endoloops with scissors or an electrosurgery device to cut instead of the linear cutter. This then lowered the cost of the laparoscopic approach to less than that of the open method (*Paschall*, 1995).

Camera drapes are also now being used to minimize the cost of reprocessing and prolong the life of the camera. With the use of these drapes, infection control and processing are simplified. One study showed that the cost of disposable camera drapes was less than the cost of the time and the supplies needed to reprocess the camera. The repair bills were minimized, too, because the camera was not then continually being reprocessed (*Laparosc Surg Update*, 1993a).

Another cost-control measure has been to do away with an assistant during less complicated endoscopic procedures. To accomplish this, physicians are learning to operate one-handed during such procedures. This may require reorganization of the surgical room and setup. The most frequently used instruments can be kept on the over-table stand within reach of the operating physician. Less used instruments can remain on the back table. The video monitor may also have to be repositioned, so that the physician can easily view the procedure.

If an assistant is needed, a registered nurse first assistant (RNFA) may be a cost-effective option, as he or she can assume many different responsibilities. Being a registered nurse, the RNFA can function not only as the first assistant but also can provide nursing assessment competencies and skills that other first assistants cannot. When a physician uses the same first assistant for every endoscopic procedure, a consistency is fostered that can translate into quality care, fewer complications, and a shortened operative time.

Endoscopy Benefits

Endoscopy techniques continue to have a great impact on surgery today, as open procedures are quickly being converted into more minimally invasive methods. The benefits of endoscopy continue to be realized as new techniques are accepted and integrated into practice. The following are some of the proven benefits of various endoscopic procedures:

For the patient

- Patient selection criteria have been broadened to include those who normally would not qualify for an open procedure (e.g., people with diabetes, pregnant women, debilitated patients).
- Less surgical preparation for the patient.
- Less intraoperative blood loss.
- Intraoperative time may be decreased.
- Other organs and structures can be inspected during endoscopy.
- Less postoperative pain.
- Fewer postoperative complications.
- Fewer postoperative infections (especially important to diabetic or immunocompromised patients).
- Superior cosmetic results.
- Decreased hospitalization.
- Normal food intake resumed sooner after surgery.
- Quicker return to normal activities.
- Recurrence rates may be lessened. (One study showed that the open approach for hernia repair was associated with a 10% failure rate, whereas the laparoscopic approach was associated with a failure rate of only 4% [*Laparosc Surg Update*, 1994]).
- The costs of the entire endoscopic experience is often less than that of the open procedure.

Because of these numerous benefits, many patients prefer to have an endoscopic procedure instead of the open procedure, even if the direct cost of the procedure is more. For example, a laparoscopic hernia repair may allow the patient to return to normal activities within days, whereas a patient who undergoes open herniorrhaphy may have to limit his or her activities for 4 weeks or more. Third-party reimbursers may not fully pay for the endoscopic methods; therefore, the patient who desires the laparoscopic procedure may have to pay for more of the cost.

For the physician

- Physicians other than surgeons are now performing endoscopic procedures (e.g., gastroenterologists).
- Endoscopy provides excellent exposure and visibility of different structures and organs for diagnostic and operative interventions.
- Endoscopy allows unsuspected problems to be identified that may not be discovered during an open procedure. (For example, liver problems may be noted during a laparoscopic appendectomy that may have gone unnoticed.)
- Offers a marketing edge to skilled physicians as more patients demand endoscopic procedures.
- Provides a learning environment in which to continually expand surgical skills.
- Allows entrepreneurship in product and instrument development.

For the perioperative nurse

- Greater career opportunities as the use of endoscopy expands to other specialties (e.g., plastic surgery, neurosurgery) and is moved to other surgical sites (e.g., physician offices, mobile surgical units). Because every surgical patient deserves the care of a registered nurse, there are greater employment opportunities in these new surgical arenas.

- Provides an area in which nursing expertise and skill are critical to the safe care of the patient.
- Allows entrepreneurship in product and instrument development.
- Offers a challenge to the perioperative nurse to provide complete patient education during a very short time with the patient.
- Provides a continuous learning environment for the perioperative nurse because endoscopic technology frequently changes.
- Allows the nurse to more readily anticipate surgical needs and the needs of the patient because the surgical field is often displayed on a monitor for the endoscopic team to view.

For the surgical technologist

- Provides an opportunity to learn new skills and advance into other specialty areas.
- Provides a continuous learning environment because new devices and techniques are continually evolving.
- Allows entrepreneurship in product and instrument development.
- Allows the technologist to more readily anticipate the physician's instrumentation needs because the surgical field is often displayed on a monitor for the endoscopy team to view.

FUTURE TRENDS IN ENDOSCOPY

Many new frontiers and challenges in the surgical environment have appeared as endoscopy has evolved. Dramatic changes in practice, surgical devices, and patient demands will continue to greatly affect the field of endoscopic surgery. One can only hope that these changes are being made so that the patient benefits either directly or indirectly from them. The patient must continue to be the focus of any decisions that influence the care provided and the advancements made. So, what can be expected of endoscopy in the future?

New Procedures and Endoscopic Sites

Many different endoscopic procedures have now been accepted as the treatments of choice. For example, the preferred method to remove a gallbladder is now through the laparoscope, as opposed to performing an open procedure. This was not the standard in 1990. The trend to convert open procedures to new endoscopic methods will continue as positive outcomes are documented.

The continued development of endoscopic techniques can be directly linked to the acceptance for payment of the procedures by third-party carriers. Reimbursement codes are slowly changing and expanding as certain endoscopic procedures are becoming more widely approved. Codes that correspond to specific endoscopic procedures will continue to be developed so that fair and appropriate remuneration can be provided.

Because of the increase in the volume of endoscopic procedures, other clinical sites providing endoscopy have emerged, and this trend will continue. Yesterday the only place where endoscopy was performed was in the hospital operating room. Now it is being done in hospital endoscopy laboratories, cardiac catheterization laboratories, emergency rooms, hospital clinics, and even at the patient's bedside.

Hospitals are now separating these outpatient services from the inpatient ones and providing them with their own surgical suites and areas specifically geared toward ambulatory services, including endoscopy. These outpatient surgical centers have aesthetically pleasing suites, with the emphasis placed on convenience, quality, efficiency, and service.

Often hospitals hire consultants to act as the non-threatening agent of change if difficult decisions need to be made involving the segregation of operating room services. During such shifts, endoscopic procedures are even being moved out of the hospital environment and into outpatient clinics and physician's offices. Mobile units that can provide increased patient access are being proposed as future endoscopy sites. Soon endoscopic procedures may even be performed in the patient's home. However, because endoscopic procedures provide access to internal structures, infection control must not be overlooked. Endoscopy can be performed in many different settings, as long as the environment can be controlled and infection prevented.

Because recovery after endoscopic procedures is quicker than that after open procedures, postoperative recovery centers are being constructed that provide skilled nursing care for patients who should not be sent home immediately after an endoscopic procedure. The care rendered at this type of extended care facility is usually less expensive than hospital care and such facilities represent another effort to control costs. The recovery center concept will survive only if these centers are cost-effective and become an accepted method for postoperative care (*Laparosc Surg Update*, 1993b).

Advanced Instrumentation and Devices

During endoscopy, the physician's tactile sense is lost because tissue cannot be directly palpated. Currently, enhanced video imaging compensates for some of this loss, but simulators are being designed to provide ways of actually feeling the tissue.

Simulators are also being developed to provide a virtual reality experience. This technology will have a tremendous impact on training because during the computer-generated simulation a three-dimensional environment is provided that mimics an actual endoscopic procedure. The challenges involved in simulated surgery are comparable to those experienced during some of the computerized games available today. It has been said that today's computer game experts will be tomorrow's surgeons because of the acute hand-eye training and coordination that are acquired.

In the future, physicians may have to graduate through a series of virtual reality experiences before they are allowed to attempt an endoscopic procedure on a human patient. Unexpected complications can be presented during the simulation, and the physician must prove that he or she is able to handle these different situations. This training would be similar to what pilots must go through before they are allowed to actually fly a jet.

Robotics are also being developed that will assist physicians and soon be able to perform the procedure with physician guidance. Current models are capable of making predetermined movements that are manually controlled. One robotic that is being used today is the camera holder, which eliminates a team member at the surgical table. Research is being done to develop robotics that can be activated by voice or physician eye movements.

Advanced optics and imaging systems are continually being introduced into surgical use. Cameras are getting smaller and require less lighting to produce a clear, distinct image. Three-dimensional systems are available that can provide depth perception. These systems are now being refined to produce more clear images with greater resolution (Fig. 2-1).

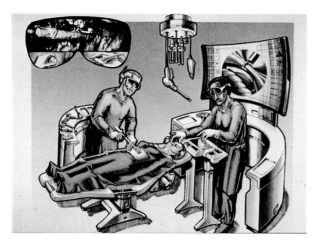

Fig. 2-1 Advancements in optics and video equipment are expanding the capabilities of endoscopy. (Courtesy Ethicon Endo-Surgery, Inc., Cincinnati, Ohio.)

Videoconferencing is now available that provides audio- and video-interactive communication during endoscopic procedures. A physician at a different site can now observe and interact with another physician performing an endoscopic procedure. This technology enhances education and allows one physician to precept and guide another. This technology is the precursor of telepresence surgery, in which the physician is not at the patient's side but at a remote site controlling the robotics that actually perform the procedure (Fig. 2-2). The health care professional at the bedside may be a nurse who observes and assists with the procedure.

Advancements in instrument design have allowed more difficult surgical techniques to be attempted. This progress will continue as the surgical instrument industry works closely with physicians and nurses to develop instruments that meet the requirements of various surgical techniques. Endoscopic staplers have been refined so that they can be passed through small trocar sites. Instruments have been devised to assist with complex suturing. The development of right-angled and articulating instruments, as well as other advances in technology, are continually occurring to supply more user-friendly endoscopic tools. Nontraumatic retractors and graspers are being developed that can be used to move and hold delicate tissue so that visibility is enhanced during endoscopy. The product development of endoscopic instruments will continue to be a focus of surgical manufacturers because advancements in this area naturally lead to an increased volume of endoscopic procedures and, hence, increased sales.

New energies are also being introduced that can be used in the performance of operative endoscopy. For example, endoscopic cryoblation and cryonecrosis technology is now available to treat liver cancer (Frantzides, 1995).

Energy sources and instruments are also being combined to create valuable surgical tools. Laser energy may soon be delivered through an endoscope to weld tissue that is being stabilized with an approximator tool.

Optical biopsy technology introduced through an endoscope is being refined to help locate malignant cells in the bladder and colon. This is done by bouncing light waves through an endoscope. The light waves normally scatter in different patterns when they hit healthy tissue but not when they hit malignant tissue. The light pulses are delivered through the endoscope as the physician examines an organ. The scatter pattern then is transmitted back to the computer analyzer for comparison with the database of patterns for normal tissue. Through this computerized analysis, the physician can determine whether the cells are malignant or healthy. If cancer is indicated, then a biopsy specimen of the pathologic tissue would be obtained for confirmation (*OR Manager*, 1995).

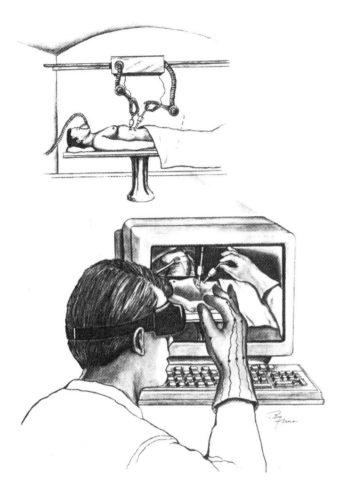

Fig. 2-2 Telepresence surgery being remotely controlled. (From Frantzides CT: *Laparoscopic and thoracoscopic surgery*, St. Louis, 1995, Mosby.)

Dramatic changes in surgical instrumentation and devices will continue to spawn alterations in procedures and changes in patient selection criteria. Because recovery is faster and the complications fewer in patients who have endoscopic procedures, endoscopic techniques will be developed and successfully used in debilitated patients or patients who normally would not have been considered for surgery.

Expansion into Other Surgical Specialities

Innovative surgical techniques will be introduced as the less invasive approach offered by endoscopy is accepted by more specialties. The main applications of endoscopy are not confined anymore to intraabdominal, intrathoracic, or intrajoint procedures. Even plastic surgeons are realizing the potential merits of the endoscope for gaining access to subcutaneous and muscle tissue. With the better cosmetic results and the smaller scars that result from its use, endoscopy has become a favored method among plastic surgeons. For example, during a brow-lift the endoscope can be used to access the surgical area. An ear-to-ear incision made across the top of the head has now been replaced by the creation of three very small incisions hidden behind the hair line. One plastic surgeon has predicted that soon all brow-lifts will be done through an endoscope (*Laparosc Surg Update*, 1994e).

Endoscopy can also be used for a variety of other procedures, including face-lifts and the harvesting of muscle tissue, because dissection can safely be performed under direct endoscopic visualization. However, new instruments need to be developed for these types of procedures, because the general surgical and gynecologic instruments physicians are trying to adapt for use in specific endoscopic plastic surgery procedures are not working well. Manual retractors must also be developed because insufflation cannot be used for many of these operations.

New techniques to replace other open procedures are also being explored. For example, cardiac surgeons are investigating the use of endoscopy to harvest veins during cardiac bypass procedures. The patient would then experience less postoperative pain because smaller incisions would be made instead of the large, lengthy incisions now needed to access the vein graft.

Advancements in endoscopic fetal diagnostics and surgery are also becoming a reality. Ultrathin scopes are being designed to assess the growing fetus. A very small, 0.5-mm endoscope that can fit through a 21-gauge needle is being refined for use in looking inside the uterus. The images yielded are not as clear as those produced by larger diameter scopes, but this technology is progressing. The procedure is similar to amniocentesis in that local anesthesia is administered around the proposed puncture site and then the needle is inserted. Upon withdrawal of the needle, the small hole is self-sealing. This procedure has been called *embryofetoscopy* or just *fetoscopy* because it should not be attempted before 10 weeks' gestation, when the embryo becomes a fetus. Fetal monitoring is provided throughout the procedure. As this technology progresses, fetoscopy will come to be used to perform operations on the fetus (*Laparosc Surg Update*, 1993).

To conclude, the future of endoscopy holds promise, challenge, compromise, and excitement for surgical teams and patients alike. Creativity, enthusiasm, and a willingness to explore beyond the boundaries of today's ideas will ensure the continued advancement of this great surgical method.

REFERENCES

Ball KA: *Lasers: the perioperative challenge*, St. Louis, 1995, Mosby, p 342.

Frantzides CT: *Laparoscopic and thoracoscopic surgery*, St. Louis, 1995, Mosby, p 287.

Laparosc Surg Update, Fetus is newest patient for diagnostic laparoscopy, 1(6):62, 1993.

Laparosc Surg Update, Camera drapes gaining interest as alternative to reprocessing, 1(10):115, 1993a.

Laparosc Surg Update, Laparoscopy expansion via post-surgical recovery center uncertain as California project ends, 1(10):109, 1993b.

Laparosc Surg Update, How to read lap research with a skeptical eye, 2(1):8, 1994a.

Laparosc Surg Update, Does cheaper lap surgery raise healthcare costs? 2(1)4, 1994b.

Laparosc Surg Update, Patient follow-up can be weak factor in success rates, 2(1):7, 1994c.

Laparosc Surg Update, Approach surgeons carefully, but expect cooperation, 2(10):111, 1994d.

Laparosc Surg Update, Plastic surgeons seen next big field for endoscopic surgery, 2(11):12b, 1994e.

Laparosc Surg Update, Lap hernia repair: wave of future or just today's folly?; 2(12):134, 1994f.

Laparosc Surg Update, Hospital saves $14,000 a year by switching to trocar kits, 3(1):75, 1995a.

OR Manager, Fiberoptics may replace biopsy to diagnose cancers, 11(7/8):44, 1995.

Paschall V: Lap appendectomy not that much more expensive, *Laparosc Surg Update*, 3(7):84, 1995b.

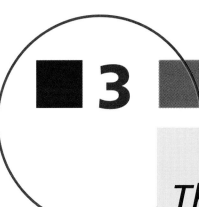

3

The Endoscopy Team

Surgical teams are confronted with many challenges as endoscopic technology changes and evolves. Consistency within a team provides stability during turbulent times of change. Ideally the members of an endoscopic team are the same persons who work together over and over, thus forming the foundation for a successful endoscopy program. The team members must be able to coordinate the care of their patients, as well as manage the ever-changing techniques, instrumentation, and equipment involved in the performance of endoscopy. Careful plans must be made and implemented regarding not only the direct care delivered to the patient but also the physical layout of the endoscopy room, the devices and supplies required, and the number of staff members needed.

Often new endoscopic techniques are only performed on day shifts when the experienced staff is available. Now with the popularity and success of endoscopy, staff members must be able to provide endoscopic expertise during all shifts. Staffing must therefore be reviewed and policies written so that quality and safe care can be delivered whenever and wherever endoscopy is performed.

The different endoscopic team members, including the physician, nurse, anesthesia provider, surgical technologist, and biomedical engineers and technicians, have varying roles and responsibilities within the endoscopy program (Fig. 3-1).

PHYSICIAN

Today endoscopy has transcended all surgical specialties. The gynecologists were the first surgeons to put this technology into practice, followed quickly by the urolo-

gists. Other surgical specialists, such as orthopedic, colorectal, and ENT surgeons, have now adopted different endoscopic procedures to enhance their practice of surgery. Currently some plastic surgeons are using endoscopy during face-lifts because of the better visibility and superior cosmetic results it provides. Endoscopy has truly become a standard way of performing many procedures that were once performed using open techniques.

Other physicians, who are not surgeons, have also come to realize the successful results and benefits conferred by endoscopy. Internal medicine specialists, including gastroenterologists and cardiologists, have mastered the endoscopic skills needed to diagnose and treat diseases. Many general practitioners are beginning to perform diagnostic endoscopy in the office using a small-lumen endoscope to access internal structures and identify pathologic conditions or problems.

Almost all physicians today have been affected by endoscopic technology. In turn, physician education and credentialing protocols have been adjusted to accommodate the learning experiences needed to perform endoscopy safely. These issues are discussed in more detail in Chapter 4.

The responsibilities of the physician are to determine the patient's diagnosis based on objective and subjective symptoms. The next step is to discuss the treatment options with the patient. If an endoscopic procedure is recommended, the physician is responsible for explaining the procedure and the anticipated outcome. Procedural risks, complications, and alternative treatments also must be discussed, so the patient can make an informed decision about the endoscopic procedure. After the patient has consented to the endoscopic procedure,

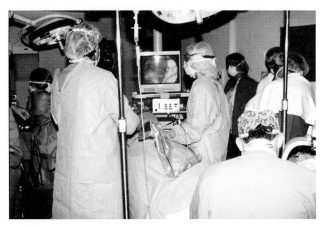

Fig. 3-1 An endoscopic team consists of many different professionals with varying responsibilities. (Courtesy Wendy K. Winer RN, BSN, Atlanta, Ga.)

he or she must sign a consent form. Sometimes the consent form is signed at the place where the endoscopic procedure is performed, as long as the patient has not already received a preoperative medication.

The physician also is responsible for performing the endoscopic procedure and discharging the patient (Fig. 3-2). Sometimes standardized patient discharge criteria are developed. If the patient meets these criteria, then the nurse is responsible for discharging the patient in accordance with the standardized physician orders. The physician usually requests a follow-up visit with the patient to evaluate the patient's recovery and the effectiveness of the procedure. Further plans for follow-up may be discussed with the patient at this time.

NURSE

Many exciting professional opportunities for perioperative nurses have recently been spawned as a result of the continued expansion of endoscopy. Some of these

opportunities include endoscopy nurse, endoscopy coordinator, and registered nurse first assistant (RNFA).

Endoscopy Nurse

An endoscopy nurse may practice in the surgical suite, endoscopy laboratory, outpatient clinic, physician's office, or wherever endoscopy is performed. Because endoscopic procedures require a combination of nursing talent and technologic skills, the role of the endoscopy nurse is very diverse and can be very demanding. Some of the responsibilities of the endoscopic nurse include maintaining a thorough understanding of endoscopic procedures and patient care, designing a plan of care for each patient, ensuring patient safety, documenting perioperative patient care, mastering the endoscopic technology involved, and providing comprehensive patient education (Fig. 3-3).

The endoscopy nurse must first, however, possess a thorough understanding of the care needed to support the patient during an endoscopic procedure. Basic perioperative nursing competencies mandated for such nurses include a knowledge of surgical sterility, infection control, medications, patient positioning, endoscopic techniques, endoscopic complications, and other perioperative patient care measures.

The focus of any endoscopic procedure must be on the safety and welfare of the patient. Therefore, endoscopic nurses must be involved in developing the patient's plan of care, as already noted, and in the policies that govern this care. After these protocols have been established and communicated to the nursing staff, the focus can turn to the endoscopic equipment, instrumentation, and supplies to be used.

An endoscopy nurse also must be technologically adept. Endoscopic instrumentation and equipment have to be incorporated into the procedure as the nurse continues to provide comprehensive perioperative

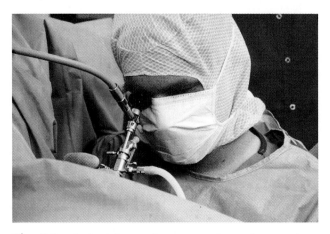

Fig. 3-2 A physician performs an endoscopic procedure. (Courtesy Karl Storz, Culver City, Calif.)

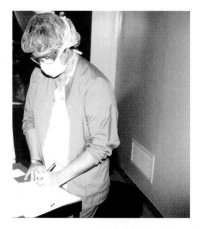

Fig. 3-3 The endoscopic nurse documents the perioperative patient care on the surgical record. (Courtesy Wendy K. Winer RN, BSN, Atlanta, Ga.)

nursing skills. Rapid changes and different routines often pose a challenge to the nurse, who must then alter traditional plans of care while assimilating new techniques or devices into practice. For example, some endoscopic procedures, such as gastroscopy, may not require sterile instrumentation, but the nurse still needs to understand the concept of surgical sterility and the conditions in which it is needed. Even though the technical aspects of endoscopy are extremely important, the nurse must always guarantee that endoscopic technology never overshadows the maintenance of patient-focused care.

The endoscopy nurse is also confronted with the challenge of providing comprehensive patient education. Often, the nurse has limited contact with the patient, because most endoscopic procedures are now performed on an outpatient basis. Creative patient teaching tools, such as booklets, brochures, and videotapes, have been developed to enhance this experience by providing the patient with pertinent information before the procedure. On the day of the scheduled endoscopy, the patient is then better prepared and usually more relaxed. The nurse can then focus on the patient's questions and determine his or her understanding to ensure compliance before, during, and after the procedure.

Endoscopy Coordinator

An endoscopy coordinator may be needed to perform the administrative and clinical responsibilities pertaining to an endoscopic program (Fig. 3-4). It may be a challenge for a hospital to validate the need for and the financial expense of a dedicated position for an endoscopic coordinator, but cost comparison can help in this effort. For example, the costs of endoscopic instrument repairs per year can be compared with the cost of employing an endoscopic coordinator. If the costs of instrument repair are excessive, endoscopic coordinators may prove their worth by reducing the costs for repairing and reprocessing instruments by monitoring the breakage and reprocessing of instruments and also by conducting ongoing training programs on instrument care for the staff. Other justifications will likely be required to verify the need for a dedicated position, however.

An endoscopy coordinator must be very enthusiastic about and interested in endoscopy to be successful in handling the multiple responsibilities of this position. In today's cost-conscious health care environment, however, the nurse who serves as the endoscopy coordinator probably will have other expanded responsibilities. Following are some of the duties that may be assigned to an endoscopy coordinator:

- Serves as an endoscopic resource person to staff and physicians
- Develops the infrastructure of the endoscopy program

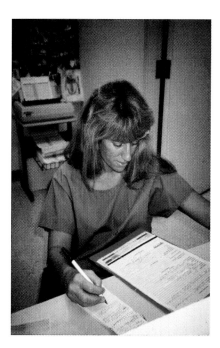

Fig. 3-4 An endoscopic coordinator may assume the administrative and clinical responsibilities pertaining to an endoscopic program. (Courtesy Wendy K. Winer RN, BSN, Atlanta, Ga.)

- Develops policies and procedures involving endoscopy
- Coordinates device evaluation
- Participates in equipment and instrumentation purchases
- Conducts in-service and hands-on training for the endoscopic team (including staff, physicians, and residents)
- Participates in endoscopy research
- Monitors advancements in endoscopy
- Designs perioperative patient education plans and tools
- Coordinates new endoscopic applications
- Monitors credentialing
- Networks with other facilities and endoscopy professionals
- Translates and communicates new information to surgical staff
- Maintains endoscopy inventory
- Oversees the proper reprocessing and care of endoscopic devices and equipment
- Communicates with endoscopic sales representatives
- Provides cost-containment ideas
- Coordinates activities with other specialty area managers who have responsibilities overlapping with those of the endoscopy coordinator
- Participates in long-term planning

Nurses interested in becoming an endoscopy coordinator must have a basic understanding of endoscopic equipment and instruments, the techniques, and patient care. He or she must be dedicated to pursuing more education about endoscopy because of the constant changes in the field. This professional must also have good rapport with staff members and surgeons, because a lot of time is spent giving advice, teaching, and coordinating the endoscopic procedures. An endoscopy coordinator should be good at networking with others who are in the specialty, because a lot can be learned and gained from listening to the experiences of others in endoscopy programs around the country.

Serving as the endoscopy coordinator also requires a keen awareness of cost containment, because health care funds have become very limited during the past few years. Being able to organize and manage an abundant inventory of instruments, supplies, and equipment is paramount. Finally, any nurse who becomes an endoscopy coordinator must be empowered to create and maintain a successful endoscopy program (*Laparosc Surg Update*, 1994).

The endoscopy coordinator must be given the responsibility and the authority to coordinate and support the endoscopy program. Often responsibility is granted to an employee but then the authority to ensure compliance with written procedures is not provided. This can diminish the significance of this position and lead to the confusion that often accompanies a technology that is continually changing.

The endoscopy coordinator must have ample time to pursue educational opportunities to stay current with endoscopic technology. Updates are frequently offered at seminars and professional organization meetings, in publications, and through visits to other facilities. Staying on the "cutting edge" is often recognized as a characteristic of a successful endoscopic program.

Because staffing is limited in many endoscopy programs, one challenge that often surfaces is that the endoscopy coordinator may also be expected to assume other responsibilities. For example, the endoscopy coordinator may be asked to temporarily work in the holding room when staffing is not available. If this situation becomes common, the person may be prevented from coordinating and advancing the endoscopy program, and this can be a source of frustration. Open communication with the supervisor may help the coordinator in prioritizing the needs of the program so that the most critical ones can be temporarily met. If these added responsibilities persist, then the endoscopy coordinator's assignments and title may need to be changed.

An industrious endoscopy coordinator can help validate the need for a full-time employee by noting the achievements of the program, cost-efficiency activities, and successful endoscopy projects. This can be communicated in an annual report, in written device-procurement evaluations, and by noting the achievement of the goals that were set for the program.

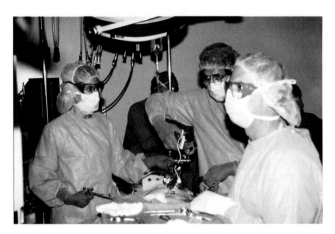

Fig. 3-5   A registered nurse first assistant (*left*) assists the surgeon with a laparoscopic procedure. (Courtesy Wendy K. Winer RN, BSN, Atlanta, Ga.)

Registered Nurse First Assistant

A perioperative nurse can also serve as an RNFA, whose function it is to help the physician perform the endoscopic procedure (Fig. 3-5). The general duties and responsibilities of the RNFA have been defined in a statement promulgated by the Association of Operating Room Nurses (Box 3-1).

The RNFA provides the extra hands needed to perform an endoscopic procedure, including holding and positioning the camera, manipulating tissue, cutting, coagulating, suturing, and retracting (Fig. 3-6).The RNFA also may close the trocar sites at the completion of a laparoscopic procedure (Fig. 3-7).

The specific qualifications of the person who serves as the first assistant during an endoscopic procedure have been a controversial issue since the time endoscopy became so popular. There is a wide range of people who call themselves first assistants, including surgeons,

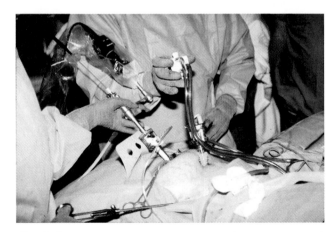

Fig. 3-6   During a laparoscopic procedure, a registered nurse first assistant positions the camera and manipulates instrumentation to assist the physician. (Courtesy Wendy K. Winer RN, BSN, Atlanta, Ga.)

Box 3-1   *AORN Official Statement on Registered Nurse First Assistants*

Definition of RN First Assistant

The RNFA at surgery collaborates with the surgeon in performing a safe operation with optimal outcomes for the patient. The RNFA practices perioperative nursing and must have acquired the necessary specific knowledge, skills, and judgment. The RNFA practices under the supervision of the surgeon during the intraoperative phase of the perioperative experience. The RNFA does not concurrently function as a scrub nurse.

Scope of Practice

The scope of practice of the nurse performing as first assistant is a part of perioperative nursing practice. Perioperative nursing is a specialized area of practice. The activities included in first assisting are further refinements of perioperative nursing practice which are executed within the context of the nursing process. The observable nursing behaviors are based on an extensive body of scientific knowledge. These intraoperative nursing behaviors may include:

- Handling tissue
- Providing exposure
- Using instruments
- Suturing
- Providing hemostasis

These behaviors may vary depending on patient populations, practice environments, services provided, accessibility of human and fiscal resources, institutional policy, and state nurse practice acts.

The decision by an RN to practice as a first assistant must be made voluntarily and deliberately, with an understanding of the professional accountability that the role entails.

Qualifications of the RN First Assistant

Qualifications for RNFAs should include, but not be limited to:

- Certification in perioperative nursing (CNOR)
- Documentation of proficiency in perioperative nursing practice as both a scrub and circulating nurse
- Ability to apply principles of asepsis and infection control
- Knowledge of surgical anatomy, physiology, and operative technique related to the operative procedures in which the RN assists
- Ability to perform cardiopulmonary resuscitation
- Ability to perform effectively in stressful and emergency situations
- Ability to recognize safety hazards and initiate appropriate preventive and corrective action
- Ability to perform effectively and harmoniously as a member of the operating team
- Ability to demonstrate skill in behaviors unique to the RNFA (as defined)
- Meets requirements of statutes, regulations, and institutional policies relevant to RNFAs

Preparation for the RN First Assistant

AORN has stated, "The complexity of knowledge and skill required to effectively care for recipients of operating room nursing services compels nurses to be well educated and to continue their education beyond generic nursing programs."

Perioperative nurses who wish to practice as RNFAs must develop a set of cognitive, psychomotor, and affective behaviors that demonstrate accountability and responsibility for identifying and meeting the needs of recipients of their nursing services.

Development of this set of behaviors begins with and builds upon the education program leading to licensure as an RN, which provides basic knowledge, skills, and attitudes essential to the practice of perioperative nursing. Further preparation for the RNFA includes perioperative nursing practice with diversified experience in scrubbing and circulating. This should culminate in the nurse achieving certification as a CNOR. Additional preparation is then acquired through completion of formal education programs including didactic instruction and supervised clinical learning activities.

These programs should consist of curricula that address all of the content areas of the modules in the *Core Curriculum for the RN First Assistant*, take place in institutions approved by The Association of Higher Education (or its equivalent), and award a degree or certificate upon successful program completion.

Establishment of Clinical Privileges for the RN First Assistant

To determine if an RN qualifies for clinical privileges as a first assistant, an approval process must be established by the institution in which the individual will practice.

The process of granting clinical privileges should include mechanisms for:

- Assessing individual qualifications for practice
- Assessing continuing proficiency
- Evaluating annual performance
- Assessing compliance with relevant institutional and departmental policies
- Defining lines of accountability
- Retrieving documentation of participation as first assistant
- Establishing systems for peer review

Each RNFA demonstrates behaviors that progress on a continuum from basic competency to excellence. Once having met the educational and experiential requirements, the RNFA is encouraged to attain a bachelor of science in nursing degree and to achieve and maintain certification (CRNFA) for this specific role.

Modified from the Association of Operating Room Nurses: AORN standards and recommended practices for perioperative nurses, Denver, 1993, AORN.

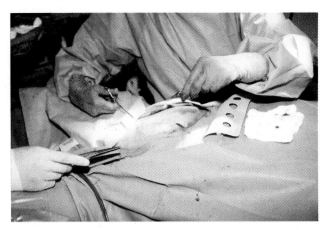

Fig. 3-7 The assistant closes the trocar sites at the completion of a laparoscopic procedure. (Courtesy Wendy K. Winer RN, BSN, Atlanta, Ga.)

general practitioners, nurses, physician assistants, and technologists, but they are not always the people best qualified to perform this function. The formal training and experience of the people being considered for the position must therefore be reviewed closely. They should be credentialed by the hospital or clinic to perform assistive duties. Many physicians, such as general practitioners, may not have received formal endoscopic training and therefore may not be the best choice for first-assistant duties for reasons of safety, among others. Pursuant to this, hospitals need to develop education and qualification guidelines for first assistants.

Some insurance carriers and managed care organizations are now refusing to provide reimbursement for the first assistant during certain endoscopic procedures, claiming that this position is not necessary. Most of the time, this has occurred when the first assistant has been another physician. If the procedure is really challenging and complex, then reimbursement for the cost of another physician may be granted. Some hospitals are responding to this problem by providing a nonphysician first assistant from the surgical staff.

If hospital management is unable or unwilling to assign a first assistant to a procedure for financial reasons, then the operating physician may want to inform the patient of the situation. However, this tends to be a very political issue, and the physician should think the matter through carefully before proceeding. If told of the situation, the patient may opt to directly pay for the first assistant or may complain to the third-party carrier for nonpayment. Insurance carriers and managed care organizations tend to pay more attention to the complaints of patients than to those of physicians in cases in which first assistant reimbursement has been denied (*Laparosc Surg Update*, 1995b).

If there are assistants available from the hospital staff, determining those endoscopic procedures for which an assistant is needed is often a challenging task. Following are the different factors that must be taken into consideration in determining this need:

- Skill level of the operating physician (an inexperienced physician usually asks for a first assistant)
- Patient's condition
- Complexity of the endoscopic procedure

If a physician asks for an assistant but this request cannot be met because of staffing problems, then the hospital will receive most of the blame if complications should arise during the procedure. Surgical administrators need to negotiate with physicians in determining those procedures for which a first assistant is truly required, and this discussion should include informing the physician of the cost of providing a first assistant. Openly discussing the rationale for needing the first assistant will either reveal reasons justifying the expense or reveal that the physician is asking for the assistant merely for arbitrary reasons.

If a physician requests a first assistant, the OR director should consider more than just the cost of the assistant. For instance, the endoscopic procedure will probably take much less time and the incidence of complications be lower with a skilled first assistant in attendance, and this will translate into indirect savings that can offset the cost of the first assistant. It has been estimated that when a qualified first assistant is in attendance, the length of an endoscopic procedure can be decreased by as much as 20% (*Laparosc Surg Update*, 1995a).

The RNFA is most effective when he or she is consistently assigned to certain endoscopic procedures and physicians. The physician then feels more secure because the RNFA understands exactly the surgical process to be employed. The physician can also be reassured that the RNFA will function appropriately and immediately in any emergency situation. When surgical directors randomly assign RNFAs to procedures, the operating physicians often feel that they are at the mercy of this decision. Physicians should be allowed to actively participate in the decision regarding the most qualified and available RNFA to assist during endoscopic procedures.

If the hospital is not financially able to provide an assistant, then the physician has to assume the responsibility of providing one, if needed. The assistant is then reimbursed or paid by the physician, depending on the contractual agreement between the two professionals. Often physicians hire an RNFA to help assess patients in the office, assist during the endoscopic procedure, provide perioperative patient education, and assist with follow-up care.

There are tremendous opportunities today for skilled RNFAs to become part of endoscopic teams, although many health care facilities require that RNFAs be certified before they can receive full privileges to assist with endoscopic procedures. Usually the RNFA must show documentation of attendance at a specialized training session focusing on the duties of the first assistant. This includes education about procedure techniques, appropriate use of instrumentation, patient safety, perioperative patient education, and specific perioperative activities.

The National Certification Board, Perioperative Nurses Inc. offers a certification examination for RNFAs. The following requirements must be met, however, before the candidate can take the examination (National Certification Board, Perioperative Nurses, Inc., 1995):

- Must be a CNOR (certified nurse in the operating room).
- Must have served as a first assistant for 2000 hours, with the last 500 documented hours being within 2 years of the date of application.
- Must be currently licensed as a registered nurse with no provisions.
- In 1998 the candidate must have a bachelor of science in nursing degree to qualify for the examination.

The candidate who passes the certification examination is granted the title of certified registered nurse first assistant (CRNFA) and must go through a recertification process every 5 years.

ANESTHESIA PROVIDER

Anesthesia for the endoscopic procedure can involve general anesthesia, regional anesthesia, conscious sedation, local anesthesia, topical anesthesia, or even no anesthesia. The providers administering anesthesia (i.e., physician anesthesiologist, nurse anesthetist, registered nurse) also vary depending on the type of anesthesia administered and the patient monitoring needed (Fig. 3-8).

The anesthesia provider is responsible for monitoring the patient and assisting with proper positioning before and during the procedure. Open communication with the operating physician is mandatory throughout the procedure to ensure that the appropriate amount of medication is being administered, depending on the course of the procedure.

If the endoscopic procedure is to be performed with the patient under conscious sedation, then the professional monitoring the patient must be proficient in patient monitoring and knowledgeable about the medication dosage, the route of administration, contraindications, potential complications, side effects, and emergency care. Sometimes a registered nurse has to monitor the patient receiving intravenous conscious sedation during an endoscopic procedure. Because of this, the Association of Operating Room Nurses has developed a recommended practice for "monitoring the patient receiving intravenous conscious sedation." The nurse providing the patient care and monitoring must review this recommendation to determine the scope of his or her practice. This recommendation is found in the appendix.

SURGICAL TECHNOLOGIST

A surgical technologist can be an integral part of the endoscopy team. The following are some of the overall responsibilities of the surgical technologist are to (Habgood, 1996):

- Provide a safe surgical or endoscopy environment
- Ensure that equipment and instruments function properly (Fig. 3-9)
- Promote patient safety

Technologists are usually graduates of postsecondary education programs in surgical technology offered at universities, community colleges, vocational-technical schools, and hospital-based programs (Habgood, 1996).

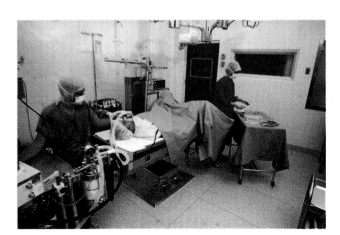

Fig. 3-8   An anesthesia provider delivers the anesthesia and monitors the patient throughout the endoscopic procedure. (Courtesy Karl Storz, Culver City, Calif.)

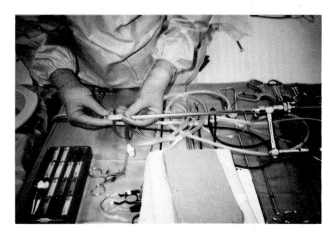

Fig. 3-9   A surgical technologist checks the working condition of an instrument. (Courtesy Wendy K. Winer RN, BSN, Atlanta, Ga.)

The Liaison Council on Certification for the Surgical Technologist grants the title of certified surgical technologist (CST) to surgical technologists who pass the credentialing examination.

A surgical technologist is an extremely important member of an endoscopic program because of the amount of technology involved. Surgical technologists can provide the technical skill needed to select and maintain endoscopic devices, but to do so, they need to receive ongoing education about these devices that focuses on the operation and care of the equipment.

Most surgical technologists function under the direction of the registered nurse in the operating room and other endoscopy areas. Any responsibilities delegated to the technologist must not conflict with the duties and the role expectations of the professional registered nurse. Usually the surgical technologist functions as scrub person (handles the instruments, supplies, and equipment during the procedure) (Fig. 3-10), second assisting technologist (assists the physician by providing retraction for exposure, suctioning, and so on), and first assistant technologist (assists the physician with draping, exposure, hemostasis, and wound closure).

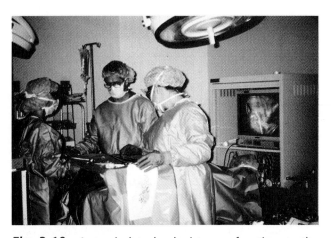

Fig. 3-10 A surgical technologist may function as the scrub person during an endoscopic procedure. (Courtesy Wendy K. Winer RN, BSN, Atlanta, Ga.)

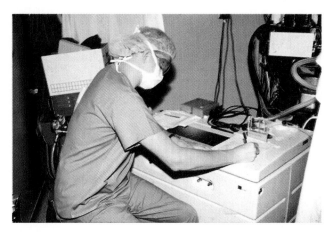

Fig. 3-11 A biomedical technician checks the performance of a laser while doing preventive maintenance. (Courtesy Wendy K. Winer RN, BSN, Atlanta, Ga.)

BIOMEDICAL ENGINEER AND TECHNICIAN

Because most endoscopic equipment and instruments are highly technical, hospitals are developing biomedical engineering departments to properly maintain and service these devices. The biomedical engineer works closely with the other endoscopic team members (Fig. 3-11). Many manufacturers of endoscopic equipment and devices offer biomedical training during the sale of the equipment to ensure its proper maintenance. This usually leads to increased use of and a longer life expectancy for the equipment. Satisfied customers then freely share their positive experiences with others who are considering the purchase of such a product.

REFERENCES

Habgood C: Statutory declaration seeks to improve recognition, *Surg Tech*, Jan 1996.

Laparosc Surg Update, Endoscopy coordinator's role clarified, 2(12):137, 1994.

Laparosc Surg Update, Question: does standard of care require assistant for surgeon?, 3(1):11, 1995a.

Laparosc Surg Update, MCOs refusing to pay for surgeon's own first assistant, 3(7):75, 1995b.

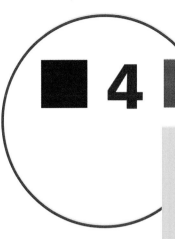

4

Professional Education

Proper professional education is the foundation of a successful endoscopic program. It helps to ensure patient safety, proper use of the equipment and instrumentation, and positive patient outcomes. However, physicians are not the only ones who need to be educated about the complexities and details of endoscopic procedures; nurses and technologists must also participate in continuing education programs.

NURSE AND SURGICAL TECHNOLOGIST EDUCATION

Endoscopy Education

Nurses and technologists involved in an endoscopic program should attend formal education sessions on endoscopic surgery. The nurse needs to learn about perioperative patient care, endoscopic techniques, safety issues, and the instrumentation and equipment; the technologist needs to learn mainly about the technology. Education gives nurses and technologists the means with which to help make endoscopy programs successful.

Physicians performing the endoscopic procedures come to value the nurse or technologist who possesses great endoscopic skill and knowledge because the procedures he or she attends tend to run more smoothly. If the hospital education budget is limited, many times a physician will offer to pay for an endoscopic training program to update and maintain the nurse's and technologist's level of expertise.

There are many different well-orchestrated endoscopic courses for physicians throughout the United States. Unfortunately, there are not as many such courses for nurses and technologists. Therefore, many nurses and technologists must settle for attending courses intended for physicians. These courses do not always meet the nonphysician professionals' expectations unless they include a special breakout session in which the role of the nurse or technologist is discussed. In turn, a physician who attends a nonphysician endoscopic course would not have all of his or her needs met either. Nurses and technologists do not need less education about endoscopy, they need different education. Nurses must learn about such topics as endoscopic instrumentation and equipment, patient positioning, the content and approach to patient education, intraoperative nursing considerations, intravenous conscious sedation, and other patient care details. Technologists need to learn about the endoscopic instrumentation and equipment, reprocessing, and the other technical components of the procedure.

On-the-job training is often the only means of education that is available to the endoscopy team. This is not ideal, but at least education is provided. A more extensive educational format, such as courses, seminars, or workshops, is usually preferred to ensure the safe performance of endoscopic procedures.

Endoscopy Courses

Many endoscopic courses for nurses and technologists have been patterned after nursing laser seminars. The registrant first attends a didactic session in which the evolution of endoscopy, the instrumentation and equipment, patient care, and specific surgical procedures are reviewed. Then the registrant may attend a hands-on laboratory where he or she is actually able to handle and operate instruments and other devices.

Endoscopic course topics may include the following:

Patient care
  Patient education
  Preoperative evaluation and preparation
  Discharge instructions
  Follow-up care
  Cultural diversity
  Psychological and social implications
Endoscopic technique
  Patient selection criteria
  Patient positioning
  Intraoperative care
  Anesthesia
  Complications
  Research—patient outcomes
Technology
  Equipment—proper operation, care, and maintenance
  Instruments—proper use, processing, quality checks
  Supply management—standardization
  Evaluations—disposables versus reusables
  Management of inventories
  Computerization of inventory
  Troubleshooting equipment
Management of the endoscopic program
  Policy and procedure development
  Management of change
  Maintenance of a total quality management program
  Financial issues and limitations
  Staffing
  Scheduling
  Marketing
  Legal ramifications

Endoscopy training for nurses must include technical and professional components. Often perioperative nurses are already expected to have mastered the professional component, so training is then focused on the technical aspects of endoscopy.

It is extremely important for both the nurse and technologist to understand the technology. The technical component of training may include instruction in the way to troubleshoot a video camera or a monitor to obtain a clearer image. Many conferences only focus on and teach the technical aspects, because this is the most complex component. Company representatives are usually very good at explaining the technology of their products but generally are not qualified to provide education on the nursing care required during an endoscopic procedure.

After attending a course or inservice, the endoscopic team member is often then partnered with a more experienced person who helps him or her apply the newly acquired information to the clinical setting. This one-on-one experience is vital to ensuring competency. Competency checklists can be designed to determine the learner's weaknesses and strengths. These lists can also trace the endoscopic experience of the team member. If a nurse or technologist has not participated in a specific endoscopy procedure or worked with a particular product for awhile, then he or she may be partnered once again with an experienced staff member until the procedure or the operation of the equipment is mastered. A nurse or technologist should always let the surgical manager or endoscopy coordinator know if he or she feels unqualified to participate in an endoscopy procedure. This may be difficult to do, but the patient always should be provided with the highest level of experienced care available.

The operating room manager must ensure that appropriate funds are available in the operating budget for staff education and courses on endoscopy, nursing care, program planning, and device management. Nurses and technologists sent to these programs should be required to provide education to other staff members upon their return. This train-the-trainer type of education has gained a lot of popularity because many more people can then participate in and benefit from this learning process.

Records of the training received and the dates of instruction need to be kept for all members of the program. A review of such records can quickly reveal a deficiency in education. These records may also be used by attorneys in malpractice litigation to show that the staff either had or had not received proper education about a technique or device.

Even though education courses are attended and guidelines are developed, some hospital staff members may take shortcuts that can compromise patient safety. The reprocessing of endoscopic instrumentation is one area in which this can easily occur. For example, a cleaning technician who attends an education class about bloodborne pathogens and the use of protective equipment during the cleaning of endoscopy instruments may refuse to follow the written guidelines that require protective attire to be worn and instruments to be thoroughly cleaned. In such a situation, the manager is then confronted with having to take disciplinary action. Any employee who subjects himself or herself to avoidable hazards and possibly compromises the reprocessing must never be tolerated. The manager should make sure that the staff member understands the consequences of not following hospital policy. The facility's risk manager may also be involved so that potential litigation is avoided should the staff member be harmed or a patient acquire an infection. Statistical analysis has shown that the treatment for an average hospital-acquired infection costs a health care facility approximately $14,000 (*Laparosc Surg Update*, 1995c).

Continuing Education

The constantly changing endoscopic technology mandates that all involved in it participate in continuing education. Changes in procedural techniques and instrumentation must be communicated continually among the members of the endoscopy team. For example, laparoscopic procedures are now performed at the bedside of critically ill patients too sick to be moved to an operating room. Nurses and technologists who participate in such bedside laparoscopies must be educated regarding the proper preparations to be made for these procedures. A laparoscopy cart can be used to move needed instruments and devices to the patient's bedside. The team approach, involving the perioperative nurse, technologist, surgeon, anesthesia personnel, and other health care professionals, is mandatory because the laparoscopy is being performed outside of the normal surgical environment. Everyone must be able to handle any emergencies and know where lifesaving equipment is located in these nonsurgical areas.

Continuing education can be obtained by means of courses, seminars, professional journal articles, computerized learning programs, videoconferences, monographs, and other sources. The acquisition of further experience in endoscopy through continuing education is the professional obligation of the nurse and technologist; it is not the responsibility of the hospital to see that this occurs.

PHYSICIAN EDUCATION

Perioperative nurses should have an awareness and understand the importance of the training physicians go through because they work so closely with them and each depends on the other's skill and knowledge.

Endoscopy has become an educational challenge to physicians because the technology is constantly changing. Surgeons who have been performing open procedures now have to learn new ways of doing these procedures using endoscopic technology. This requires a major shift from the accepted methods that many physicians have used for years. No longer can the surgeon directly see the internal structures during the operation. He or she must learn to operate in two dimensions from a video monitor image using instruments that are manipulated differently. The expertise that is needed to perform an operative endoscopy can be likened to mowing the grass with a riding lawn mower but doing it backward at full speed while watching through a mirror.

Physicians must stay continually abreast of new surgical techniques and instrumentation. Continuing education is critical to their remaining current regarding new advancements. Physicians can achieve this by attending postgraduate courses and other continuing medical education (CME) programs, reading publications, participating in computerized learning programs, and observing actual procedures. Physicians should also objectively and critically compare results and outcome data before incorporating new techniques into their practices.

Education in endoscopy can also be acquired in academic settings, but an interesting trend that has been observed is that most academic institutions are not always the first to jump into endorsing or teaching new technology. They appear to be more interested in becoming involved after the new advancements have been widely accepted. This trend was noted in the late 1980s and early 1990s when laparoscopic cholecystectomy techniques were otherwise being rapidly accepted. The academic community watched the evolution of these techniques and the interest that emanated from the smaller community hospitals. Numerous nonacademic training programs were initiated, and acceptance of the procedure was widespread, even though the academic community provided little input. After the popularity of the laparoscopic approach to cholecystectomy appeared to be established, universities then began to provide education courses on endoscopy. Now education on many endoscopic procedures is part of academic programs. Medical students, interns, and residents attend classes, participate in animal laboratory experiences, and then assist with endoscopic procedures on humans.

Today many nurses and technologists attend endoscopic courses designed for physicians. A variety of such courses have been developed since the endoscopic explosion first began during the early 1990s. Usually an endoscopic course for physicians offers category I CME credits, meaning that the course has been preplanned, has specific objectives, and meets the requirements of CME accreditation. Ideally the course should include a didactic session and a laboratory experience in which endoscopic technique and instrument usage are taught. Animal laboratories are being conducted in conjunction with many didactic courses, but antivivisectionist groups have been effective in limiting the animal models that are acceptable for this type of training. The porcine (pig) model is now used by many endoscopic laboratories for physician practice and education.

Some educational courses provided by hospitals allow physicians to actually scrub in during the procedures so that they can have a close look at what is being done. The visiting physician learner must receive temporary privileges to participate, however, and the patient must be informed of this added person at the surgical table. Because this arrangement is very difficult to orchestrate, videoconferencing is becoming a more acceptable way to achieve the same end. It allows many physician learners at a distant site to closely observe the surgery while interacting with the surgeon.

CREDENTIALING

Credentialing Overview

The perioperative nurse must understand the physician credentialing process to appreciate its complexity. Sometimes nurses themselves are involved with the credentialing process, either when applying for RNFA credentials or when assisting with the routing of the paperwork and the documentation required for physician credentialing.

Physicians and other professionals who have been credentialed are granted privileges and are considered qualified to perform or participate in surgical procedures. As new endoscopic procedures are introduced and older ones expanded and refined, credentialing processes have become quite complicated and confusing. Because so many endoscopic procedures have been initiated recently, even seasoned practitioners have had to attend specialized training programs to learn about the new techniques and instrumentation required. Setting standards and developing policies addressing education and experience needed for credentialing have posed interesting challenges. There currently is no consensus on the criteria for credentialing.

Professional organizations have offered guidelines to help hospitals develop credentialing policies. For example, the American College of Surgeons in a 1990 statement recommended that "For optimal quality patient care, laparoscopic cholecystectomy should be performed by surgeons who are qualified to perform open cholecystectomy." The college believes that these surgeons must have the skill and experience to treat complications, to perform biliary tract procedures, and to determine the best method of gallbladder removal (White and Klein, 1991).

Health care facilities have formed credentialing committees to oversee this process and to establish standards and protocols. According to the Joint Commission on the Accreditation of Healthcare Organizations (JCAHO), hospitals must follow their own written policies. For example, it may be a hospital credentialing policy that the medical staff office have a copy of a physician's certificate of attendance at an endoscopy conference to validate that the physician attended it. If a joint commission inspector reviews the files and a credentialed physician's certificate is not there, then the hospital would not be considered to be following its own written policies. This would be deemed as an infraction by the JCAHO but could also be the source of potential litigation if that physician were ever a defendant in a lawsuit involving an endoscopic procedure.

Administrators of endoscopic programs must beware of the opportunists who want to try a new procedure only because they have been attracted to the new instrumentation or equipment that may have been purchased. Surgical staff members must continually monitor the physicians who have received final approval to perform any new procedures.

When new endoscopic procedures are introduced, records may be kept by credentialing committees to document surgical outcomes. This information can be periodically compared with the results of the conventional treatments. This information will either prove or disprove the safety and appropriateness of new applications and will show whether expected results are consistently produced. The credentialing committee can then determine if credentialing should be awarded, allowing the new procedure to be performed.

Usually hospital bylaws state that credentialing privileges awarded to physicians, RNFAs, advanced practice nurses, physician assistants, surgical technologist first assistants, and other providers must be preempted if a review of the education and training (including any preceptorships) received raises any questions about its quality. The particular credentialed practitioner must then be monitored to ensure that safe and quality care is being delivered.

Those physician specialists who will actually be credentialed to perform a particular endoscopic procedure continues to be a controversial issue. Physicians in overlapping specialties may want privileges to do the same procedure. For example, cardiologists, radiologists, general surgeons, and vascular surgeons all want to be able to perform percutaneous endoscopic transluminal angioplasty. In situations such as this, collaboration and not competition is needed. Some procedures, especially new ones, may require the skills of two different specialists. Patient safety again must be the primary determinant of the decisions regarding these matters.

Managers must communicate the updated credentialing status of each physician to the staff. Staff members need to know the procedures that can be performed by a physician and should have ready access to this information. For example, if a noncredentialed physician performs an endoscopic procedure in the surgery or endoscopy suite during off-shift hours and injures the patient, the facility also has to assume some of the blame because hospital employees participated in the procedure and the endoscopy was performed in the hospital. Under the legal doctrine of corporate liability, the hospital can be held liable for this type of patient harm. The facility's lawsuit usually can be separated from the physician's lawsuit, however, to minimize the hospital's liability (Gruendemann and Fernsebner, 1995).

Preceptorships

After the basic course work has been completed by a physician, the credentialing policy may then require that a physician have one or more procedures preceptored (proctored) before privileges can be awarded.

The puzzling questions that have to be answered are how many cases need to be proctored and what are the actual role and responsibilities of the preceptor?

Physicians should be willing to share their expertise with others, but this may not always be the case. Sometimes a physician may want to be the only one who offers a particular procedure, or a physician may not have time to serve as a preceptor to others. To obtain privileges the learning physician must then find someone outside of the hospital to precept him or her.

The actual number of preceptored procedures a physician needs to perform has become a very controversial topic for many credentialing committees. Is only 1 enough or are 10 too many? Should the number of proctored cases be decided by the preceptor after he or she observes the first procedure? If the preceptor subjectively determines that the physician performed the procedure safely and appropriately in the first case, should others then be required? If multiple preceptored cases are required (e.g., more than 10), are credentialed physicians on the committee trying to keep others from obtaining privileges? Are many of the physicians not making themselves available for preceptorships? These are just some of the questions that have been asked as credentialing committees develop protocols.

The Society of American Gastrointestinal Endoscopic Surgeons (SAGES) has stated that proctoring is desirable but does not state that it must be done. These details are left to the hospital to determine (Gruendemann and Fernsebner, 1995).

Another controversial issue is the actual role of the preceptor. Is it merely to observe the procedure being performed and report back to the credentialing committee? Should the preceptor intervene if the physician being observed makes a blatant mistake or is about to cause the patient injury? Is the proctor authorized to assist? What are the legal ramifications of a preceptor intervening during a procedure? The credentialing committee should specify the exact role of the preceptor. If the preceptor is not allowed to participate in the procedure in any way, even if an untoward outcome is imminent, then this must be written into the hospital policy and communicated to the preceptor (*Laparosc Surg Update*, 1994a).

There is a difference between teaching and preceptoring. A teaching physician is more apt to intervene during a procedure if the patient's safety is compromised. A true preceptor's function, on the other hand, is only to observe the physician's technique to determine the safety of the procedure and the competency of the physician. The preceptor is not present to ensure that the patient is not harmed. Because no patient-physician relationship is established, the preceptor has no obligation to the patient. The preceptor is considered a bystander, not an active participant in the procedure. If the preceptor intervenes, the relationship to the patient changes and the preceptor is then liable for the outcome of the procedure.

On the other side of this controversial issue, plaintiff attorneys may challenge the nonparticipation of a preceptor if he or she observes gross neglect or malpractice taking place. The fact that a preceptor is usually present to ensure that a physician is meeting the standard of care may be interpreted to mean that the preceptor is in attendance to intervene and protect the patient in the event the physician is observed to be unskilled. The real reason for the preceptor being present therefore needs to be determined and whether he or she *is* there to protect the patient.

A preceptor should have a written document outlining the proctoring agreement with the physician. It should explicitly state whether the preceptor is expected and authorized to intervene should the patient's safety be compromised or an emergency situation arise.

The dilemma posed by this situation will continue to be a source of argument. In one legal case tried in Pennsylvania (*Clarke* v. *Hoek*, 1985), it was decided that the preceptor could not be sued because he did not intervene in an orthopedic case. The decision of the court was that the preceptor did not have a patient-physician relationship established, so he was not expected to intervene. A further argument in the preceptor's defense was that the patient was not billed for the proctor's services. Some attorneys have challenged this attitude, claiming that giving verbal advice could be construed as actually performing the procedure. Laws in regard to this issue differ from state to state, however.

A possible solution to this dilemma would be to have a physician educator also present during the preceptorship. If the learning physician gets into difficulty, then the teaching physican could step in to help instead of the proctor.

A further problem arises, however, when a new endoscopic procedure is first introduced. This often leads to credentialing confusion because if, for example, a hospital requires that a physician be preceptored by a qualified staff physician for two procedures, this requirement could not be met because there would be no qualified physicians on staff who already perform the procedure. A process therefore needs to be developed and put into effect that allows a physician to be the first to become credentialed to perform a particular endoscopic procedure. Such a process might require that the first physician seeking credentialing observe at least two procedures at another facility. Or, it might allow for a visiting physician from another hospital to be granted temporary privileges to precept the staff physician performing the new procedure. The visiting physician may only be needed to observe and not participate in the procedure. Once one physician is credentialed, then he or she can function as the preceptor of others.

The actual role of the preceptor will continue to be a source of legal and ethical controversy. Ultimately it may be decided that physicians must rely on their own common sense and do what they feel is right for the patient.

The following qualifications may be considered when developing guidelines for a preceptor:

- Has performed the particular procedure many times
- Is recognized as a skilled endoscopist
- Has no fiduciary relationship with the physician being proctored
- Will have no actual involvement in the procedure
- Should be objective and uninvolved with the physician's credentialing approval
- Should report the results of the preceptorship back to the credentialing body in writing

Points that the preceptor should note about the physician being observed may include the following:

- Familiary with the endoscopic instrumentation and equipment
- Competence during the procedure
- Appropriate surgical decisions
- Safety
- Appropriateness of patient selection
- Duration of the procedure
- Success of the procedure

If a surgeon is a skilled endoscopist and has mastered the basic competency required for endoscopy, then it should not be necessary for him or her to go through a preceptorship for each different laparoscopic procedure he or she wishes to offer. For example, the skills needed to perform a laparoscopic lysis of adhesions are very similar to those needed to perform a laparoscopic vaporization of endometrial implants. If a physician wants to do something that is completely different from a basic endoscopic procedure, however, then a review board should evaluate the proposed procedure. For example, a surgeon who has been credentialed to perform a laparoscopic cholecystectomy may need to obtain additional specific credentialing and privileges to perform a laparoscopic bowel resection.

Preceptorships may also be necessary for surgeons who are experiencing quality assurance problems. If a physician is noting an increased incidence of complications or undesirable outcomes in his or her patients during or after endoscopic procedures, then a preceptorship may be needed to explore the reasons for these results. Sometimes physicians are not eager to accept another physician from their own facility to serve as the preceptor in these situations. In this event, a preceptor may be brought in from another facility to provide an unbiased opinion. Some professional organizations have established registries of qualified preceptors that can be used as a source of outside preceptors.

RESIDENT EDUCATION

Because many perioperative nurses work in teaching institutions, they need to understand the credentialing or certification process for residents. Often the endoscopy team is involved in the routing of the documentation of residents' learning experiences pertaining to endoscopy procedures.

Endoscopy is now being taught in academic settings, usually in conjunction with training at an animal laboratory. Simulators are also being developed that will decrease the reliance on animal laboratories as practice settings. In addition, residents may receive education about the newer endoscopic procedures at ongoing continuing education conferences and may participate in these training sessions along with the staff physicians.

Many facilities do not actually credential a resident because they only credential physicians and other permanent providers on staff. However, facilities should certify residents to perform endoscopic procedures. Certification requirements are often the same as the requirements for actual credentialing. Resident certification usually requires proof of academic education or attendance at a formal endoscopic course.

For residents to be certified to perform certain endoscopic procedures, they should be able to perform the respective open procedures, should conversion to these prove necessary. However, endoscopic training has become so advanced and so much a focus of training that many residents are not getting the training and experience in performing the traditional open procedures.

Creative and innovative ways of teaching endoscopic skills are now being explored for use in resident training programs. An Alabama hospital has developed a simple, reproducible examination to objectively test the laparoscopic skill level of their residents (*Laparosc Surg Update*, 1994b). The test has not actually been used to certify residents but could be used for this.

Practice and testing stations were set up in the residents' quarters. An objective hands-on examination tested the resident's dexterity, hand-eye coordination, and ability to work with both hands. The time it took for the resident to perform the different tasks was recorded, but the quality of the resident's skill was not assessed.

The following supplies were provided at the testing sites:

- Trocars and sheaths
- Laparoscopy training boxes
- Instruments (e.g., needle holders, suture passers, dissectors, forceps, and so on)
- Cameras
- Monitors
- Laparoscopes
- Small beads or other items to use to practice hand-eye coordination

The examination objectively measured the essential laparoscopic skills the resident would need to master more complicated endoscopic procedures. Some of the skills tested were knot tying, the proper use of instruments, the endoscopic use of different needles, loop tying, stapling, tacking mesh, and excising tissue.

The residents began to compete with each other for top test scores, which caused them to practice more and more and which naturally increased their endoscopic skill.

The surgical team and staff physicians also began to practice using these testing models. The laparoscopic examination requirements were found to be very successful in promoting self-improvement. The test motivated all members of the laparoscopy team because the scores of all were compared. This type of skill challenge was tremendously successful not only in refining surgical coordination but also in enhancing the comradery among team members.

PRODUCT AND SKILLS DEVELOPMENT

Any new technology goes through a series of laboratory and clinical investigation stages before being integrated into practice. All members of the endoscopy team should understand the details of this process because nurses and technologists may be involved at any stage of product development.

The procedure involving product development for endoscopic procedures follows the generic process described below (White and Klein, 1991):

1. In vitro feasibility testing. During this initial phase, products are reviewed to determine their ease of use and any limitation of use.

2. In vitro investigation on animal models. During this stage, any device hazards are noted, along with the short-term effects and results of animal studies.

3. Open clinical trials on selected patients. This stage involves the development of a comprehensive plan for using the device on humans. The investigational review boards of the participating facilities must review and approve the plan before the investigational device is used on their patients. The review board is responsible for ensuring that the plan is adhered to closely and results are monitored. Patients asked to participate in the studies are counseled so that they can make a knowledgeable decision about whether to do so.

Results of the study will either show or not show the effectiveness of the device. In this regard, subjective data are not as important as objective data. For example, a patient may subjectively note relief of the symptoms from occluded femoral arteries after laser endovascular therapy, but hemodynamic studies may show objectively that the procedure has not been a success. Because the objective results are more important, the likelihood of

this procedure being accepted would diminish. (It actually did happen that, although laser endovascular procedures performed in animals were successful, the human clinical studies did not replicate the animal study results.)

The U.S. Food and Drug Administration (FDA) is involved in this third stage of product development. The goal of this stage is to confirm a product's safety and to determine whether its use is associated with successful patient outcomes. If the outcomes and results are positive, then the FDA grants marketing approval and the next stage can begin.

4. Randomized trials to compare procedures involving the new device with those involving standard methods. This stage usually involves a multicenter study. Usually a lot of excitement about a product is generated at this point. However, many physicians want to get involved before the results of multicenter studies are published to make sure that they are not left out. This is illustrated by the fact that physicians were buying lasers to perform laparoscopic cholecystectomies before studies had shown that electrosurgical units could also be used safely and appropriately for this procedure.

There needs to be enough patients in these multicenter studies to ensure that the results are statistically meaningful. The demographics, symptomatology, site and severity of the disease, and other such factors must be examined to make sure that the patient population is truly randomized, that is, that it is a representative sample of patients. This is needed to further validate the results of the study.

Physicians, nurses, and other endoscopy team members should evaluate the data and results of the investigational studies from the following three standpoints (White and Klein, 1991):

1. What are the results of the trials versus those of standard therapies?

2. Would the results of these trials be applicable to the patient population the physician serves?

3. What is the impact of other competing alternative treatments?

Advancements in endoscopy will continue to be a source of turmoil and confusion for physicians and the endoscopic team. To help reduce this turmoil and confusion the following plan can be used to assess new endoscopic technology and to incorporate it into practice (White and Klein, 1991):

1. Evaluate the stage of development of the endoscopic technology and assess its impact to date.

2. Participate in training and practice sessions to learn safe techniques and become competent in using the technology.

3. Develop guidelines for credentialing physicians and first assistants and determine requirements for preceptors.

4. Monitor the ongoing effectiveness of and the patient outcomes from the new endoscopic technology.

5. Integrate the education about the new endoscopy advancement into residency and nursing programs.

As endoscopic procedures are incorporated into practice, the endoscopic team members must realize that the learning curve for physicians is usually longer for more complicated procedures. Initial procedures also may be associated with a higher complication rate than that for the respective open procedures (Gruendemann and Fernsebner, 1995).

The operating time is often used to measure the learning curve for similar endoscopic procedures. For example, a retrospective study was performed to determine the learning curve for laparoscopic-assisted colectomies. It was found that the mean operating time for the first 25 procedures was 250 minutes but leveled off to 140 minutes after 75 procedures had been performed. It was also found that the rate of conversions to open procedures declined as the surgeons gained more experience. No significant trend could be detected with regard to intraoperative complications (*Laparosc Surg Update*, 1995a).

The rate of conversion to an open method is not a gauge of the skill or qualifications of the physician or endoscopy team. Conversion to an open procedure is also not necessarily regarded as a failure, because there may be sound reasons for doing this. Although a significantly higher conversion rate may prompt a review of a particular surgeon's techniques and skill, again there may be factors not entirely under the surgeon's control necessitating these conversions. For example, the physician may be operating on more critically ill patients who may not totally meet the selection criteria for endoscopy, or it may be that a surgeon is just learning a new technique.

If the reasons for a high conversion rate are being sought, then other factors that more appropriately reflect the physician's skill should be reviewed, too. The surgeon's operative technique could be observed by a preceptor, or the surgeon's postoperative results could be examined. If corrective action is indicated, then the decision should be made not just on the basis of the surgeon's rate of conversion.

Patients should be informed about the possible need to convert an endoscopic procedure to the open method. This allows the patient to make a more knowledgeable decision about whether to have a particular procedure attempted endoscopically.

After attending an educational session on endoscopy, conquering new techniques may be easier if the team approach is used. One group of surgeons and endoscopy team members divided a laparoscopic method of Nissen fundoplication into the following four different areas to master:

1. Dissection of the esophagus from crural structures

2. Suture closure of the crura

3. Creation of the wrap

4. Suturing of the wrap

Each surgeon became an expert in one area. When the first procedures were done, each of the four surgeons performed his or her assigned part of the operation. The surgeons then attempted other segments of the surgery in subsequent procedures after successfully conquering one part, until they had mastered all four areas. By becoming skilled in each aspect of the surgery, the learning curve for the physicians was altered as experience and skill were segmentally acquired. The nonphysician endoscopy team members were the same for each procedure. This team approach works especially well for procedures not performed frequently at hospitals (*Laparosc Surg Update*, 1995b).

REFERENCES

Clarke v. Hoek. 174 Cal. App. 3d 208, 219 Cal. Reporter 845. Nov. 8, 1985.

Gruendemann BJ, Fernsebner B: *Comprehensive perioperative nursing*, vol 2, *Practice*, Boston, 1995, Jones and Bartlett Publishers, 457.

Laparosc Surg Update, Proctors warned on intervention perils, 2(3):28, 1994a.

Laparosc Surg Update, Simple exam tests skill of laparoscopic surgeons, 2(7):77, 1994b.

Laparosc Surg Update, Learning curve for colectomy longer than supposed, 3(4):46, 1995a.

Laparosc Surg Update, Team approach reduces learning curve for Nissen fundoplication, 3(4):45, 1995b.

Laparosc Surg Update, Question: What to do when equipment techs won't clean properly, 3(5):59, 1995.

White RA, Klein SR: *Endoscopic surgery*, St. Louis, 1991, Mosby, p 274.

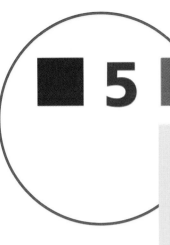

Preoperative Assessment and Planning

The perioperative nurse is responsible for making clinical decisions throughout the patient's endoscopy experience. The foundation for this role is the nursing process, which consists of assessment, diagnosis, outcome identification, planning, implementation, and evaluation. Throughout the nursing process the nurse must continually focus on the care of the patient and avoid approaching patient care from the perspective of all of the technology involved in the endoscopic procedure. The phases of the nursing process as they pertain to patient care during an endoscopic procedure are explained in more detail in the following sections.

PREOPERATIVE ASSESSMENT

Before the endoscopic procedure, the patient must be assessed so that an individualized plan of care can be formulated. Information about the patient can be obtained from several sources, including a preoperative interview with the patient, family members and friends, and hospital records and other health care reports (Fig. 5-1). Often the patient has already undergone diagnostic tests, such as an ultrasound or a barium enema radiologic examination, to validate the need for the endoscopic procedure.

The perioperative nurse interviews the patient to determine the plan of care to be implemented. This interview can take place in the physician's office, the operating room suite, an inpatient unit, an outpatient center, or some other area. Privacy must be maintained, especially if sensitive issues are addressed. The nurse is responsible for minimizing or eliminating any environ-mental distractions so that the patient feels comfortable during this interview.

The patient's history provides valuable information about the patient, including the symptoms of the condition, the effect of the disorder on the patient's functional and emotional status, past conditions and surgical procedures, medications currently being taken, any disabilities or limitations that would necessitate an alteration in the surgical plan of care for the patient, and other notable details. Information about past surgical procedures should include the type of procedure, the date performed, the patient's response to the anesthetic, the postoperative recovery course, and the impact of the procedure on the patient.

Often questionnaires are used to facilitate this assessment (Fig. 5-2). After the patient completes the questionnaire, the nurse reviews the information provided with the patient to formulate a nursing diagnosis and a plan of care. This interview should reflect a holistic attitude, in that the patient must be treated as a whole person, not just as a condition that must be treated. A thorough interview with the patient assists in determining the patient's desired outcomes.

Once the patient's history is obtained, a physical assessment is performed to review the patient's current health status. A head-to-toe examination of the patient's body systems is completed. The patient's physical conditions, including vital signs, range of motion, height, weight, congenital or acquired impairments, nutritional status, and cardiovascular and respiratory status, must be included in the assessment (Fig. 5-3). Limitations or alterations in the patient's physical well-being must be noted, since they will have an impact on the plan of care.

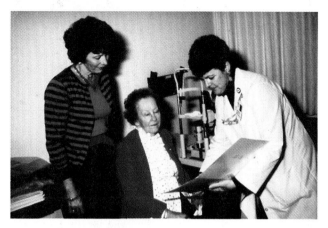

Fig. 5-1 Preoperative assessment of the patient usually includes the patient's support person.

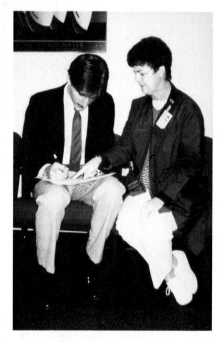

Fig. 5-2 Patient completes preoperative questionnaire.

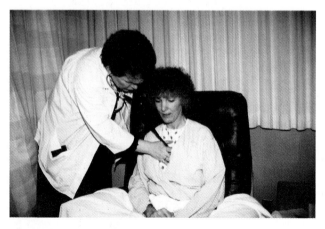

Fig. 5-3 The nurse performs a preoperative physical examination.

Recovery may be delayed if these concerns are not addressed adequately.

Laboratory tests or studies may be ordered by the physician to further determine the patient's condition before the endoscopic procedure. Often these tests can be done just before the procedure if the results can be obtained immediately. It may take more time for the results of other tests to become available, so preplanning must be done to coordinate such tests.

Often the perioperative nurse who obtains the history and performs the physical examination is not the same nurse who accompanies the patient to surgery. The nurse who cares for the patient in surgery must review the record of the preoperative assessment findings to understand the patient's physical and emotional condition so that he or she can design an appropriate care plan. The continuity of nursing care is extremely important to help the patient feel comfortable about the impending procedure. Therefore the nurse who performs the preoperative assessment should communicate his or her findings to the intraoperative nurse.

During the initial assessment of the patient, the nurse must verify that the patient understands the procedure and has given written consent for it. At this time the nurse must also determine whether the patient understands the type of anesthesia to be used. If the endoscopic procedure is to be performed using general or regional anesthesia, then the anesthesiologist or nurse anesthetist also assesses the patient. Because many endoscopic procedures are less invasive, only local anesthesia may be administered while the nurse monitors the patient. The patient needs to understand the type of anesthesia to be administered and the expectations during the procedure. For example, if intravenous sedation is planned for a colonoscopy, the patient should realize that he or she may feel sleepy but also may be asked to move to different positions during the procedure.

During the preoperative assessment, the nurse also must evaluate the patient's psychologic health. This includes the patient's response to and understanding of the impending endoscopic procedure. This response may have a bearing on the patient's willingness to participate in the rehabilitation process. For example, the understanding of the procedure should include the ways in which pain is controlled postoperatively. By involving the patient's family or designated friends preoperatively, they can then know the kind of support that they will need to provide during the postoperative phase.

Videotapes about specific endoscopic procedures are often available for patients and their support system. This added educational tool assists in promoting a complete understanding of the perioperative course. Often a videotape is sent to the patient before the procedure so that realistic expectations can be fostered. The patient can then be shown the preoperative preparations, the intraoperative procedure, and the anticipated postoperative course. Once the patient has a basic understanding of the endoscopic procedure, then he or she can ask specific questions about the procedure during the assessment interview with the nurse. Allaying anxiety and fulfilling the patient's need to understand will facilitate a more smooth performance of the procedure.

Preoperative preparation for the endoscopic procedure is critically important and usually depends on the patient's condition, the endoscopic procedure to be performed, the physician's preference, and the hospital or outpatient clinic's protocols. For example, patients may be instructed not to eat or drink after midnight before the day of surgery. Some patients, such as those with mitral valve prolapse, may also need to begin taking antibiotic medications 2 to 3 days before the procedure.

NURSING DIAGNOSES

After the perioperative nurse analyzes the preoperative assessment information, nursing diagnoses can be made. These diagnoses should be validated with the patient and his or her support system. The nurse should then document the nursing diagnoses so that appropriate outcomes can be expected and an individualized nursing care plan can be designed.

Nurses may choose to use the North American Nursing Diagnosis Association (NANDA) diagnoses for patients scheduled for an endoscopic procedure. Following are some examples of the nursing diagnoses relevant to patients scheduled for an endoscopic procedure:
- Anxiety
- Risk for altered body temperature
- Fear
- Risk for fluid volume deficit
- Fluid volume excess
- Altered health maintenance
- Hypothermia
- Hyperthermia
- Risk for infection
- Risk for injury (related to perioperative positioning, the use of electrical equipment, physical surroundings, and so on)
- Knowledge deficit
- Impaired physical mobility
- Noncompliance
- Pain
- Powerlessness
- Sensory/perceptual alterations
- Risk for impaired skin integrity
- Ineffective thermoregulation
- Impaired tissue integrity
- Altered tissue perfusion
- Risk for trauma
- Altered urinary elimination
- Urinary retention

OUTCOME IDENTIFICATION

Expected outcomes that are unique to the patient scheduled for the endoscopic procedure are identified after the nurse has formulated the nursing diagnoses (Fig. 5-4). Patient outcomes are determined with the patient and are derived from the nursing diagnoses. Outcomes should be realistic and attainable, taking into consideration the patient's resources and support available after the procedure. The outcomes must also be measurable so that achievement of the identified outcomes can be determined during the evaluation phase.

Nursing diagnoses and identified outcomes help to guide the nurse in developing the plan of care for the patient having an endoscopic procedure. Specific nursing interventions can then be planned that promote the achievement of the goals set, which in turn determine the outcome of the procedure.

The nurse must continually involve the patient during this phase of the nursing process. Joint agreement on the expectations of the endoscopic procedure helps the patient understand the importance of his or her active participation to ensure that the anticipated recovery progresses as expected.

PLANNING

Care Plans

Appropriate planning identifies actions to be implemented that ensure the achievement of the desired patient outcomes. Care plans are developed on the basis of

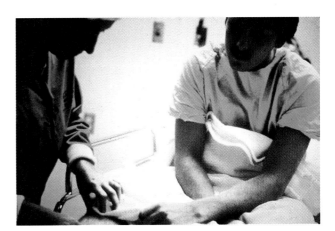

Fig. 5-4 The patient and nurse identify the expected outcomes of the endoscopic procedure.

Box 5-1 *Sample care plan for laparoscopic procedure*

Nursing diagnosis

Anxiety related to apprehension about the laparoscopic procedure and/or the perioperative experience.

Patient outcome

Symptoms of anxiety (e.g., increased heart rate, elevated blood pressure, restlessness, sweating, increased respiratory rate, minimal eye contact, agitation) are reduced.

Interventions

Assess anxiety level, as revealed by the patient's vital signs and verbal and nonverbal communication.
Assess patient's understanding of the laparoscopic procedure to be performed.
Discuss patient's anticipated outcomes from the procedure.
Provide education about the procedure, as needed.
Involve the patient's support system.
Answer patient's questions honestly.
Encourage the patient to verbalize his or her feelings and concerns.
Orient the patient to the laparoscopic room and carefully describe what the patient will see, hear, or feel.
Stay with the patient and provide comfort measures as needed (e.g., hold patient's hand, provide warm blankets or soothing music).

Nursing diagnosis

Risk of injury related to patient positioning.

Patient outcome

The patient is free from injury related to positioning during the laparoscopic procedure, as evidenced by an absence of neuromuscular impairment and tissue necrosis.

Interventions

Have adequate positioning devices available for the patient, as needed, to provide safety and comfort (e.g., pillows, pressure point pads).
Have appropriate number of personnel available to position the patient.
Lift the patient, rather than pulling or sliding him or her.
Avoid shearing forces or friction during patient transport and positioning.
Maintain patient's proper body alignment.
Maintain patient's airway at all times.
Monitor vital signs to note any changes as a result of positioning.

Nursing diagnosis

Risk for injury related to electrical hazards.

Patient outcome

The patient is free from injury related to electrical hazards, as evidenced by an absence of skin redness or blistering after the laparoscopic procedure is completed.

Interventions

Ensure the appropriate location of the electrosurgery dispersive pad. (Place pad on clean, dry skin, over a muscular area. Avoid bony prominences or areas of broken skin.)
Ensure that the pad adequately adheres to the skin.
Protect the electrosurgery active electrode (laparoscopic probe) when not in use.
Inspect laparoscopic instruments to ensure that they are well insulated.

Continued

---

the preoperative assessment findings, the nursing diagnoses formulated and the outcomes identified. Sample nursing diagnoses, outcomes, and a plan of care for a patient undergoing a laparoscopic procedure are given in Box 5-1.

The patient or his or her support system is involved in developing the care plan to foster acceptance and compliance. Designing an organized plan also minimizes the complications that may be associated with an endoscopic procedure. Safety concerns noted in the nursing diagnoses automatically alert the nurse to plan to implement activities to minimize and even eliminate these risks.

The nurse must continually prioritize the activities in the plan of care. Interventions must be reassessed in terms of their appropriateness and effectiveness. If complications do arise, the nurse must rearrange the plan so that potential problems are immediately addressed. Sometimes this requires collaboration with other nurses, physicians, or endoscopic team members.

The care plan may be written or unwritten. Many hospitals are decreasing the need to document the care plan because the patients move so quickly through the endoscopic area. Other hospitals still require that care plans be written as evidence of the nurse's judgment and knowledge of the care needed for the patient undergoing an endoscopic procedure. Some agencies or regulating bodies require written nursing care plans so that the health care facility can be licensed or accredited. Model computerized care plans for different endoscopic procedures can also be used and modified for each patient.

A plan of care identifies the nursing interventions that will achieve expected outcomes. Developing a care plan helps the nurse organize his or her thoughts and activities before implementing the plan. A plan of care developed in advance also helps to minimize the intraoperative time spent doing this, so that often the patient is provided with safer care. In addition, a care plan serves as the basis for the evaluation of nursing implementations.

Box 5-1   *Sample care plan for laparoscopic procedure—cont'd.*

Avoid situations in which direct or capacitive coupling could occur. (Do not activate an electrosurgical instrument near a metal instrument that could cause direct coupling. Do not mix metal trocars with plastic stability sleeves, which could result in capacitive coupling.)

Nursing diagnosis
Risk for wound infection related to surgical incisions made for trocar sites.

Patient outcome
The patient is free from infection related to breaks in asepsis, as evidenced by an absence of skin redness, swelling, or other signs of infection.

Interventions
Avoid shaving over the intended trocar sites. Use depilatories or electric clippers, if needed.
Ensure and monitor surgical asepsis throughout the endoscopic procedure.
Appropriately dress all surgical incisions after closure.

Nursing diagnosis
Risk for injury related to physical hazards.

Patient outcome
The patient is free from injury related to physical hazards, as evidenced by the use of properly functioning and appropriate instruments, equipment, and supplies.

Interventions
Ensure that equipment (e.g., insufflator, light source, endoscope) is working safely and appropriately before the laparoscopic procedure.

Inspect reusable laparoscopic instruments to assess their appropriate function and integrity (e.g., inspect for insulation breaks, misalignments, or malfunctions). Replace instruments as needed.
Ensure that needles and instruments are accounted for or intact at the end of the procedure.
Have backup instruments, equipment, and supplies available in the event of a device failure during the procedure.

Nursing diagnosis
Risk for altered participation in recovery process.

Patient outcome
The patient will participate in the recovery phase, as evidenced by his or her performing activities related to postoperative care.

Interventions
Assess the patient's understanding of the postoperative activities required for recovery.
Involve the patient's support system in the patient's care during recovery.
Assess the patient's feelings about the laparoscopic procedure.
Encourage the patient and his or her support system to verbalize their concerns and request more information if desired.
Verify the patient's and his or her support system's understanding of the early signs and symptoms of postoperative complications and the proper way to report them.
Assess the patient's and his or her support system's ability to comply with the postoperative instructions at home.

The plan of care for patients scheduled for endoscopic procedures may involve the following tasks:

- Verifying the endoscopic application to be performed and the patient's understanding of the procedure.
- Confirming the patient's expectations of the procedure.
- Developing perioperative patient education materials to ensure that patients understand the procedure, comply with intraoperative and discharge instructions, and understand the nature of the anticipated recovery course.
- Identifying the appropriate anesthesia to be administered.
- Providing competent nursing support.
- Ensuring the availability of functional equipment and appropriate instruments and supplies.
- Providing nursing care that promotes safety, prevents infection, and delivers quality services.
- Documenting the perioperative patient care activities.

Special Considerations

Standard nursing care plans must be altered to address the individual needs of the patients undergoing an endoscopic procedure. Many patient conditions or populations require special considerations that necessitate the formulation of a unique, distinctive plan of care. Some of these specific groups include pediatric, geriatric, pregnant, disabled, immunocompromised, and trauma patients.

Pediatrics

Pediatric surgery has now become a recognized specialized field of surgery. A definite distinction must be made between the surgical treatment of children and that of adults (Meeker and Rothrock, 1995). Therefore, endoscopic procedures and techniques performed in children and infants must be altered so that they are safe and effective. Many hospitals classify pediatric patients according to the following age groups (Meeker and Rothrock, 1995):

Premature infant: less than 37 weeks' gestation

Neonate, or newborn: birth to 1 month of age (in certain circumstances a premature infant may remain in this group until 3 months of age)

Infant: up to 1 year old

Toddler: 1 to 3 years old

Preschooler: 3 to 6 years old

School-age child: 6 to 11 years old

Adolescent: 11 to 18 years old (some hospitals consider 11- to 16-year-old patients to be in this group).

With the advances made in endoscopic equipment and instrumentation, along with the refinement in surgical techniques, endoscopic approaches have been increasingly used in the treatment and diagnosis of pathologic conditions in pediatric patients. Development of this less invasive method of surgery has been encouraged because endoscopy is often less traumatic to the patient and recovery from the procedure quicker. Following are some of the key perioperative nursing considerations that apply to pediatric patients scheduled for endoscopic procedures:

- Involve the family and support system of the pediatric patient in the preoperative assessment and postoperative care. They are critically important during the preoperative assessment because the patient may be too young to participate. They are also important in providing postoperative care because the patient may not be able to care for himself or herself. The family and support system must be involved as much as possible with every phase of the pediatric patient's care (Fig. 5-5).
- Realize the patient's growth and developmental stage and alter the nursing care accordingly.
- Implement a preoperative program to educate the patient and family or support system that may include a tour of the endoscopic suite to help provide the preoperative education needed to allay anxiety.

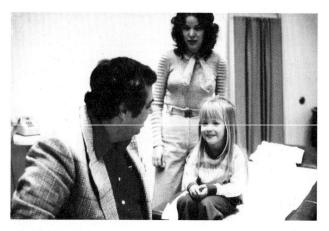

Fig. 5-5 The family or support system must be involved as much as possible with every phase of the pediatric patient's care.

Medical play items, such as puppets, audiovisual aids, and pictures, can be used during this process.

- Allow the pediatric patient to bring his or her favorite security object into the endoscopy room.
- Carefully verify that the patient has had nothing by mouth for the time before the procedure ordered by the physician.
- Determine the presence of the signed consent form on the chart and verify that the signature is that of the responsible party.
- Ensure that the appropriate doses of medications are administered by the perioperative nurse.
- Use age-appropriate communication during implementation of the nursing plan of care.
- Closely monitor the pediatric patient's temperature to ensure that effective thermoregulation is provided.
- Closely monitor the pediatric patient's fluid intake to prevent overload and dehydration.
- Determine the appropriate length of surgical instrumentation to be used during the endoscopic procedure.
- Ensure that the appropriate amount of irrigation or insufflation is used, depending on the size of the patient.
- Closely inspect the patient's skin after the procedure to determine whether any injury has been sustained during the endoscopic procedure.
- Reunite the pediatric patient with his or her support system as soon as possible after the endoscopic procedure.

Following are tips for performing a laparoscopy procedure on a pediatric patient:

- Space the trocars farther apart than they would be in adults to provide more working space. The trocar site also needs to be farther away from the target area. Plan to use about a 30-degree entry angle to best manipulate instruments at the target site.
- Ensure that the layers of tissue at all trocar sites are closed adequately. If a site is not closed sufficiently, the trocar site scar will enlarge as the child grows. This could leave a potentially significant defect in the abdominal wall.
- The child's abdomen is more pliable than an adult's, making it easier to manipulate instruments. However, care must be taken not to accidentally damage organs because instruments can be moved so freely.
- During a laparoscopic cholecystectomy, obtain a cholangiogram in all pediatric patients to determine the anatomy and find out whether there are any common bile duct stones (*Laparosc Surg Update*, 1994b).
- Nitrous oxide is often given to calm a pediatric patient during intravenous line insertion. Do not use nitrous oxide for anesthesia after line insertion because it causes distention of the bowel, making it more difficult to visualize organs and structures.

- An open procedure may be used to insert the trocar because a blind puncture with a Veress needle is more risky.
- The CO_2 pneumoperitoneal pressure is decreased, depending on the size of the pediatric patient. Children usually require only 7 mm Hg (*Laparosc Surg Update*, 1994a).

Geriatrics

The over-65-year age group is the fastest-growing segment of the population in the United States (Meeker and Rothrock, 1995). The Census Bureau has predicted that there will be more than 1 million centenarians (people over 100 years old) in the United States by the year 2050 and almost 2 million by the year 2080 (Meeker and Rothrock, 1995).

Less invasive surgical procedures are preferred for geriatric patients to promote quicker recovery. In a study conducted by Gross and Kammerer in 1990, the overall mortality rates for patients in different age groups undergoing any surgery were as follows:

1% in patients less than 65 years old

5% to 10% in 65- to 80-year-old patients

10% in patients older than 80 years

Because of the concerns specific to geriatric patients, continual attempts are being made to develop less invasive procedures for use in the elderly.

Following are special considerations that pertain to the care of geriatric patients scheduled for endoscopic procedures:

- The physician will closely assess the patient to determine whether the risk of surgery, either using the open or the endoscopic approach, outweighs the potential risk of not doing the surgery at all. Age alone should not be used as a contraindication to the performance of an endoscopic procedure. Studies have confirmed that even very old patients can benefit from surgical procedures (Meeker and Rothrock, 1995). In fact, the chronologic age of the patient does not necessarily determine the condition of the patient. A 75-year-old man may be in better physical condition than a 35-year-old man.
- The patient's understanding of the procedure must be carefully assessed to determine his or her level of awareness so that appropriate perioperative education can be planned for the patient and the support system (Fig 5-6).
- Nurses should be aware of the implications of surgery in geriatric patients. Factors to be considered when evaluating a geriatric patient for surgery include (Meeker and Rothrock, 1995):
  1. The life expectancy of the patient if the surgical procedure is performed versus that if the disease is allowed to take its natural course.

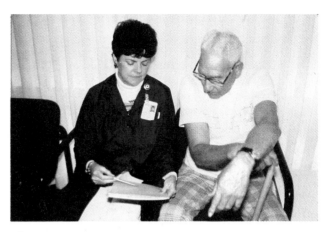

Fig. 5-6   The nurse must ensure that the patient understands the nature of the endoscopy procedure that will be performed.

  2. The independence versus dependence of the patient after the procedure if complications or incapacitation are anticipated.
  3. The motivation of the patient to want to undergo the pain or discomfort associated with the endoscopic procedure and the rehabilitation necessary for recovery.
  4. The risk of nonoperative management versus surgical risks. The patient must determine whether the endoscopic procedure is worth the risks involved. If a condition continues to worsen and the endoscopic procedure is needed later, the mortality rates for emergency surgery may be double those for elective surgery in the elderly.
- Extra time must be taken during the preoperative assessment so that the patient does not feel rushed.
- Allow the geriatric patient time to respond to questions instead of communicating only with the patient's support system. This promotes the patient's dignity, self-respect, and control of the situation.
- Normal physiologic changes can be expected with the aging process, so the care plan must be altered to accommodate these needs. Following are some of these changes and the alterations in the plan of care necessary to deal with them:
  1. The skin loses elasticity and subcutaneous fat; therefore the skin must be handled carefully, inspected regularly, and padded as needed.
  2. Vascular circulation may be impaired, thus external means of maintaining thermoregulation must be provided as needed (e.g., warm blankets).
  3. Respiratory muscles weaken, decreasing the ability to breathe deeply.
  4. Peristalsis decreases and salivary secretions become thickened, thus altering the patient's response to oral medications.

5. Elasticity of the urinary structures may be lost, thus causing difficulty in voiding.
6. Bone mass is decreased, thus causing skeletal instability and an increased risk of broken bones.
7. Neurons are lost, thus causing the geriatric patient to respond more slowly.
8. Changes in vision and hearing occur, thus the geriatric patient may become disoriented or confused, especially after general anesthesia has been administered.

There are many risk factors associated with surgery in elderly patients. Some of the more common ones are listed in Box 5-2. (Meeker and Rothrock, 1995)

Pregnant Patients

Endoscopy performed on the pregnant woman has lately been a controversial and evolving issue. The endoscopic procedure to be performed, the type of anesthesia to be administered, and the general health of the mother and developing fetus help to determine whether endoscopy should be performed.

Laparoscopy has been widely accepted for the diagnosis and treatment of many diseases in a variety of patients, but its use in pregnant women is still met with skepticism. However, techniques are being refined so that the risks to the pregnant woman and her unborn child are decreased. An experienced surgeon and a skilled laparoscopic team can safely perform laparoscopy in a pregnant woman, but care must then focus on not one but two patients, the mother and the unborn child.

The nurse must ensure that the patient and her family are involved in the decision to have the surgery and the decision to perform the procedure laparoscopically, since the threat of lawsuits can extend for years after the child is born and grows up. Therefore, documentation of the patient and family's full knowledge of the procedure and their consent to it is critical.

First it must be determined that surgery is really needed; then the type of surgical procedure can be determined. If surgery is needed, then the fact that an open procedure often causes the release of large amounts of adrenaline that can harm the fetus must be considered (*Adv Technol Surg Care*, 1995). Advantages to laparoscopic surgery of particular relevance to pregnant women are that it often takes less time, so the patient is anesthetized for less time; the smaller laparoscopic incisions are more cosmetically acceptable; and the chance of wound infection is less.

A survey conducted by the Society of Laparoscopic Surgeons revealed that laparoscopy has been performed safely during all trimesters of pregnancy. The most common procedure performed has been laparoscopic cholecystectomy, accounting for 48% of the cases (*Laparosc Surg Update*, 1995c).

Box 5-2	*Risk factors for surgery in elderly patients*

General
Dehydration
Anemia
Malignancy
Recent stroke
Acute confusion, depression, dementia, pseudodementia

Cardiovascular
Recent myocardial infarction
Unstable arrhythmias
Decompensated congestive heart failure
Unstable angina
Uncontrolled hypertension

Pulmonary
Infection
Decompensated chronic obstructive pulmonary disease
Smoking

Gastrointestinal/Nutritional
Active peptic ulcer disease
Hepatic insufficiency
Severe malnutrition

Endocrine
Adrenal insufficiency
Hypothyroidism or hyperthyroidism
Uncontrolled diabetes

Genitourinary
Infection
Obstruction

From Barry PP: Primary care evaluation of the elderly for elective surgery, *Geriatrics* 42:77, 1987.

Laparoscopy is often preferred to laparotomy in a pregnant woman needing surgery. However, following are different considerations that apply to pregnant women undergoing laparoscopic procedures that have a bearing on the plan of care and the surgical technique used:

- CO_2 insufflation should be done at low pressures (10 to 12 mm Hg).
- The laparoscopic procedure should be relatively simple and short to avoid prolonged anesthesia times that could lead to complications.
- The second trimester is usually the best time to perform a laparoscopy, because surgery in the first trimester often leads to miscarriage (*Laparosc Surg Update*, 1995c).
- Laparoscopy in the third trimester poses more risks because the uterus is larger, and the procedure is technically more difficult as a result. It has been recommended that laparoscopy not be performed after

24 weeks' gestation, unless absolutely necessary (*Laparosc Surg Update*, 1995c).

- An ultrasound scan should be obtained before the procedure to reveal the existence of any fetal abnormalities.
- Continuous fetal monitoring should be performed during the laparoscopy, but sometimes this is difficult to do because the pneumoperitoneum can interfere with the function of the monitoring devices.

Studies are being conducted to determine the effect of CO_2 insufflation on the placenta and fetus, but more studies need to be conducted to determine whether the CO_2 has an effect on the enteroplacental circulation. One preliminary study in sheep has shown that CO_2 insufflation causes an increase of 10% in the fetal pulse rate. Insufflation performed with nitrous oxide was noted to cause no change in fetal pulse rate (*Laparosc Surg Update*, 1994c).

- Special laparoscopic abdominal wall–lifting devices may be used in place of CO_2 insufflation to minimize injuries stemming from a pneumoperitoneum.

Controversy has also surfaced regarding the performance of laparoscopy on patients in the immediate postpartum period. Arguments against it are that the uterus is still large and the pelvic viscera displaced, thus increasing the chance of injury. Patients having cesarean deliveries could also be at increased risk of adhesion formation, and some physicians have noted that CO_2 insufflation may hinder the healing of the cesarean incision. Proponents of the performance of laparoscopy in the immediate postpartum period suggest that for such procedures to be successful experience is necessary, trocar sites should be placed to avoid organ injury, and Veress needle placement for insufflation is best in the right upper quadrant (*Laparosc Surg Update*, 1995a).

Laparoscopic diagnostic procedures performed on developing fetuses represent a new, evolving area of surgery. It involves the introduction of an endoscope with a very small diameter lumen (approximately 0.5 mm) through a needle insertion port. The physician searches for fetal abnormalities such as extra toes or neural tube defects that cannot be diagnosed using ultrasound. This procedure has been named *transabdominal thin-gauge embryofetoscopy* or *fetoscopy* and is performed after 10 weeks' gestation, when the embryo becomes a fetus (*Laparosc Surg Update*, 1993).

Extremely Obese or Thin Patients

Special considerations apply to the planning of care for the endoscopic patient who is either obese or extremely thin.

Positioning problems may be encountered in the obese patient. Because of this the nurse should ensure that positioning devices and an adequate number of personnel are available for positioning such patients.

Longer instruments may be needed, especially in laparoscopic procedures. In addition, postoperative recovery may take longer because obesity complicates a quick return to activities.

There are also specific concerns that pertain to the thin patient. The nurse must ensure that bony prominences are padded well to prevent skin breakdown. In addition, during laparoscopic procedures, trocar insertion may injure underlying structures that are not far from the skin surface. For example, the aorta and vena cava can usually be palpated in thin patients. The fascia therefore may be carefully dissected during trocar insertion to provide better control and offset the amount of force needed. Many thin patients may also be athletic and therefore have a very rigid abdomen. This may make it difficult to insert the Veress needle because the anterior abdominal wall cannot be elevated easily. The thin patient should also undergo a thorough bowel preparation and be catheterized preoperatively so that a full bowel or bladder does not reduce the space in the abdominal cavity needed for the adequate manipulation of instruments.

Immunocompromised Patients

The care implemented in immunocompromised patients must include constant attention to asepsis and infection prevention. As part of this effort, it is recommended that sterile rather than disinfected instruments be used in such patients because sterilization destroys all microorganisms on the instruments. Possible breaks in sterile technique must be closely watched for and addressed immediately to prevent the introduction of any pathogens into the surgical area. Often prophylactic antibiotics are administered.

Laparoscopy has been used in the diagnosis of TB peritonitis in patients with acquired immunodeficiency syndrome (AIDS) who have fever of unknown origin and ascites. Early diagnosis of this condition is critically important so that immediate treatment can be initiated, because tuberculosis frequently causes early death in AIDS patients (*Laparosc Surg Update*, 1995d).

Disabled Patients

When endoscopy is performed in disabled patients, proper communication is critical to ensure patient compliance. The patient needs to understand the endoscopic plan of care and his or her responsibility before, during, and after the procedure. The patient's limitations must also be discussed openly so that appropriate alterations in the normal plan of care can be made. For example, the proper positioning is of paramount importance in visualizing the colon during colonoscopy especially if the patient has sustained a spinal cord injury and cannot move.

Trauma Victims and Critically Ill Patients

Patients who are victims of trauma often undergo an open procedure, such as a laparotomy or thoracotomy. However, one study showed that laparoscopy may be a reliable way to detect internal injuries. It was found that unnecessary laparotomy was avoided in 38% of patients with penetrating thoracoabdominal trauma through the use of preliminary diagnostic laparoscopy. Laparoscopy has been performed to evaluate peritoneal penetration or diaphragmatic and upper abdominal solid organ injuries. It is probably the best choice for the evaluation of suspected pancreas, kidney, or hollow organ injuries (*Laparosc Surg Update*, 1995e).

Laparoscopy is now even being performed on trauma patients in emergency rooms, especially on those with penetrating abdominal wounds. It may come to replace diagnostic peritoneal lavage and computed tomographic scanning, the primary diagnostic tools and techniques now used. Physicians have complained that these standard diagnostic tools can miss injuries such as internal bleeding or organ ruptures that laparoscopy can identify (*Adv Technol Surg Care*, 1995a).

Some trauma patients are prone to shock, so it has been recommended that laparoscopy only be performed on trauma patients in stable condition. Laparoscopy will not entirely replace exploratory laparotomy, but its use may eliminate the need for laparotomy in some patients whose injuries would otherwise necessitate the open approach.

Researchers are studying the effects on animals of introducing fibrin glue into the abdomen during laparoscopy to stop hemorrhages. Results have shown that the glue promotes normal coagulation in animal spleen and liver hemorrhaging, with a 100% survival rate in the treated animals. This technique may be useful for the management of trauma patients in stable condition who are showing signs of intraperitoneal hemorrhage resulting from injury to a solid organ (Salvino et al, 1993).

Bedside laparoscopy is now being performed on patients who are not in stable enough condition to be transported to the operating room. Often a condition cannot be diagnosed on the basis of laboratory, radi-ology, and physical examination findings. Diagnostic laparoscopy may be the only means of arriving at an accurate diagnosis in such patients. Some critically ill patients who cannot be moved would be excellent candidates for such bedside laparoscopy. Intravenous sedation could be used for anesthesia, if needed.

A mobile laparoscopy cart can be used to transport all of the essential equipment and instrumentation needed for bedside laparoscopy. Some of the items that should be included are a small monitor, insufflator, light source, trocars, laparoscope, camera, light cables, other needed instrumentation, and basic sterile supplies. One expert noted that bedside laparoscopy is as safe as peritoneal lavage in critically ill patients (*Laparosc Surg Update*, 1995b).

REFERENCES

Adv Technol Surg Care, Laparoscopy moving from OR to ED 13(5): 65,1995.

Adv Technol Surg Care, Tips for safe laparoscopy in pregnant patients.

Gross RF, Kammerer WS: Special topics. In Kammerer WS, Gross RD (eds): *Medical consultation: the internist of surgical, obstetric, and psychiatric services*, ed 2, Baltimore, 1990, Williams & Wilkins.

Laparosc Surg Update, Fetus is the newest patient for diagnostic laparoscopy, 1(8):61,1993.

Laparosc Surg Update, Question: Differences in pediatric laparoscopy, 2(5):59, 1994a.

Laparosc Surg Update, Tips for performing laparoscopy on children, 2(6):67, 1994b.

Laparosc Surg Update, CO_2 pneumoperitoneum may endanger fetus, N_2O may be better, 2(7):83, 1994c.

Laparosc Surg Update, Laparoscopy safe for postpartum women, doesn't hinder healing, 3(2):23, 1995a.

Laparosc Surg Update, Bedside laparoscopy in ICU makes diagnosis quicker, easier, 3(6):68, 1995b.

Laparosc Surg Update, Laparoscopy for pregnant patient still met with skepticism, 3(7):73, 1995c.

Laparosc Surg Update, Laparoscopy used to diagnose TB peritonitis in AIDs patients, 3(7):83, 1995d.

Laparosc Surg Update, Diagnostic laparoscopy helps avoid surgery for penetrating trauma, 3(8):95, 1995e.

Meeker MH, Rothrock JC: *Alexander's Care of the Patient in Surgery*, ed 10, St. Louis, 1995, Mosby.

Salvino C, Esposito T, Smith D, et al: Laparoscopic injection of fibrin glue to arrest intraparenchymal abdominal hemorrhage: an experimental study, *J Trauma* 35:762, 1993.

6

Implementing and Evaluating Patient Care

IMPLEMENTATION

The next phase of the nursing process involves implementing the plan of care that has been specifically designed for the patient scheduled to undergo an endoscopic procedure. Each intervention must be implemented, evaluated, and changed as needed to provide dynamic patient care so that the predetermined outcomes are achieved.

The perioperative nurse is responsible for implementing the plan of care. Some of his or her responsibilities in this regard include patient education, positioning, and monitoring, as well as infection prevention, and these are discussed in the following sections.

Patient Education

The nurse is responsible for making sure the patient feels comfortable with his or her understanding of the impending endoscopic procedure. Usually patient teaching begins in the physician's office at the time the decision is made to perform an endoscopic procedure. This initial contact can also begin at the patient's bedside at the time it is determined the patient would benefit from an endoscopic procedure.

Patient teaching begins with the initial explanation about the procedure to the patient and the support system. Many health care professionals are involved with this education process, so continuity must be ensured. The nurse, however, is responsible for developing the individualized teaching program that provides the patient with information and emotional support.

Instructions to prepare the patient for the endoscopic surgery are given preoperatively. Sometimes the patient may have questions about these directions. For example, before a colonoscopy, the patient may have concerns about the most appropriate method of bowel cleansing. Descriptions of each method can help the patient decide on the one that is most desirable. During preoperative education, the intraoperative endoscopic procedure should be discussed and the expected postoperative instructions given to facilitate quick recovery.

During the endoscopy, the patient may be awake and may be expected to change positions to facilitate the visualization of an internal structure. For example, during gastroscopy, the patient may have to change position so that the endoscope can be guided through the pyloric or cardiac sphincters. The nurse may be responsible for ensuring that the patient complies with the physician's instructions during the procedure. Sometimes patients want to be able to see the monitor so they can actually observe the endoscopic procedure as it is being performed. Therefore, before the procedure, the nurse should ask the patient if this is desired so that the monitor can be positioned within the patient's view. If the patient does not want to see the monitor, the nurse should make sure the monitor is positioned so that only the endoscopic team can see it.

Postoperative patient education is critical to ensure that recovery proceeds without untoward incidents. Because many endoscopic patients are sent home after the procedure, the patient and his or her support system need to understand the discharge instructions. Written explanations and directions provide an easy reference for the patient once he or she is at home (Fig. 6-1). Often videotapes are used to provide visual coaching to ensure that instructions are followed. The patient and support

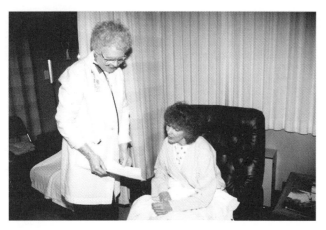

Fig. 6-1 Written explanations and directions provide easy reference for the patient once at home.

system must be given specific contact telephone numbers to call should questions or problems arise after he or she returns home.

Positioning

The perioperative nurse, along with the physician, is responsible for implementing appropriate and safe positioning of the patient during the endoscopic procedure. If general anesthesia is administered, the anesthesiologist or the nurse anesthetist shares this responsibility. Positioning aids should be available to stabilize the patient in a particular position. The preoperative assess-

ment will identify any limitations or special conditions in the patient that may necessitate a change in the standard position. Padding bony prominences or protecting compromised areas is required for every patient. The prevention of peripheral nerve injury is also a priority in every patient undergoing an endoscopic procedure.

Positioning varies depending on the area being examined during the endoscopic procedure. The ideal position for the patient must meet each of the following objectives (De Rome, 1995):

- It must allow optimal airway and monitoring access.
- It must be physiologically safe.
- It must provide the best access to the area to be examined.

Some of the more common positions are described in the following sections.

Supine (dorsal recumbent) position

In the supine or dorsal recumbent position, the patient is lying on his or her back with the face upward (Fig. 6-2). The patient's head may rest on a small pillow to prevent neck strain. The patient's arms are secured along his or her body with the palms against the body, or they are pronated (palm down) against the mattress. The patient's arms may also be extended on an armboard at less than a 90-degree angle with the palms up. The mattress and armboard pad should be the same height to prevent nerve damage, and the patient's head,

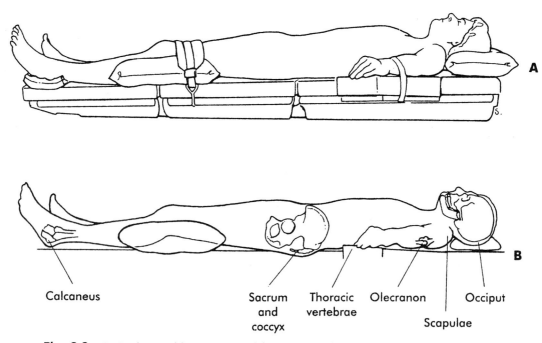

Fig. 6-2 **A,** Supine position. **B,** Potential pressure points. (From Meeker MH, Rothrock JC: *Alexander's care of the patient in surgery*, ed 10, St. Louis, 1995, Mosby, p 101. Courtesy David Schumick, Ohio State University Biomedical Communications, Columbus, Ohio.)

Calcaneus   Sacrum and coccyx   Thoracic vertebrae   Olecranon   Scapulae   Occiput vertebrae, and legs should be in alignment. A restraint can be loosely placed along the lower portion of the patient's thighs (approximately 2 inches [5 cm] above the knees) so that circulation is not compromised.

This position can be altered, depending on the endoscopic procedure to be performed. For example, the patient may be placed in a modified supine position for a knee arthroscopic procedure (Fig. 6-3). After anesthesia has been administered, the lower portion of the hinged surgical table is then lowered to allow the patient's knees to bend 90 degrees. A knee holder may be used to secure the operative knee. The security strap is placed above the other knee.

The supine position may have certain physiologic effects. The patient may experience reduced respiratory vital capacity and diaphragmatic movement. Obese patients especially may need to receive supplemental oxygen. This position may also cause a lowered heart rate, reduced diastolic blood pressure, and a greater potential for venous pooling in the extremities. A sandbag can be placed under the right abdomen of a pregnant patient to reduce uterine pressure on the inferior vena cava.

Trendelenburg's position

Trendelenburg's position is a variation of the supine position in which the patient's body is tilted with the head downward (Fig. 6-4). This position is used to better visualize abdominal organs during laparoscopy.

It, too, has certain physiologic effects. It causes a reduction in the diaphragmatic expansion and lung volume as abdominal contents press against the diaphragm, which may lead to pulmonary congestion. Blood from the lower extremities may also pool in the upper torso, thus causing blood pressure to be elevated. This may be hazardous to patients with cardiac problems. When the

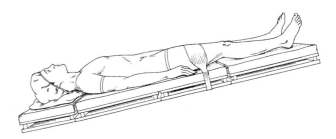

Fig. 6-4 Trendelenburg's position. (From Meeker MH, Rothrock JC: *Alexander's care of the patient in surgery*, ed 10, St. Louis, 1995, Mosby, p 102.)

patient is returned to the supine position, there may then be a risk of hypotension. Trendelenburg's position may also cause an increase in intracranial pressure, so this position may pose a risk to patients who have undergone neurosurgical procedures.

Often the reverse Trendelenburg's position is used during laparoscopy to provide optimal visualization of the upper abdominal organs. If the patient is placed in this position, appropriate precautions must be taken, however, so that he or she does not accidentally slide off the operating table.

In a study that examined the effects of the combination of CO_2 insufflation and reverse Trendelenburg positioning, it was found that the cardiac index was decreased by 3%, the heart rate was increased by 7%, and the mean arterial pressure was increased by 16% in such patients. Even though these changes would be relatively insignificant for healthy patients, they may produce untoward effects in high-risk patients. It has been suggested that biplane transesophageal echocardiography be used in high-risk patients undergoing laparoscopy to assess cardiac function during the procedure and thereby minimize complications (*Laparosc Surg Update*, 1994).

Lithotomy position

In the lithotomy position, the patient lies supine with the legs elevated, flexed, and abducted (Fig. 6-5). Stirrups are used to support the legs and feet and must be well padded to prevent nerve damage. The nurse should monitor the color and pulse of the patient's feet during prolonged procedures to ensure that adequate circulation is occurring. The patient's hips should be symmetrical, and the patient's calves should be parallel to the surgical table. To prevent kinking of the femoral nerve, the thighs must not be overabducted with external rotation. The patient's fingers must also not extend past the table break, because they could then be injured during repositioning of the table. In addition, the patient's buttocks must not extend past the table break, because this can cause undue stress to be placed on the

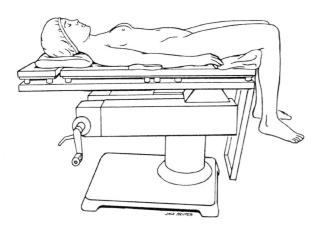

Fig. 6-3 Modified supine position for knee arthroscopic procedures. (From Gregory B: *Orthopaedic surgery*, St. Louis, 1994, Mosby, p 30.)

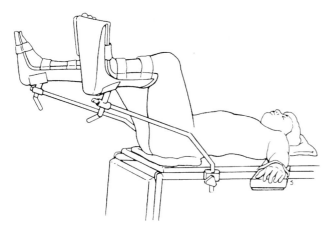

Fig. 6-5 Lithotomy position. (From Meeker MH, Rothrock JC: *Alexander's care of the patient in surgery*, ed 10, St. Louis, 1995, Mosby, p 104. Courtesy David Schumick, Ohio State Biomedical Communications, Columbus, Ohio.)

patient's lower back when the legs are lowered. Two people should be used to place the patient's legs in the stirrups and then to lower them at the completion of the procedure (Fig. 6-6).

Many laparoscopic procedures are performed with patients in this position, and, like the other positions, it also has certain physiologic effects. Respiratory efficiency and diaphragm movement may be restricted when the patient's legs are elevated. This problem may be more likely if gas insufflation is used during laparoscopy. The resulting pressure on the vena cava exerted by the abdominal contents may also compromise circulation. Blood may pool in the lumbar region, and if this occurs and the legs are lowered too rapidly, sudden hypotension may develop.

Lateral position

In the lateral position the patient is lying on his or her side (Fig. 6-7). The patient may be placed in the left or right lateral position, and the table may be bent in the middle to provide more access to the flank area.

During colonoscopy, the patient is usually placed in the left lateral position on a flat table for endoscope insertion. Positioning devices help to stabilize the patient's position. Even if the patient is awake, a pillow may be used to maintain this position and a restraining strap may be used to provide patient security.

Prone position

The prone position is used to access posterior parts of the body (Fig. 6-8). The modified knee-chest position (jackknife position) is used for procedures such as sigmoidoscopy (Fig. 6-9). Pillows and positioning devices are used to help maintain patients in this position. If the endoscopy is performed while the patient is awake, the patient must be moved slowly out of this position to prevent hypotension or dizziness.

Patient Monitoring

A variety of anesthetic agents, from general anesthesia to no anesthesia at all, can be used in patients undergoing endoscopic procedures. The nurse is often responsible for monitoring patients receiving intravenous (IV) conscious sedation or local anesthetics. Because of this the nurse must know the actions of the drugs, expected patient response, doses, routes of administration, duration of action, contraindications, and complications of the anesthetic preparations used. Nurses must also follow hospital protocols closely when administering a drug before or during the endoscopic procedure. Some hospitals require that these nurses attend a special training program before they assume responsibility for administering IV anesthetic drugs (e.g., meperidine hydrochloride, diazepam, midazolam hydrochloride) to patients.

Patient monitoring during endoscopic procedures includes the provision of adequate oxygenation, ventilation, circulation, and temperature control. A pulse oximeter, a heart monitor, and blood pressure equipment are used to detect any significant changes during the procedure. The nurse needs to understand the monitoring equipment to be used, know how to connect the piece of equipment to the patient, and how to interpret the data. (Usually an IV line is started before an endoscopic procedure begins, even if IV anesthesia is not planned to provide access to the patient's bloodstream in case emergency medications need to be administered.)

Many endoscopic procedures are performed with patients under monitored anesthesia care using local anesthesia and possibly an IV analgesic supplement (e.g., fentanyl) or sedative or amnesic drugs (midazolam

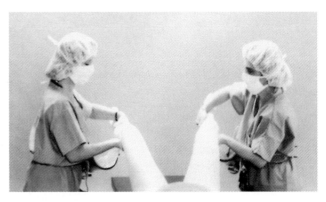

Fig. 6-6 Two people should be used to place the patient's legs in the stirrups and then lower the patient's legs at the completion of the procedure. (From Meeker MH, Rothrock JC: *Alexander's care of the patient in surgery*, ed 10, St. Louis, 1995, Mosby, p 104. Courtesy Allen Medical Systems, Cleveland, Ohio.)

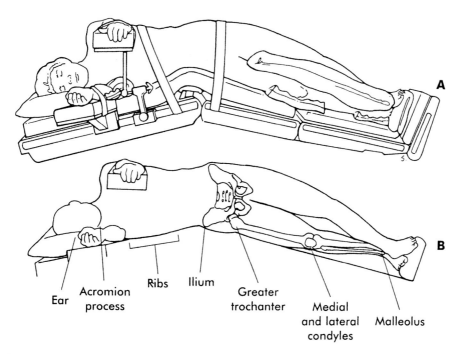

Ear   Acromion   Ribs   Ilium   Greater   Medial   Malleolus
        process   trochanter   and lateral   condyles

Fig. 6-7 **A,** Lateral position. **B,** Potential pressure areas. (From Meeker MH, Rothrock JC: *Alexander's care of the patient in surgery*, ed 10, St. Louis, 1995, Mosby, p 109. Courtesy David Schumick, Ohio State University Biomedical Communications, Columbus, Ohio.)

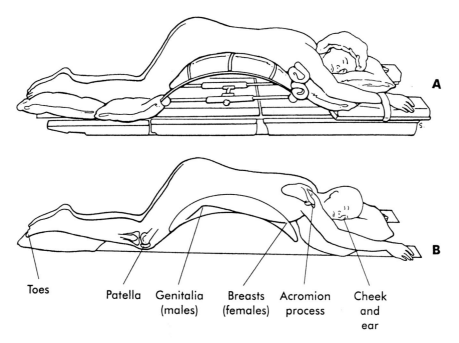

Toes   Patella   Genitalia   Breasts   Acromion   Cheek
                       (males)   (females)   process   and
                                                             ear

Fig. 6-8 **A,** Prone position. **B,** Potential pressure areas. (From Meeker MH, Rothrock JC: *Alexander's care of the patient in surgery*, ed 10, St. Louis, 1995, Mosby, p 107. Courtesy David Schumick, Ohio State University Biomedical Communications, Columbus, Ohio.)

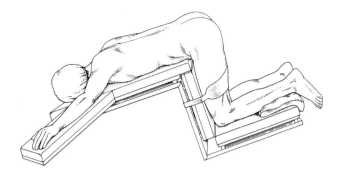

Fig. 6-9 Jackknife position for proctologic endoscopy. (From Meeker MH, Rothrock JC: *Alexander's care of the patient in surgery,* ed 10, St. Louis, 1995, Mosby, p 108.)

or propofol). Local anesthesia may also be used to infiltrate an area where the endoscopic procedure is to be performed. The nurse is expected to frequently assess the patient; vital signs should be taken and recorded at least every 15 minutes.

The nurse is responsible for documenting the patient's status, the nursing care delivered, and the medications administered perioperatively during the endoscopic experience. Many endoscopy suites are beginning to use computerized patient charting systems for the purpose of documentation. Some computer systems are even connected to the family waiting room, so the nurse can leave messages to be delivered to the patient's support system during the procedure. This type of communication allows the support system to constantly know the patient's status during the procedure. If the patient's care is transferred to another nurse for postoperative recovery, the surgical nurse is also responsible for communicating a complete report of the patient's endoscopic experience to that nurse.

Infection Prevention Measures

Infection prevention is the responsibility of the entire endoscopic team. However, patients with certain conditions may be at particular risk of infection during and after endoscopic procedures. Following are the surgical infection rates noted for specific patient populations (Drez et al, 1991):

    Markedly obese patients—18%
    Malnourished patients—22.4%
    Diabetic patients—10.4%

With appropriate aseptic techniques, appropriate care on the part of the surgical team, and appropriate use of antibiotics, the surgical infection rates can be reduced to 1% to 1.5% (Drez et al, 1991). A particular advantage of endoscopic procedures is that surgical incisions are minimized or eliminated, thereby decreasing the risk of postoperative infections.

The place where the endoscopic procedure is performed often determines the level of sterility observed. For example, laparoscopic procedures are usually performed within the sterile environment of an operating room. Gastroscopy, colonoscopy, and other similar endoscopy procedures can be performed in endoscopy laboratories or physicians' offices, where disinfected instrumentation is used within a "clean" environment.

Antibiotics may be administered prophylactically, usually immediately before the procedure, to reduce the chance of infection. A broad-spectrum antibiotic is often recommended. The use of antibiotics has become controversial, however, with some physicians now stating that prophylactic antibiotics are unnecessary for most patients. Sometimes the use of antibiotics also has the drawback of masking problems with intraoperative asepsis, such as the inadequate reprocessing of reusable instruments.

EVALUATION

The final step of the nursing process is the evaluation phase, which notes the patient's progress toward achievement of the predetermined outcomes. The evaluation step continually changes, however, as the patient's status changes or goals are achieved, thus requiring that the plan of care also be altered. The evaluation process is ongoing during the patient's endoscopic experience as each implementation activity is continually reviewed to determine its effectiveness. Evaluation starts during the immediate postoperative phase and extends through the recovery phase at home. Perioperative nurses often call patients at home after their discharge to answer questions, evaluate the outcome of the care delivered, and determine the patient's compliance with the postoperative instructions (Fig. 6-10).

The evaluation phase also offers a way for nurses to provide quality management and improved care. The Association of Operating Room Nurses has provided quality improvement standards for perioperative nurses that can be applied to nurses involved with endoscopic surgery (Box 6-1). Specific quality indicators that denote the important aspects of care delivered during endoscopic procedures can be identified in a quality improvement program. Data for each indicator can be collected and evaluated to determine ways to provide improved patient care. The benefit of using a quality improvement tool and ongoing monitoring and evaluation is that better patient care is provided.

The recovery time should not be determined solely by the amount of time it takes for the patient to return to work. Sometimes patients enjoy being off of work for the extended time necessitated by the recovery from a

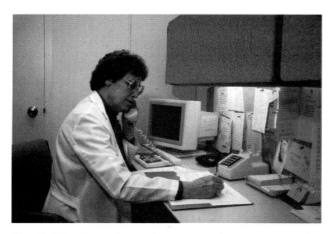

Fig. 6-10 The perioperative nurse makes a postoperative phone call to evaluate the care delivered during surgery and the patient's compliance with the discharge instructions.

Box 6-1	*AORN quality improvement standards for perioperative nursing*

Standard I: Assign responsibility for monitoring and evaluation activities

Standard II: Delineate the scope of patient care activities or services

Standard III: Identify important aspects that impact the quality of patient care

Standard IV: Identify quality indicators for each important aspect of care

Standard V: Establish thresholds for evaluation of indicators

Standard VI: Collect and organize data for evaluation

Standard VII: Evaluate care based on cumulative data

Standard VIII: Take actions to improve care and services

Standard IX: Assess the effectiveness of action(s) and document outcomes

Standard X: Communicate relevant information to organization-wide quality assessment program

From Association of Operating Room Nurses: *Quality improvement in perioperative nursing*, Denver, 1992, AORN.

surgical (or endoscopic) procedure. If a workplace benefit covers the employee for a prolonged recovery period, the patient is usually inclined to take advantage of this benefit. A better measure of recovery is therefore the amount of time it takes for the patient to return to full activities of daily living. A patient is usually considered fully recovered when he or she is able to drive a car, perform housekeeping duties, engage in yardwork, or resume sexual relations.

Complications

Complications may occur when least expected, even during or after the most successful endoscopic procedures. Some of the more common complications associated with endoscopy are described in the following sections.

Positioning problems

The different positions a patient may need to assume to provide optimal visualization during an endoscopic procedure may have untoward effects on the patient, as discussed earlier in this chapter. Close monitoring of the patient's status can ensure the early recognition of problems so that preventive measures can be instituted in a timely manner.

Tissue or organ injury

During an endoscopic procedure, there is always a chance that an organ or structure will be injured. Because endoscopic surgery is performed with the physician looking through a lens or watching a monitor, it is particularly easy for an accidental injury to occur. For example, sharp laparoscopic scissors could accidentally perforate an organ or structure during insertion of the instrument into the abdominal area. Electrosurgical energy could escape from a break in instrument insulation, causing a bowel burn. A laser tip could inadvertently touch adjacent tissue, causing a coagulative impact.

Because accidents leading to patient injury can easily occur during laparoscopy, the surgical team must be constantly vigilant to prevent them. Untoward events resulting from laparoscopy often have led to patient complications and lawsuits. For example, a patient's iliac artery was lacerated during elective laparoscopic bilateral tubal ligation, resulting in the loss of a lot of blood and no pulse for 12 minutes. She suffered a stroke and was left with brain damage, renal failure, and a loss of cognitive abilities. The family sued for $2.8 million, but the case was settled for an undisclosed amount (*Laparosc Surg Update*, 1995b).

Bowel injuries have also been on the increase as laparoscopy has grown in popularity. Sometimes these injuries are difficult to detect postoperatively, but there are some telltale signs. For example, the presence of free air in the abdominal cavity after laparoscopy is evidence of possible bowel injury and should not just be considered residual CO_2 (*Laparosc Surg Update*, 1995a).

Equipment or instrumentation hazards

The nurse should continually monitor the functioning of equipment and the integrity of endoscopic instruments to ensure that hazards are minimized. For example, reusable biopsy forceps must be checked before each procedure to confirm that they are functioning appropriately and will not cause injury to the patient. The insulation on electrosurgery tools must also be inspected to ensure that there are no breaks that could allow the escape of electrosurgery energy. (See Chapters 7, 8, and 11 for more information.)

Anesthetic or medication complications

During the endoscopic experience, there is always the risk of complications stemming from the anesthetic or medications administered. The nurse must therefore constantly evaluate the effects of the medications administered and be prepared to alter the plan of care if unexpected complications arise. For example, 50% of the morbidity and 60% of the mortality associated with upper gastrointestinal endoscopy are related to hypoxemia caused by conscious sedation medications which may lead to cardiopulmonary complications, among others (*Today's OR Nurse*, 1995).

Trocar site hernias

If trocar sites are not completely closed, a hernia may develop after a period of time. This complication is easily prevented by ensuring that the tissue layers at the trocar site are completely closed. New devices have been developed to assist in the complete closure of trocar sites. For example, there is now a device that facilitates the placement of a pursestring suture that secures the tissue layers and thereby minimizes the risk of a trocar site hernia.

Hypotension

Excessive bleeding can occur if a structure is inadvertently punctured or lacerated. This would lead to hypotension and must be managed immediately.

Hypertension

Patient positioning may cause increased intraabdominal pressure that would lead to hypertension. The increased absorption of CO_2 introduced for insufflation can cause increased blood pressure. Constant monitoring of the patient's vital signs can alert the provider to blood pressure increases. Precipitating factors must be eliminated or medications given to decrease hypertensive periods during the endoscopic procedure.

Gastric reflux

Sometimes obese patients experience gastric reflux during endoscopic procedures, especially if pressure from a pneumoperitoneum becomes excessive. Patients with hiatal hernias may also exhibit signs of gastric reflux. A nasogastric tube may need to be inserted to relieve gastric distention, but if the patient is awake during the procedure, then a nasogastric tube is inserted only if the distention becomes severe.

Gas embolism

Overinsufflation is one of the leading causes of a gas embolism during laparoscopic procedures. The risks associated with such overinsufflation can be minimized through constant monitoring of the insufflation gas flow and the abdominal pressure.

A gas embolism can also result from the use of the argon-enhanced coagulator during laparoscopy, because it may cause an unexpected rise in the gas pressure within the abdominal cavity. This happens because the argon gas stream, emitted to form an ionized arc to achieve better coagulation during electrosurgery, constitutes an additional gas flowing into the abdominal cavity. Further, because argon gas is less soluble in blood than CO_2, an embolism may form that could then last long enough to reach the heart. In one case an argon-enhanced coagulator was used during a laparoscopic procedure to control bleeding on the liver bed. The intraabdominal pressure rose to 33 mm Hg, an embolism formed, and the patient died. Extreme caution must therefore be used whenever an argon-enhanced coagulator is employed during laparoscopy. Following are some suggested ways to decrease the chances of embolism formation during the use of the argon-enhanced coagulator in laparoscopic procedures (Health Devices, 1994):

- Set the argon flow at the lowest setting, usually less than 4 liters per minute.
- Purge the electrode and the argon gas line of air before the procedure.
- Hold the electrode tip more than several millimeters from the surgical site.
- Flush the abdominal cavity with several liters of CO_2 insufflation gas between extended periods of argon-enhanced coagulator use.
- Leave one instrument cannula vent open while using the argon-enhanced coagulator to minimize the chance of overpressurization.
- Use an insufflator with an audible and visual overpressurization alarm.
- Closely monitor the patient for early signs of venous or pulmonary gas embolism.

There is also a risk of gas embolism formation if a catheter laser fiber is used in a fluid environment, such as that present during a cystoscopy or hysteroscopy. If the laser fiber is purged with a gas, an embolism can easily form that could be fatal to the patient.

Conversion to Open Procedure

Often endoscopic procedures must be converted to open approaches if the surgery cannot be performed using the endoscopic method. Some surgeons state that it should be possible to determine within 15 minutes of the start of a laparoscopic procedure whether conversion is needed, unless an unexpected event occurs later during the operative laparoscopy. Like the golden hour involved in trauma care, there is also a golden 15 minutes that can be used as a guide in the performance of laparoscopy (Greene, 1995).

The need to convert to an open procedure should not be construed as an indication of the surgeon's expertise, however. Sometimes a more experienced surgeon may attempt an endoscopic approach when others would immediately proceed with the open technique. A physician may also still be learning an endoscopic technique and thus may convert more procedures to open ones until experience is acquired.

Often physicians disclose their conversion rates to their patients if they are trying to point out the benefits of a particular endoscopic procedure. The patient must also fully understand that the risk for conversion is higher for certain endoscopic procedures. For example, surgeons may more readily convert a laparoscopic bowel resection than a laparoscopic cholecystectomy to an open procedure.

REFERENCES

DeRome S: Patient positioning for endosurgery, *ACORN J* 8(2):25, 1995.

Drez D, Finney TP, Roberts TS: Sepsis on orthopedic surgery, *Orthopedics* 14:157, Feb 1991.

ECRI: Fata gas embolism caused by over-pressurization during laparoscopic use of argon-enhanced coagulation, *Health Devices* 23(6):257, 1994.

Greene FL. Minimal access surgery and the "golden period" for conversion, *Surg Endosc* 9:11, 1995.

Laparosc Surg Update: CO_2 and reverse Trendelenburg adversely affect cardiac function, 2(10):112, 1994.

Laparosc Surg Update: Free intraperitoneal air probably sign of bowel injury, 3(1):11, 1995a.

Laparosc Surg Update: Lacerated iliac artery results in $2.8 million lawsuit, 3(3):70, 1995b.

Meeker MH, Rothrock JC: *Alexander's care of the patient in surgery*, ed 10, St. Louis, 1995, Mosby.

McConnell EA: By the way, *Tod OR Nurse* 17(4):45, 1995.

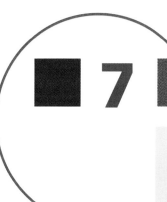

Endoscopic Instruments

Endoscopy requires a variety of instruments, each serving a different purpose. Instruments are used to:

- Access the target area
- Establish and maintain visualization
- Perform the diagnostic or operative intervention

Many of the instruments described in this chapter are used during rigid endoscopic procedures, such as laparoscopy. More common instruments, such as scissors, graspers, and biopsy forceps, have been adapted for use in flexible endoscopic procedures.

VERESS NEEDLES

The Veress needle was initially developed during the 1930s to induce a pneumothorax in patients with tuberculous lungs (White and Klein, 1991), but then as laparoscopy became more popular in the 1970s, physicians discovered that it could also be used to establish the needed pneumoperitoneum.

A Veress needle is a double-barreled device consisting of an inner, blunt-tipped, spring-action stylet with an outer, sharply beveled needle. The outer needle perforates the tissue, and the inner blunt-tipped needle pushes tissue away (Fig. 7-1). Usually two "pops" are heard during insertion, one when the abdominal wall fascia is traversed and one when the peritoneum is entered. Once it is determined that the needle is properly positioned within the peritoneal cavity, the insufflation gas line is connected to the Veress needle hub. Gas insufflation is begun at a low-flow rate, usually 1 L/min. (See Chapter 9 for more details on insufflation techniques.)

Veress needles are available in reusable or single-use forms (Fig. 7-2). The one most commonly used is 2.1 mm in diameter, or 14 gauge. Smaller needles produce more resistance to the flow of the gas, thus causing intraabdominal pressure to be increased during insufflation. Larger needles do the opposite. Veress needles have two ports, one for the insufflation of the gas and the other for the pressure reading during insufflation.

The standard Veress needle used for infraumbilical site insertion is usually 80 mm long, so it can traverse all layers of the abdominal tissue. Longer needles are required for obese patients.

Insertion of the Veress needle begins by making a small stab wound in a strategically placed area on the abdomen. The assistant can grasp and lift the abdominal wall to facilitate the insertion, or this can be done with single-tooth skin hooks or towel clips. Skin hooks may be easier to manipulate than towel clips. The needle is slowly inserted at a 45- to 90-degree angle to the abdominal wall (Fig. 7-3). Many physicians prefer a Veress needle with a transparent hub to facilitate visualization during insertion.

To determine and validate the proper positioning of the Veress needle before initiation of the gas flow, a hanging drop test is often performed. A syringe is connected to the Veress needle and the plunger pulled back to determine whether bowel contents or blood are aspirated, indicating that the needle is positioned in a loop of the bowel or a blood vessel, respectively (Fig. 7-4). If this does not occur, then saline is instilled. If the column of saline in the syringe drops quickly and without resistance during instillation, then the needle is properly placed, and insufflation can begin. If the hanging drop test fails, the Veress needle is withdrawn and reinserted. Another site may be chosen for the Veress needle placement.

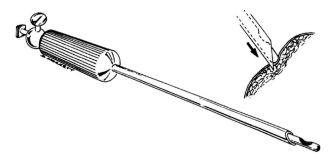

Fig. 7-1 The Veress needle, which consists of an inner blunt-tipped stylet with an outer sharply beveled sleeve. (From White RA, Klein SR: *Endoscopic surgery*. St. Louis, 1991 Mosby.)

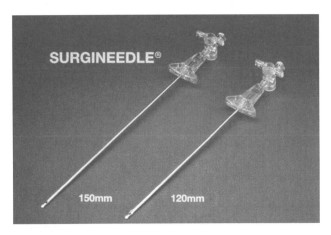

Fig. 7-2 Veress needles. (Courtesy United States Surgical Corp., Norwalk, Conn.)

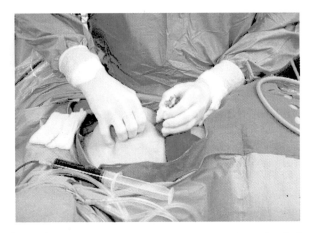

Fig. 7-3 Veress needle insertion. The needle is slowly inserted at a 45- to 90-degree angle to the abdominal wall. (Courtesy InnerDyne, Inc., Sunnyvale, Calif.)

There are several abdominal sites that can be used for Veress needle placement. Proper angling of the needle is important, however, to avoid injuring organs and structures below the site. The following guidelines can be used for Veress needle insertion, with the sites listed in order of their use, from most to least common:

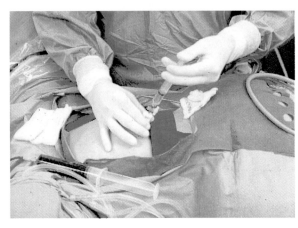

Fig. 7-4 A hanging drop test, performed to validate the proper placement of the Veress needle. (Courtesy InnerDyne, Inc., Sunnyvale, Calif.)

Supraumbilical area—Aim down and to the left to avoid the falciform ligament.

Right upper quadrant—Aim down and to the left to avoid the liver.

Right lower quadrant—Aim medially to avoid the cecum.

Left upper quadrant—Aim down and to the right to avoid the spleen.

If the hanging drop test fails at all of these sites, then a mini-incision open procedure using the blunt-nosed Hasson trocar can be done.

TROCARS AND CANNULAS

A trocar is a cutting or blunt-tipped rod that is placed through the lumen of a cannula, which is a hollow tube with a valve mechanism (Fig. 7-5). The purpose of a trocar and cannula assembly is to create an orifice through which an endoscope and the instruments needed to perform an endoscopic procedure can be introduced. The trocar is used as an obturator and is placed through a cannula to provide the portal of entry. After the entry has been made, the trocar is removed and the cannula is left in place to provide access for the endoscope and other instruments.

The trocar and cannula must be comparable in size because they are used in conjunction with each other. If smaller instruments are to be used, then a smaller trocar and cannula setup is needed. Larger units are used if larger diameter instruments or endoscopes are to be used (Fig. 7-6). If a larger trocar and cannula are used during laparoscopy to establish the access port and smaller instruments are used at different times during the procedure, then an adapter can be employed to keep the insufflation gas from leaking around the smaller instrument (Fig. 7-7). Newer cannulas are now

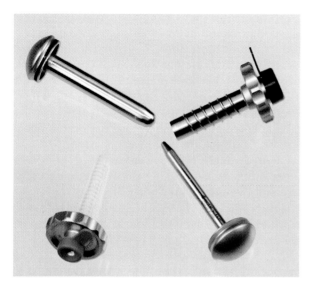

Fig. 7-5 A trocar, which is a cutting or blunt-tipped rod that is placed through the lumen of a cannula. (Courtesy Aesculap, Inc., South San Francisco, Calif.)

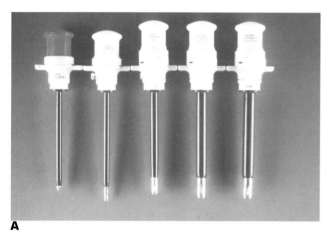

A

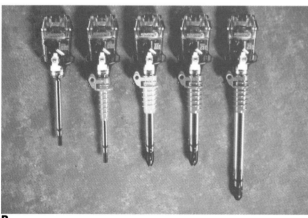

B

Fig. 7-6 **A** and **B**, Trocar/cannulas vary in size, depending on the technique and instrumentation to be used. (Courtesy United States Surgical Corp., Norwalk, Conn., and Ethicon Endo-Surgery, Inc., Cincinnati, Ohio.)

being developed, however, that can accommodate a variety of sizes of instruments without the need to use adapters. For the sake of cost-efficiency, kits are now available that contain one disposable trocar and multiple cannulas. The same trocar is then used to place each cannula needed for the procedure (Fig. 7-8).

Trocars

Trocar tips may be sharp or blunt. Blunt-tipped trocars are used to minimize the risk of injury to underlying tissues (Fig. 7-9); sharp-tipped trocars are used to create the orifice through the tissue for the access port.

Sharp-tipped trocars have either a pyramidal or conical tip (Fig. 7-10). Many physicians prefer a trocar with the pyramidal tip because it takes less force to insert it through the different tissue layers.

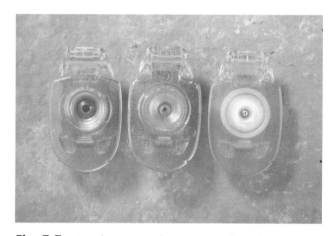

Fig. 7-7 An adapter or reducer cap, used to allow the passage of smaller instruments through a larger cannula to prevent the escape of insufflation gas. (Courtesy Ethicon Endo-Surgery, Inc., Cincinnati, Ohio.)

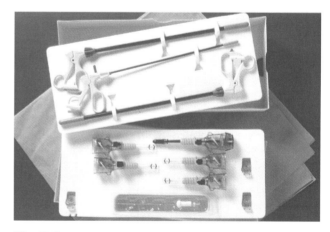

Fig. 7-8 Kits are available that contain several cannulas and one trocar. Other instruments such as the Veress needle, scissors, or graspers may also be included. Kits provide a significant cost savings. (Courtesy Ethicon Endo-Surgery, Inc., Cincinnati, Ohio.)

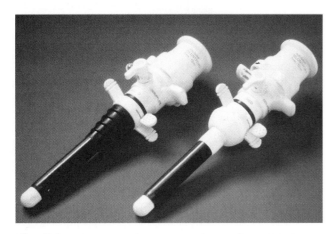

Fig. 7-9 Blunt-tipped trocars can be used to minimize injuries during insertion. (Courtesy United States Surgical Corp., Norwalk, Conn.)

Trocars may either be reusable or single use. Reusable trocars should be maintained in a sharpened condition because more force is needed to insert a dull trocar into the abdomen, thus heightening the risk of uncontrolled entry and injury to the viscera or other structures. Single-use (disposable) trocars are often preferred because of the guaranteed sharpness.

The degree of trocar sharpness has been a debated issue. Some physicians prefer very sharp tipped trocars that slide through the tissue as easily as a knife in soft butter; others prefer a duller trocar that requires more force and turning on insertion.

Most trocars also have a hollow lumen with a hole near the tip to facilitate the flow of gas once the peritoneal cavity has been entered (see Fig. 7-10).

Single-use trocars with safety shields are available today (Figs. 7-11 and 7-12). The protective shield slips

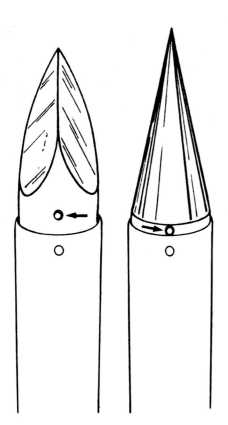

Fig. 7-10 The tips of sharp-tipped trocars can be either pyramidal, **A**, or conical, **B**. Both designs have an internal gas-escape port, as shown by the arrow. (From White RA, Klein SR: *Endoscopic surgery*. St. Louis, 1991, Mosby.)

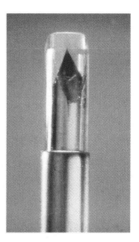

Fig. 7-11 A close-up view of the trocar safety shield in place. (Courtesy Ethicon Endo-Surgery Inc., Cincinnati, Ohio.)

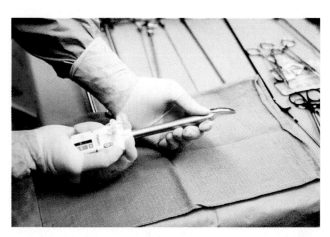

Fig. 7-12 A trocar with the safety shield retracted to expose the sharp end. When released, the safety shield falls back into place. (Courtesy Ethicon Endo-Surgery Inc., Cincinnati, Ohio.)

down over the trocar's sharp tip during insertion to prevent inadvertent injury once the tip has passed through the abdominal wall (Fig. 7-13). The justification for a safety shield has become a very controversial issue. Some say that the safety shield offers a false sense of security and that the sleeve does not slip into place as quickly as it should to be effective. Opponents also state that the safety shield increases the risk of patient harm, claiming that the shield itself could cause injury because tissue can be caught in the shield as it slides into place. Proponents of safety shields have testified that they have helped to minimize tissue trauma.

While this issue continues to be debated, and until it is known which side is right, the following technique can be used to eliminate the need for safety shields while still ensuring safe trocar insertion during laparoscopy (*Laparosc Surg Update*, 1995b):

- Elevate the umbilicus with lateral tension, using towel clips to increase the distance from the aorta.
- Make a vertical incision through the layers of skin and fascial tissue.
- Insert a hemostat and spread it into the peritoneal cavity.
- Insert a blunt pyramidal-tipped trocar (sometimes called "the nail") while rotating it until it is firmly seated within the fascial defect, causing fascial separation.
- Remove the trocar.
- Begin low-flow insufflation.
- Insert the laparoscope through the cannula and view the fascial margin. Advance the cannula with the laparoscope under direct visualization into the peritoneal cavity.

Structural balloon trocars are being developed for use in extraperitoneal procedures (Fig. 7-14). The preperitoneal distention balloon trocar is inserted and tunneled inferiorly between the posterior fascia and the rectus muscle in such laparoscopic procedures as extraperitoneal hernia repair (Fig. 7-15). The balloon trocar is advanced to the pubic bone and then slowly inflated with room air (Fig. 7-16). Usually the balloon is

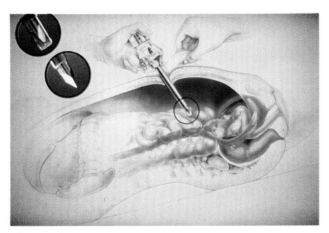

Fig. 7-13   The trocar safety shield slips over the sharp end of the trocar immediately after insertion to minimize injury to abdominal organs. (Courtesy Ethicon Endo-Surgery Inc., Cincinnati, Ohio.)

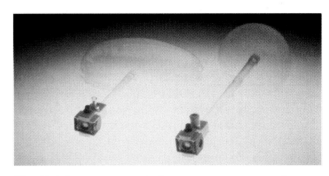

Fig. 7-14   A distention balloon trocar system, used to create a preperitoneal space for a laparoscopic hernia repair. (Courtesy Origin Medsystems, Menlo Park, Calif.)

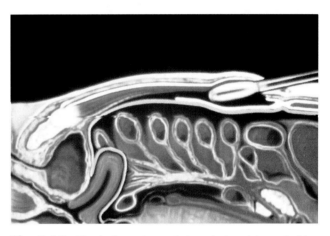

Fig. 7-15   The balloon trocar is inserted and tunneled inferiorly between the posterior fascia and the rectus muscle. (Courtesy Origin Medsystems, Menlo Park, Calif.)

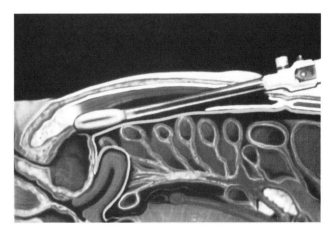

Fig. 7-16   The balloon trocar is advanced to the pubic bone and then slowly inflated with room air. (Courtesy Origin Medsystems, Menlo Park, Calif.)

transparent to permit constant visualization. An extraperitoneal space is then created by the balloon, distending the structures until an adequate space is formed (Fig. 7-17). The balloon trocar is then removed and replaced with a blunt-tipped trocar and the preperitoneal space is insufflated (Fig. 7-18).

Cannulas

The most popular cannulas available today come in diameters ranging from 3 to 12 mm. The cannulas most commonly used for laparoscopy have lumens with a diameter of 5 or 10 mm. The cannulas used for laparoscopy have valves that prevent the escape of the insufflation gas and also allow for the passage of endoscopes or instruments. There are two different types of valves most commonly used today.

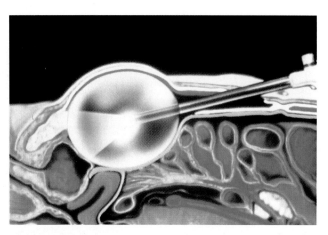

Fig. 7-17   The balloon then distends the structures, creating an extraperitoneal space. The balloon is transparent to permit constant visualization. (Courtesy Origin Medsystems, Menlo Park, Calif.)

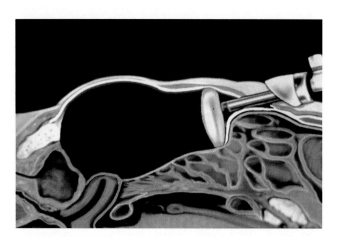

Fig. 7-18   The balloon trocar is then removed, leaving a preperitoneal space. (Courtesy Origin Medsystems, Menlo Park, Calif.)

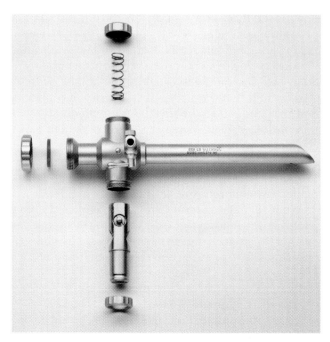

Fig. 7-19   Trumpet valve in a reusable cannula. (Courtesy Aesculap, Inc., South San Francisco, Calif.)

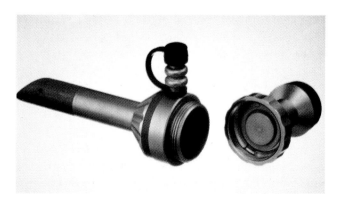

Fig. 7-20   Flap valve in a trocar/cannula system. (Courtesy Aesculap, Inc., South San Francisco, Calif.)

1. A trumpet valve consisting of an external plunger that is depressed to permit the passage of an endoscope or instruments (Fig. 7-19).
2. A trap door or flap valve that automatically opens when the endoscope or instruments are passed through the lumen of the cannula (Fig. 7-20).

Reusable cannula valves must be continually checked and maintained to ensure easy access with uninhibited movement as well as a proper seal so that no insufflation gas can escape. Cannulas also have a port with a side Luer-Lok connector to which is attached the tubing for the insufflation gas that maintains the abdominal distention.

Cannulas used during laparoscopy also have a stopcock assembly to permit the infusion of the insufflation

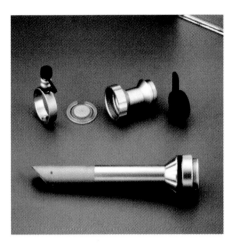

Fig. 7-21 A modular cannula system. Only broken parts have to be replaced, instead of the entire unit. (Courtesy Aesculap, Inc., South San Francisco, Calif.)

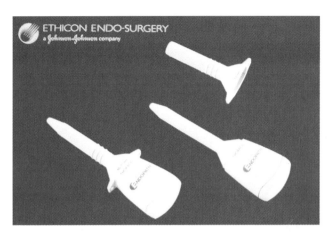

Fig. 7-22 A cannula and blunt-tipped trocar, used for thoracoscopy. Such an instrument may not need a stopcock assembly to permit the infusion of insufflation gas. (Courtesy Ethicon Endo-Surgery, Inc., Cincinnati, Ohio.)

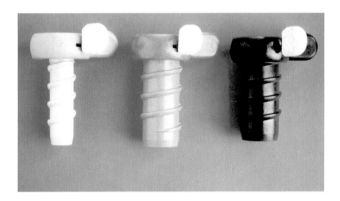

Fig. 7-23 Grippers. These can be used to stabilize an access port during laparoscopy or thoracoscopy. (Courtesy United States Surgical Corp., Norwalk, Conn.)

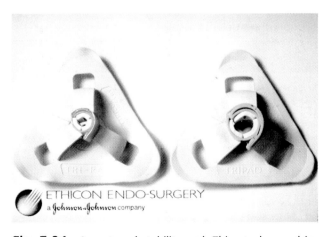

Fig. 7-24 An external stability pad. This can be used instead of a plastic, threaded gripper to stabilize the access port. (Courtesy Ethicon Endo-Surgery, Inc., Cincinnati, Ohio.)

gas during the procedure. If the cannula is reusable, the valve must be checked regularly to make sure that it is in proper working order. Many reusable cannulas have modular parts that can easily be assembled (Fig. 7-21). If one part fails or wears out, then it can be readily replaced, thus eliminating the need to replace the entire unit.

The cannula used in thoracoscopic surgery may not need to have a stopcock assembly because insufflation is usually not required (Fig. 7-22), though it may be required to help the anesthesiologist collapse the lung on the operative side. In this event a cannula with an insufflation infusion port is needed. The trocars used for thoracoscopy are blunt and short, and grippers are used to stabilize the access port cannula.

Cannulas also may incorporate a system to grip the tissue after placement, so inadvertent removal of the cannula is prevented during the endoscopic procedure (Fig. 7-23). Many disposable cannulas with such gripping devices are available, but stabilization threading devices may be needed for reusable cannulas. If the cannula is metal, then plastic stabilization devices should not be used because the mixture of plastic and metal will prevent the safe dispersion of electrical energy. This could allow capacitive coupling to occur, causing electrosurgical tissue burns. (See Chapter 11 for more details.) External stability pads are available to stabilize the port without the need for plastic threading devices, thus minimizing the threat of capacitive coupling (Fig. 7-24).

Flexible cannulas are now available that permit the passage of an endoscopic instrument at an angle (Fig. 7-25). Such flexibility facilitates access to hard-to-reach areas (Fig. 7-26).

Cannulas made of radiolucent material are often used for those procedures that are to include radiologic examinations. Radiolucent materials do not obstruct the

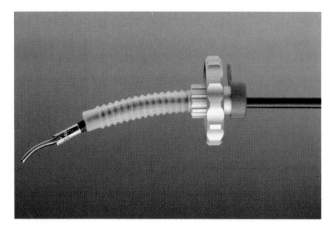

Fig. 7-25 Flexible cannula with endoscopic instrument. (Courtesy Aesculap, Inc., South San Francisco, Calif.)

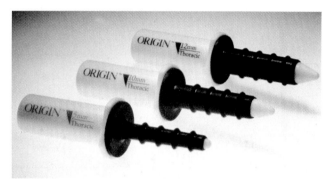

Fig. 7-26 A flexible cannula, which permits greater access to hard-to-reach areas. (Courtesy Origin Medsystems, Menlo Park, Calif.)

image, allowing structures and organs to be seen during operative radiology examinations, such as operative cholangiograms.

Optical (transparent) trocar/cannula assemblies are also available that allow entry under direct visualization, thus decreasing the risk of "blind entry" (Figs. 7-27 and 7-28). Sometimes these optical assemblies can also magnify the tissue layers.

"Open" Laparoscopy

A patient who has undergone previous abdominal operations may be scheduled for an "open" laparoscopy if extensive adhesions are anticipated. In this procedure a small incision, usually not greater than 1.5 cm in diameter, is used to dissect down and open the peritoneum. A blunt-tipped trocar/cannula assembly (e.g., Hasson cannula and trocar) is then gently inserted. Stay sutures are placed to close the excess open incision around the cannula. The pneumoperitoneum is then established, and the laparoscopy progresses as usual. The unique parts of this device are:

- A blunt obturator trocar
- A sleeve (cannula) with wings to secure fascial suture anchors on either side of the trumpet valve
- A cone-shaped sleeve to obliterate the fascial opening

Extracorporeal surgery (surgery performed outside of the body) is sometimes planned if a difficult surgical technique cannot be performed within the confines of the body. This involves bringing the organ or structure outside of the body, performing the surgical procedure on it, and then returning it back inside the body. This technique is accomplished through a large-diameter endoscopic access port. For example, during laparoscopic bowel procedures, a loop of the bowel may be brought to the outside of the body, repaired, and then returned to the inside.

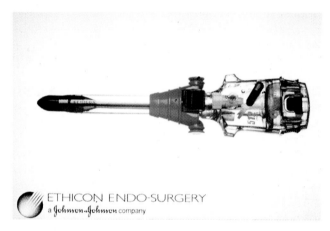

ETHICON ENDO-SURGERY
a Johnson-Johnson company

Fig. 7-27 Optical trocar/cannula assembly that provides direct visualization during entry. (Courtesy of Ethicon Endo-Surgery, Inc., Cincinnati, Ohio.)

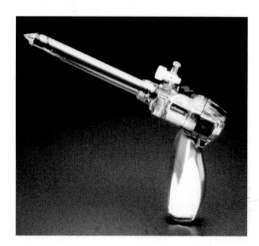

Fig. 7-28 A pistol-grip optical trocar/cannula assembly. (Courtesy Ethicon Endo-Surgery, Inc., Cincinnati, Ohio.)

Trocar/Cannula Placement

The trocar/cannula should be inserted with the patient's anatomy in mind. The trocar must be aimed away from vital structures, such as the liver, spleen, and vessels, and also away from the midline.

Proper trocar placement is extremely important during laparoscopy, thoracoscopy, or arthroscopy because it determines where instruments are inserted and hence whether the surgical procedure can be performed easily and safely (Fig. 7-29). One key point is to place the trocar adequately away from the operative area so that instruments are not positioned at right angles from the entry wall or just over the top of the target. An entry angle of about 30 degrees usually allows for the most comfortable and effective positioning of instruments.

Special consideration must be given to the trocar/cannula placement site in patients who have undergone prior open abdominal surgical procedures (Fig. 7-30). Adhesions can form after any open surgical procedure, but patients with midline incisions are more prone to adhesion formation than those with Pfannensteil incisions. A thorough bowel preparation is very important before a laparoscopic procedure in such patients to minimize bowel distention that could lead to possible perforation. The patient should understand that bowel injury is possible during laparoscopy, and consent for an open procedure should be obtained in the event conversion is necessary.

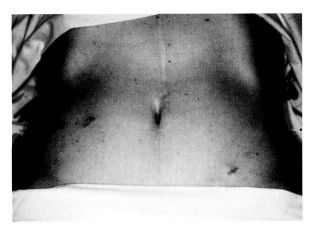

Fig. 7-30 Trocar placements for a laparoscopic cholecystectomy in a patient who has undergone previous abdominal surgery. Note the midline incision scar.

The following guidelines apply to the performance of a laparoscopic procedure in a patient who has had previous abdominal operations (*Laparosc Surg Update*, 1995a).

- Obtain documentation and information about the previous operations, which will help to determine where adhesions have probably formed.
- After insertion of the Veress needle, conduct a "hanging drop" test by aspirating with a syringe to confirm that the bowel has not been entered.
- If no fluid is aspirated, insert a small (e.g., 5-mm) trocar/cannula assembly, along with a small (e.g., 4-mm) endoscope, to examine the entry area.
- If no injury is sustained, then insert a larger (e.g., 10-mm) trocar/cannula.
- If the bowel is entered, then leave the trocar in place and enter through another laparoscopic site or through a minilaparotomy incision to repair the injured bowel.

Radially Expanding Dilator Systems

Radially expanding dilators that cause less traumatic abdominal wall entry for laparoscopy are now available. A radially expanding dilator setup has a cannula with a blunt obturator and an insufflation/access needle with a radially expandable sleeve (Fig. 7-31). It is a single-use device that creates a large working port access through a small initial puncture. The following procedure is used to place it:

- Intraabdominal entry is made using an insufflation/access needle with a radially expandable sleeve. The needle is inserted through the tissue and insufflation is achieved (Fig. 7-32).
- After insufflation, the needle is withdrawn, leaving the expandable sleeve in place. The operator's thumb

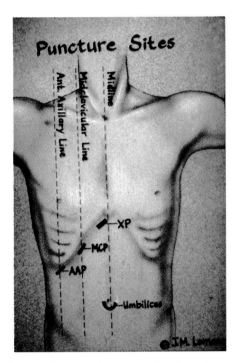

Fig. 7-29 Usual trocar placement sites for a laparoscopic cholecystectomy. (Courtesy Jack Lomano, MD, Sanibel, Fla.)

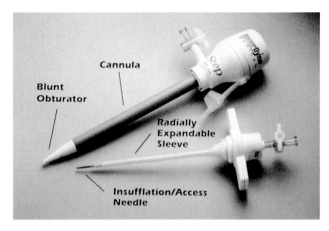

Fig. 7-31 A radially expanding dilator system. (Courtesy InnerDyne, Inc., Sunnyvale, Calif.)

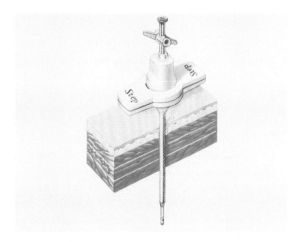

Fig. 7-32 Insertion of the insufflation/access needle. (Courtesy InnerDyne, Inc., Sunnyvale, Calif.)

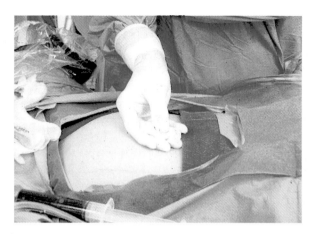

Fig. 7-33 The operator's thumb blocks the port so that no insufflation gas can escape. (Courtesy InnerDyne, Inc., Sunnyvale, Calif.)

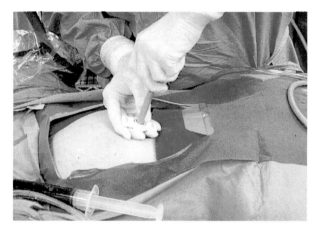

Fig. 7-34 Insertion of a tapered, blunt-tipped dilator while the sleeve and tissue tract are expanded. (Courtesy InnerDyne, Inc., Sunnyvale, Calif.)

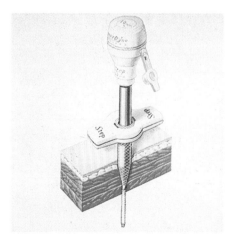

Fig. 7-35 Expansion of the sleeve and tissue tract. (Courtesy InnerDyne, Inc., Sunnyvale, Calif.)

blocks the port so that no insufflation gas can escape (Fig. 7-33).

A tapered, blunt-tipped dilator is inserted while the sleeve and tissue tract are expanded, thus providing a large working channel (Figs. 7-34 to 7-36). Dilation can be controlled to provide a 5-, 10-, or 12-mm access port (Fig. 7-37).

Because a sharp trocar is not used, the risk of trocar-related injuries is minimized. In addition, the muscle tissue is stretched, not cut, so the port has a tighter seal, causing a more stable pneumoperitoneum. Because the muscles are not punctured, the chance of postoperative hernia formation at the trocar site is also decreased. A traditional trocar puncture can cut tissue, leaving a larger hole or defect (Fig. 7-38), with herniation of the internal tissues a possible postoperative complication (Fig. 7-39). Anchors and screws are also not needed to secure the cannula in place because of the tight seal provided by the stretched tissue. Furthermore, the tight port serves as a tamponade of the area should bleeding

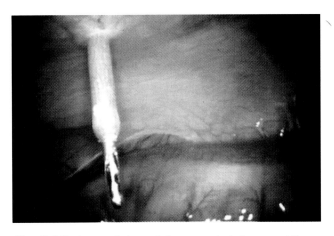

Fig. 7-36 Internal view of the expanded sleeve and tissue tract. (Courtesy InnerDyne, Inc., Sunnyvale, Calif.)

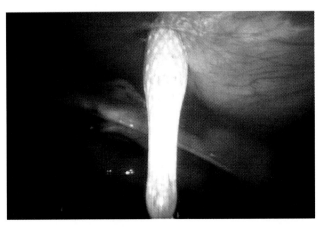

Fig. 7-37 A large working channel, created by radially dilating the tissue for the access port. (Courtesy InnerDyne, Inc., Sunnyvale, Calif.)

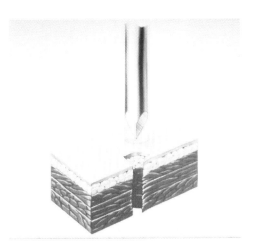

Fig. 7-38 The traditional nonexpandable cannula trocar puncture. (Courtesy InnerDyne, Inc., Sunnyvale, Calif.)

occur during insertion, thus providing better visualization. When the device is removed, the tissue contracts naturally, leaving a small slitlike wound (Fig. 7-40). A further advantage of the radially dilating system is that it can be used to gain access to hollow organs for endoscopic procedures that were previously inaccessible except by means of open surgery.

ENDOSCOPIC INSTRUMENTATION

There is an array of different instruments that can be used for endoscopic procedures (Fig. 7-41), but different factors must be considered when determining the most appropriate endoscopic instrument to be used. These include the following:

- The type of endoscope and the size of the operating channel (Fig. 7-42)
- The length and diameter of the instrument

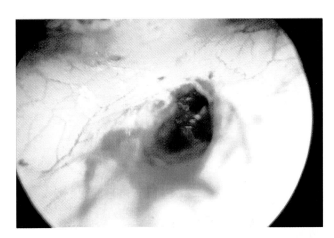

Fig. 7-39 A conventional trocar puncture can cut tissue and leave a defect that later could become herniated. (Courtesy InnerDyne, Inc., Sunnyvale, Calif.)

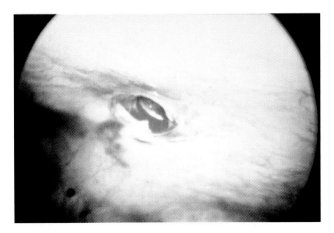

Fig. 7-40 The slitlike defect left after the use of a radially expanding dilator to stretch the trocar port site. (Courtesy InnerDyne, Inc., Sunnyvale, Calif.)

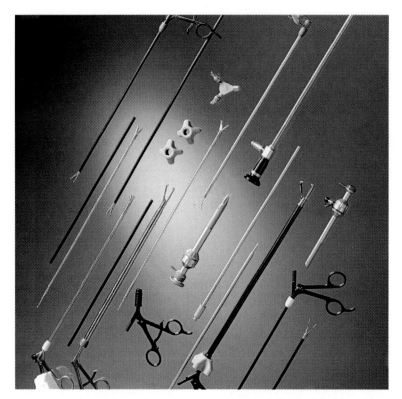

Fig. 7-41   A variety of instruments can be used for an endoscopic procedure. (Courtesy Aesculap, Inc., South San Francisco, Calif.)

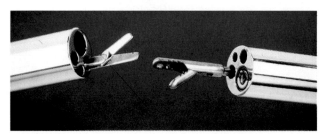

Fig. 7-42   The operating channel must be large enough to accommodate endoscopic instruments.

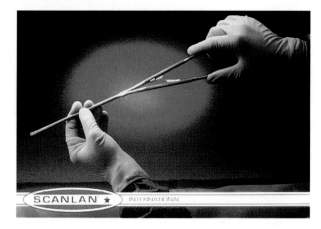

Fig. 7-44   Squeeze-action handle on endoscopic instrument. (Courtesy Scanlan International, St. Paul, Minn.)

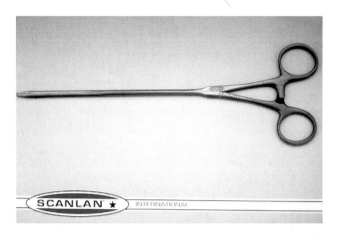

Fig. 7-43   Finger-hole handle on endoscopic instrument. (Courtesy Scanlan International, St. Paul, Minn.)

- The working end of the instrument
- The ease of use and control of the instrument

A variety of handles are available that provide efficient maneuverability and control as well as operator comfort (Figs. 7-43 to 7-45). Some handles also include a ratcheting mechanism that can provide continual closure (Fig. 7-46).

Endoscopic instruments can be reusable, single use, or reposable. Reposable (sometimes called *multi-use*) instruments have a reusable component and a single-use or limited-use component. There are many different

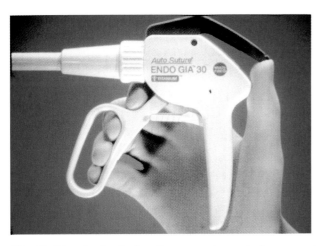

Fig. 7-45 Pistol-grip handle on endoscopic instrument. (Courtesy United States Surgical Corp., Norwalk, Conn.)

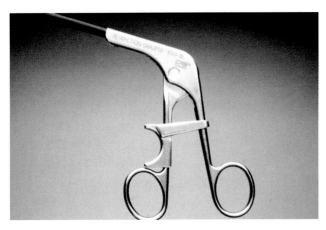

Fig. 7-46 A ratcheting mechanism, which locks the handle of the endoscopic instrument. (Courtesy Aesculap, Inc., South San Francisco, Calif.)

jaw inserts for the working end of the instrument (Fig. 7-47). Manufacturers usually recommend the number of times the jaw insert can be used safely.

Endoscopic instruments can be categorized into the following five groups:

- Dissecting instruments
- Clamping instruments
- Suturing or stapling instruments
- Rectractors
- Accessory instruments

Dissecting Instruments

Dissecting instruments are used to cut or separate tissue, and scissors, dissectors, and other types of dissecting instruments fall into this category.

Scissors

Endoscopic scissors are available in many designs (Fig. 7-48). However, regardless of the design, scissors must always be sharp to prevent the tissue trauma that can occur from the shearing produced by dull scissors (Fig. 7-49). The scissors usually have a rounded tip when closed, so they can be used to manipulate tissue without causing trauma (Fig. 7-50). When open, both jaws of the scissors should be visualized to prevent accidental tissue injury.

Straight or curved scissors are available for blunt or sharp dissection (Fig. 7-51). There are also hook scissors that are used to divide vessels or the cystic duct during laparoscopic cholecystectomies. This type of scissor must be used carefully because it has sharp tips and can easily injure nontargeted tissue. Scissors can be insulated for connection with an electrosurgical energy source, thus they can be used for cutting and electrosurgical coagulation (Fig. 7-52). Both monopolar and bipolar electrosurgery scissors are now available. Microscissors are often used for delicate techniques (Fig. 7-53).

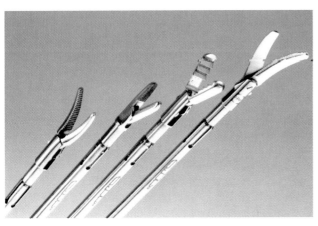

Fig. 7-47 Jaw inserts for reposable endoscopic instruments. (Courtesy Aesculap, Inc., South San Francisco, Calif.)

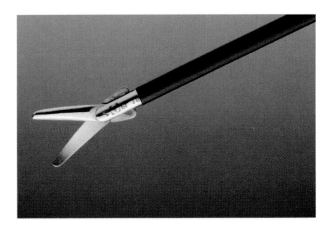

Fig. 7-48 Endoscopic scissors. (Courtesy United States Surgical Corp., Norwalk, Conn.)

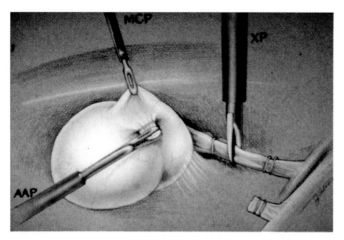

Fig. 7-49 Endoscopic scissors are used to precisely cut the cystic duct. (Courtesy Jack Lomano, MD, Sanibel, Fla.)

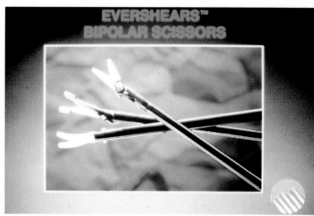

Fig. 7-52 Bipolar electrosurgical scissors. (Courtesy Everest Medical Corp., Minneapolis, Minn.)

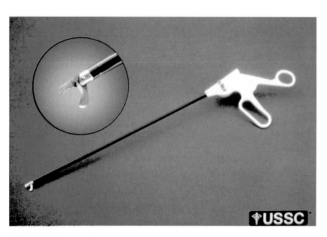

Fig. 7-50 Scissors usually have rounded tips so that when closed they can be used to manipulate tissue. (Courtesy Aesculap, Inc., South San Francisco, Calif.)

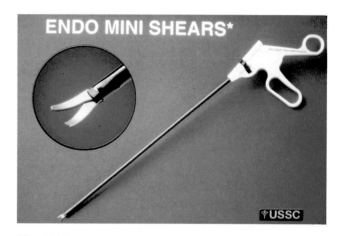

Fig. 7-53 Microscissors, designed for delicate work. (Courtesy United States Surgical Corp., Norwalk, Conn.)

However, care must be taken to avoid damage when the microscissors are moved in and out through the access sheath.

Some endoscopic scissors have a head that can be rotated to obtain better positioning (Fig. 7-54). The operator does this by rotating a control located at the proximal end of the endoscopic sheath. The distal working end of the scissors then assumes the desired angle.

Dissectors

Dissectors are used to separate or divide tissue from other tissue or structures. They can be used for grasping, precise dissection, and monopoplar or bipolar coagulation with electrosurgical energy.

Dissectors now come with many different geometrically shaped tips. Some have long, round-edged jaws with small teeth or ridges to firmly hold tissue. The tissue is separated by opening the jaws while in contact with the tissue (Figs. 7-55 and 7-56).

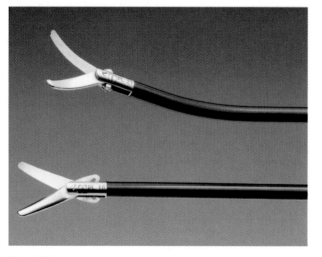

Fig. 7-51 Straight and curved endoscopic scissors. (Courtesy Aesculap, Inc., South San Francisco, Calif.)

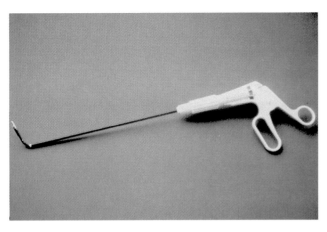

Fig. 7-54 Endoscopic scissors with a rotating head. (Courtesy United States Surgical Corp., Norwalk, Conn.)

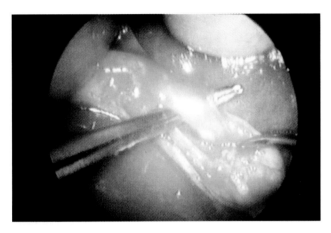

Fig. 7-55 Dissector with jaws closed. (Courtesy Origin Medsystems, Menlo Park, Calif.)

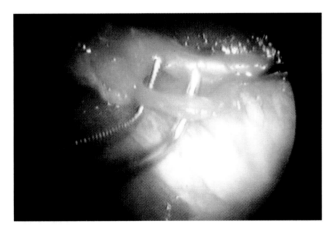

Fig. 7-56 A dissector with jaws open to divide and separate tissue. (Courtesy Origin Medsystems, Menlo Park, Calif.)

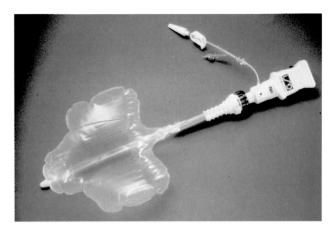

Fig. 7-57 Balloon dissecting instrument. (Courtesy United States Surgical Corp., Norwalk, Conn.)

There are also hook-and-spatula dissectors that can be insulated for use with electrosurgical energy. They are used both to separate tissue and to coagulate. These dissectors also come in designs that allow them to be connected to suction and irrigation systems.

Other dissecting instruments

Other dissecting tools have been developed for endoscopic use. Blunt dissection can be achieved by placing a small cotton pledget ("peanut") on the end of a grasping instrument. The tissue is then dissected through tissue separation. The surgeon can also use his or her fingers to bluntly dissect when establishing the access port during "open" laparoscopies. Sharp dissection can be achieved by using the edges of curettes, elevators, and knives.

Blunt dissection can also be performed with a balloon dissector that is part of the endoscopic cannula (Fig. 7-57). A balloon dissector is used to create space within an area, such as the preperitoneal space during a laparoscopic herniorrhaphy. The endoscope is then inserted into the balloon dissector for visualization during the dissection (Fig. 7-58).

Clamping Instruments

Clamping instruments are used to hold tissue or other materials and usually have the following characteristics:
- Finger rings for ease of holding
- Appropriate length for the endoscopic procedure being performed
- Ratchets to allow the distal tip to be locked onto the tissue or whatever is grasped

Clamping instruments can be graspers, forceps, and even biopsy forceps.

Graspers and forceps

Graspers and forceps are used to manipulate and hold tissue and are either traumatic or atraumatic (Fig. 7-59).

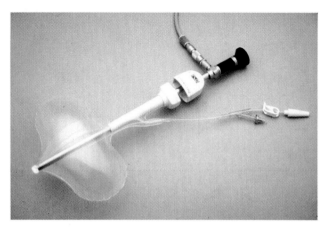

Fig. 7-58 Endoscope inserted into the balloon dissector for visualization during the dissection. (Courtesy General Surgical Innovations, Inc., Palo Alto, Calif.)

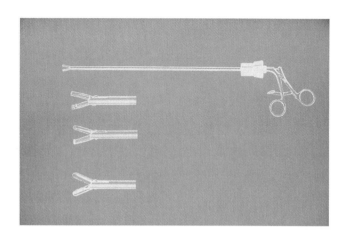

Fig. 7-60 Atraumatic Allis grasping forceps. (Courtesy Jarit Instrument, Hawthorne, N.Y.)

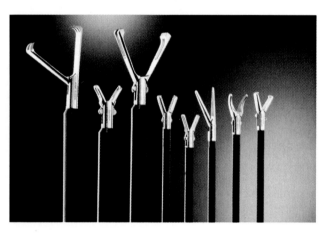

Fig. 7-59 Endoscopic grasping instruments. (Courtesy Karl Storz, Culver City, Calif.)

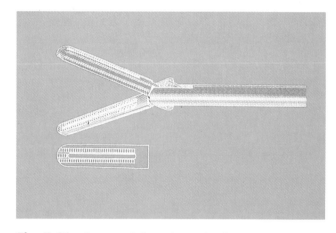

Fig. 7-61 Atraumatic bowel grasping forceps. (Courtesy Jarit Instrument, Hawthorne, N.Y.)

Atraumatic forceps have a smooth, serrated surface and an automatic spring or ratchet mechanism to control the action of the jaws at the surgical site (Fig. 7-60). The ratcheting effect allows for constant maintenance of the grip on the structure or tissue. Atraumatic forceps are used to gently hold delicate structures, such as the bowel or liver (Figs. 7-61 to 7-63). Traumatic forceps have sharp teeth, so they are customarily used on tissue that is being excised, not on healthy tissue because the teeth might injure the tissue (Fig. 7-64).

Some graspers may be insulated so that electrosurgical energy can be transmitted through them to provide coagulation (Fig. 7-65). The jaws come in different configurations so that they can be used for different types of tissue, structures, and manipulations. Graspers may also be used to dissect tissue.

Forceps may have single- or dual-action working ends (Fig. 7-66). With single-action forceps, one jaw of

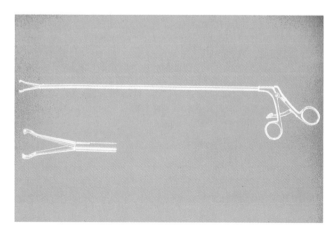

Fig. 7-62 Atraumatic Babcock forceps. (Courtesy Jarit Instrument, Hawthorne, N.Y.)

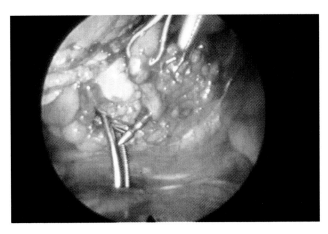

Fig. 7-63 Babcock forceps are used to gently hold tissue. (Courtesy Origin Medsystems, Menlo Park, Calif.)

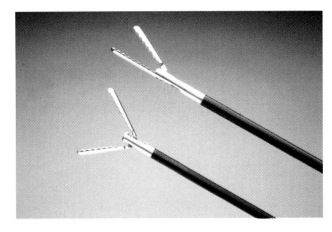

Fig. 7-66 Single- and dual-action forceps. (Courtesy Aesculap, Inc., South San Francisco, Calif.)

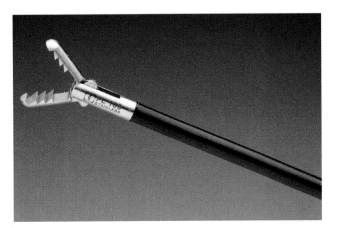

Fig. 7-64 Traumatic grasping forceps. (Courtesy Aesculap, Inc., South San Francisco, Calif.)

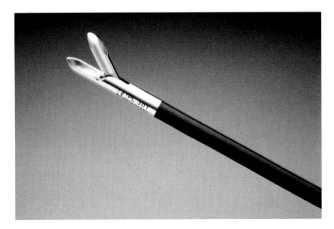

Fig. 7-67 Endoscopic biopsy forceps. (Courtesy Aesculap, Inc., South San Francisco, Calif.)

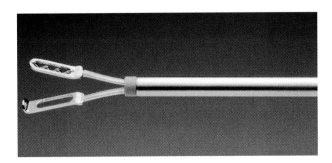

Fig. 7-65 Bipolar electrosurgical fixation forceps. (Courtesy Aesculap, Inc., South San Francisco, Calif.)

the working end moves and the other does not. Both jaws of dual-action forceps can be moved.

Biopsy forceps

Biopsy forceps come in many different designs for use in different locations and different types of tissue (Fig. 7-67). Some biopsy forceps have two movable jaws; oth-

ers have one fixed and one movable jaw. The size and design of the jaw determines the size of the biopsy specimen. Most biopsy forceps have sharp cutting edges to allow a cleaner biopsy specimen to be obtained without tearing the tissue. Usually biopsy forceps are insulated so that electrosurgical energy can be applied to coagulate the biopsy site. Biopsy forceps have either a flexible or rigid shaft for use with different types of endoscopes.

Suturing or Stapling Instruments

Suturing or stapling instruments are used to deliver sutures, staples, or clips to secure, hold, join, or combine tissue. Needle holders, clip appliers, staplers, and endoscopic linear cutters all fall in this category.

Needle holders

Endoscopic needle holders have been developed that can be used to place sutures within a body cavity (Fig. 7-68). Because needle holders grip metal needles, however, they are more apt to break down as a result of the

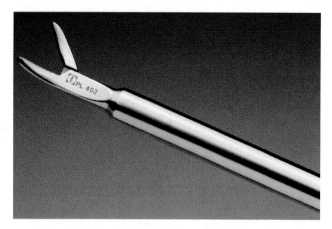

Fig. 7-68   **Endoscopic needle holder.** (Courtesy Aesculap, Inc., South San Francisco, Calif.)

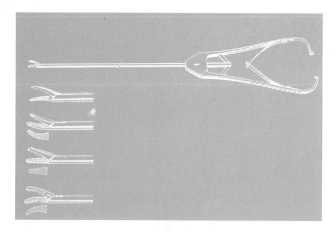

Fig. 7-70   **Left, right, straight, and micro needle holder tips.** (Courtesy Jarit Instrument, Hawthome, N.Y.)

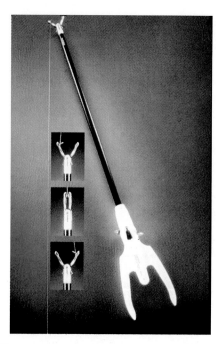

Fig. 7-69   **An endoscopic needle holder that transfers the needle from one prong of the jaw to the other.** (Courtesy United States Surgical Corp., Norwalk, Conn.)

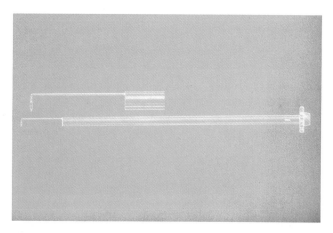

Fig. 7-71   **Endoscopic suture passer.** (Courtesy Jarit Instrument, Hawthorne, N.Y.)

increased wear and tear to which they are subjected. Some needle holders have tungsten carbide jaw inserts designed to prevent rotation of the needle. Many physicians prefer double-action needle holders with two movable jaws because of the easier manipulation afforded. There are also instruments now available to help with needle transfer during the endoscopic procedure. Such an instrument can pass the needle from one jaw to another, and this is done by squeezing its handles together (Fig. 7-69).

Because laparoscopic suturing can be tedious, needle holders and other instruments have been designed to help facilitate this process. There are now needle holders that curve right and left for easier maneuverability (Fig. 7-70). Suture passers that allow sutures to be advanced through the endoscope port to the surgical site (Fig. 7-71) and knot pushers that deliver a suture knot to the surgical area (Fig. 7-72) have been developed. There is also a knot placement device that allows the passage of a standard endoscopic needle driver. Using a standard suture and needle, the device can be used to tie, push and tighten knots (Fig. 7-73).

Surgeons, residents, and nurses can easily learn laparoscopic suturing, including extracorporeal and intracorporeal suturing and knot tying, but they need to practice with models to master the skill.

Extracorporeal knot tying is performed externally after the sutures have been placed. Essentially it involves the tying of the knot, then the introduction of the knot into the abdominal cavity and its securement in place. Specifically it consists of the following steps:

- A swaged-on suture (a suture with the needle already attached) is grasped with a needle holder just below

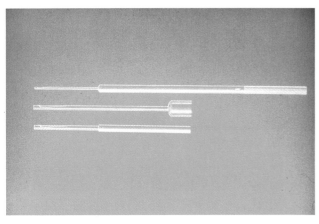

Fig. 7-72 Endoscopic knot pusher. (Courtesy Jarit Instrument, Hawthorne, N.Y.)

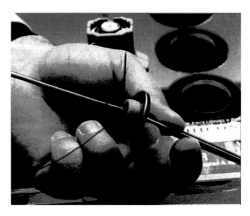

Fig. 7-74 The needle holder is inserted into the introducer cannula as the suture is held near the swage point. (Courtesy Ethicon Endo-Surgery Inc., Cincinnati, Ohio.)

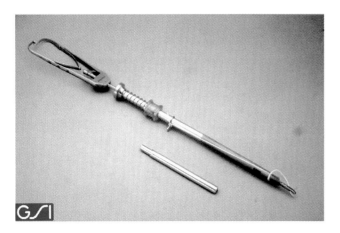

Fig. 7-73 Knot placement device. (Courtesy General Surgical Innovations, Inc., Palo Alto, Calif.)

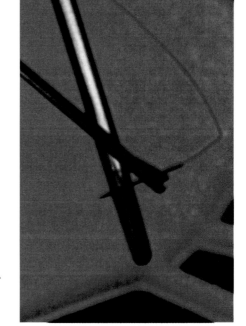

Fig. 7-75 Using the grasper, the operator repositions the needle in the needle holder jaws. (Courtesy Ethicon Endo-Surgery Inc., Cincinnati, OH)

the swage point so that a straight needle would collapse within the suture introducer and a curved needle would slightly protrude. The needle and needle holder are then placed within the suture introducer (Fig. 7-74).
- The introducer is placed through a cannula positioned to serve as the access port.
- A grasper is inserted through another port to assist with the endoscopic suturing.
- The needle is advanced through the suture introducer.
- Using the grasper, the operator repositions the needle in the needle holder jaws (Fig. 7-75).
- The needle holder is used to pass the needle through the tissue to the grasper (Fig. 7-76). If the needle tip is difficult to see, then the grasper can be used to gently depress the tissue where the needle is thought to be located, which will provide better exposure.

- The needle is then passed back to the needle holder, making sure that the needle is securely positioned within the needle holder jaws (Fig. 7-77).
- The grasper can be used to relieve the excess tension on the suture by pulling more of the suture material into the abdominal cavity.
- After suturing is complete, the suture is grasped by the needle holder just below the swage point and removed through the suture introducer (Fig. 7-78).

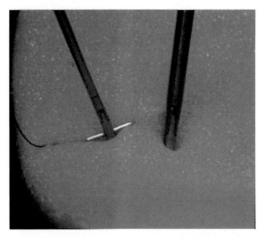

Fig. 7-76 The needle holder is used to pass the needle through tissue to the grasper. (Courtesy Ethicon Endo-Surgery Inc., Cincinnati, Ohio.)

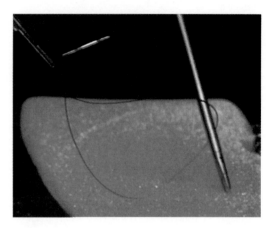

Fig. 7-78 After suturing is complete, the suture is grasped by the needle holder just below the swage point and removed through the suture introducer. (Courtesy Ethicon Endo-Surgery Inc., Cincinnati, Ohio.)

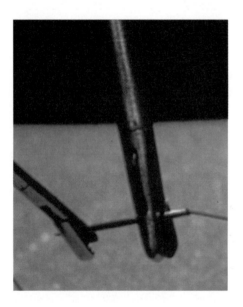

Fig. 7-77 The needle is passed back to the needle holder. (Courtesy Ethicon Endo-Surgery Inc., Cincinnati, Ohio.)

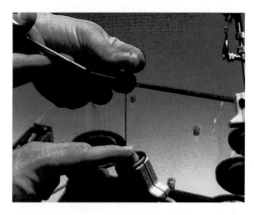

Fig. 7-79 The assistant places a finger over the suture introducer port to prevent the escape of insufflation gas while the suture is being tied. (Courtesy Ethicon Endo-Surgery Inc., Cincinnati, Ohio.)

- The assistant can place a finger over the suture introducer port to prevent the escape of insufflation gas while the suture is being tied (Fig. 7-79).
- The needle is cut off of the suture and a knot is made in the suture while the two ends of the suture are outside the body (Fig. 7-80).
- One strand of the suture is cut to leave a ¼-inch (0.60-cm) tail just above the knot (Fig. 7-81).
- A knot pusher is inserted through the access port to place the knot internally at the tissue surface (Fig. 7-82).
- The knot is tightened and the excess length of suture material is cut about ¼ inch (0.60 cm) from the knot (Fig. 7-83).

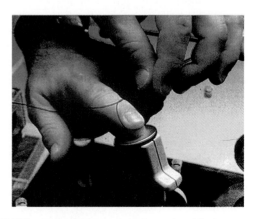

Fig. 7-80 A single-throw knot is made with the two suture ends. (Courtesy Ethicon Endo-Surgery Inc., Cincinnati, Ohio.)

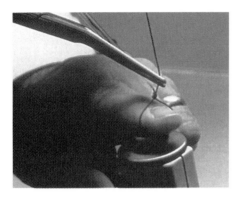

Fig. 7-81 One strand of the suture is cut approximately ¼ inch (0.60 cm) above the knot. (Courtesy Ethicon Endo-Surgery Inc., Cincinnati, Ohio.)

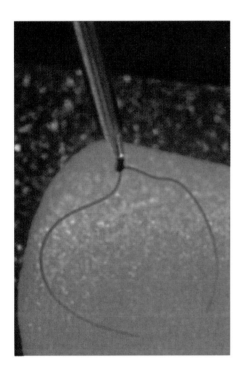

Fig. 7-82 A knot pusher is used to position and tighten the knot. (Courtesy Ethicon Endo-Surgery Inc., Cincinnati, Ohio.)

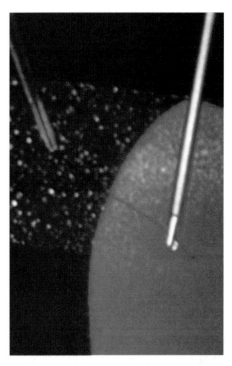

Fig. 7-83 The excess length of suture material is cut about ¼ inch (0.60 cm) from the knot. (Courtesy Ethicon Endo-Surgery Inc., Cincinnati, Ohio.)

Intracorporeal knot tying is performed inside the body. However, sometimes it is more difficult to perform than extracorporeal knot tying and practice on inanimate objects is necessary to master it. Following is a procedure for intracorporeal knot tying:

- An endoscopic needle holder is used to grasp the suture just below the swage point so that a straight needle would collapse within the suture introducer and a curved needle would slightly protrude (Fig. 7-84).
- The needle holder and suture are inserted into the suture introducer (Fig. 7-85).
- The suture introducer is advanced through the trocar cannula

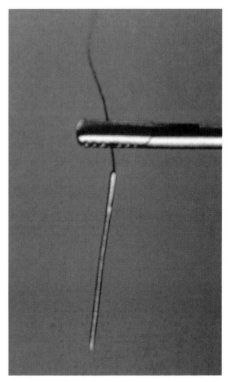

Fig. 7-84 An endoscopic needle holder is used to grasp the suture just below the swage point. (Courtesy Ethicon Endo-Surgery Inc., Cincinnati, Ohio.)

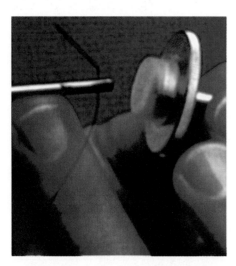

Fig. 7-85 The needle holder and suture are inserted into the suture introducer. (Courtesy Ethicon Endo-Surgery Inc., Cincinnati, Ohio.)

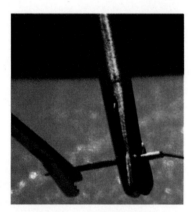

Fig. 7-86 The grasper is used to help position the needle in the jaws of the needle holder. (Courtesy Ethicon Endo-Surgery Inc., Cincinnati, Ohio.

- A grasper is introduced through another port. It is used to help position the needle in the jaws of the needle holder (Fig. 7-86).
- The suture is placed in the tissue using both the needle holder and the grasper.
- When the suturing is complete, the needle is passed to the grasper.
- The grasper is used to loop the length of suture around the needle holder shaft two times (Fig. 7-87).
- The needle holder is used to grasp the tail of the suture and pull it through the suture loops, creating a knot.
- The grasper is then used to repeat the process, but the loops are made around the needle holder in the opposite direction (Fig. 7-88).
- The needle holder is used to grasp the suture tail again to form the second knot.

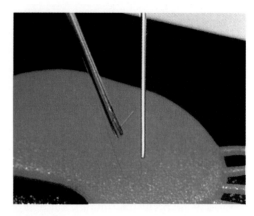

Fig. 7-87 The length of suture is wrapped twice around the shaft of the needle holder. (Courtesy Ethicon Endo-Surgery Inc., Cincinnati, Ohio.)

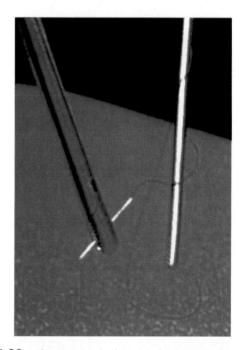

Fig. 7-88 The grasper is then used to repeat the process, but the loops are made around the needle holder in the opposite direction. (Courtesy Ethicon Endo-Surgery Inc., Cincinnati, Ohio.)

- The suture tail is pulled to tighten the knot (Fig. 7-89).
- The suture is cut, leaving ¼-inch (0.60-cm) tails (Fig. 7-90).

There are now pre-tied sutures that come in the form of a loop to ligate vessels and tissue pedicles during rigid endoscopic procedures (Fig. 7-91). Following is the procedure for placing them:

- The pre-tied knot is centered in the introducer cannula (Fig. 7-92).
- The loop is passed through the cannula and secured around a structure with the assistance of a grasping instrument introduced through another port.

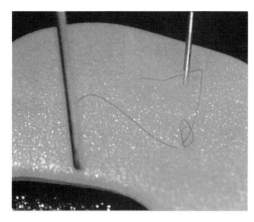

Fig. 7-89   The suture tail is pulled to tighten the knot.
(Courtesy Ethicon Endo-Surgery Inc., Cincinnati, Ohio.)

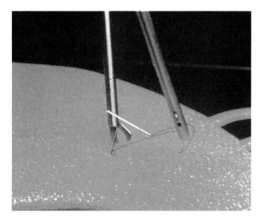

Fig. 7-90   The suture is cut, leaving ¼-inch (0.6-cm) tails.
(Courtesy Ethicon Endo-Surgery Inc., Cincinnati, Ohio.)

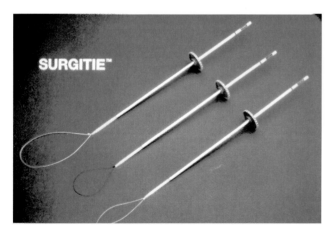

Fig. 7-91   Endoscopic ligating loops. (Courtesy United States
Surgical Corp., Norwalk, Conn.)

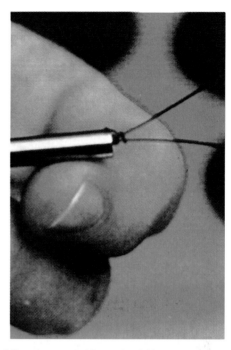

Fig. 7-92   The pre-tied knot should be centered in the introducer cannula. (Courtesy Ethicon Endo-Surgery Inc., Cincinnati, Ohio.)

- The grasper positions the tissue within the loop.
- Through manipulation of the ligature device from outside of the body, the loop is tightened around the structure and the knot is set (Fig. 7-93).
- Endoscopic scissors are used to cut the ends of the suture immediately above the suture knot, leaving approximately a ¼-inch (0.60-cm) tail.

Different devices have been developed to close the trocar site. Some devices deliver the suture material to opposite sides of the wound to close both the fascial and peritoneal layers of tissue. Sometimes skin and fat may also be closed with the same device (Fig. 7-94). Closure of the fascia minimizes the possibility of incisional hernia formation.

Other laparoscopic closure instruments have been developed to minimize fascial trocar defects and secure abdominal wall bleeders resulting from trocar injuries. Following are the steps involved in the use of one type of fascial closure system:

- The trocar/cannula is removed (Fig. 7-95).
- A special plug is placed into the incision.
- The plug is aligned with the peritoneum (Fig. 7-96).
- The special needle is loaded with a suture (Fig. 7-97).
- The threaded needle is directed through the plug guide from one side to the other (Fig. 7-98).
- The suture is released.
- The needle is withdrawn and then inserted into the opposite side of the plug. The suture is loaded into the needle within the abdomen and the suture is retrieved (Fig. 7-99).

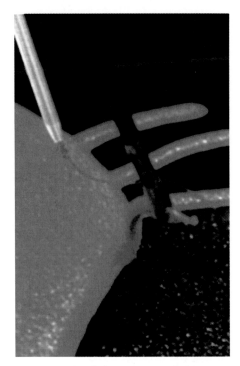

Fig. 7-93 The loop is placed and tightened while the tissue is manipulated with a grasper. (Courtesy Ethicon Endo-Surgery Inc., Cincinnati, Ohio.)

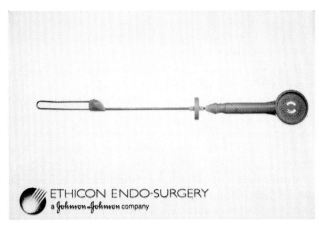

Fig. 7-94 Disposable wound-closure device. The J-shape of the suture needle on this device allows the user to reach into the trocar port and return the suture back to the surface to close all layers of the tissue. (Courtesy Ethicon Endo-Surgery Inc., Cincinnati, Ohio.)

- Suture placement is completed, with both ends extending through the fascial and other tissue to the outside of the body (Fig. 7-100).
- The plug is removed, and the sutures are tied (Fig. 7-101). The intraabdominal pressure is relieved before the suture is tied to minimize skin dimpling.

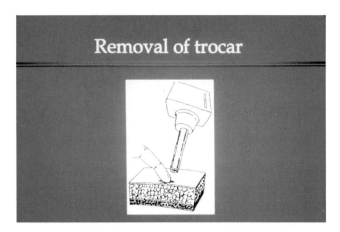

Fig. 7-95 The trocar/cannula is removed. (Courtesy R-Med, Inc., Oregon, Ohio.)

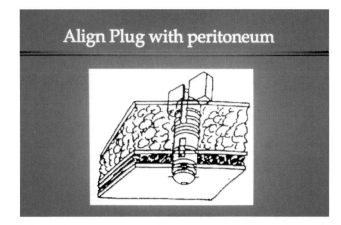

Fig. 7-96 The plug is placed in the port hole and aligned with the peritoneum. (Courtesy R-Med, Inc., Oregon, Ohio).

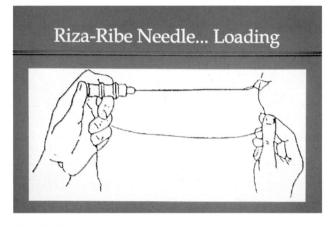

Fig. 7-97 The special needle is loaded with a suture. (Courtesy R-Med, Inc., Oregon, Ohio.)

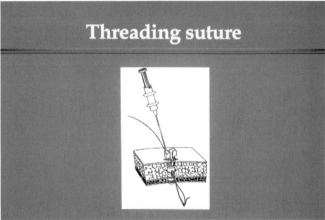

Fig. 7-98 The threaded needle is directed through the plug guide from one side to the other. (Courtesy R-Med, Inc., Oregon, Ohio.)

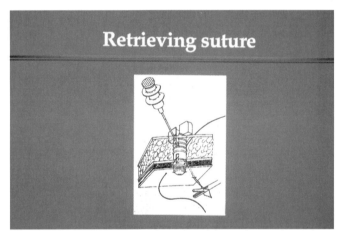

Fig. 7-99 The suture is released and brought up through the other plug hole. (Courtesy R-Med, Inc, Oregon, Ohio.)

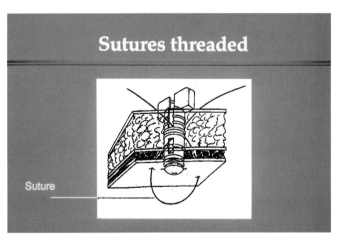

Fig. 7-100 Completed suture placement. (Courtesy R-Med, Inc., Oregon, Ohio.)

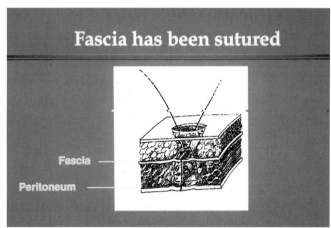

Fig. 7-101 The plug is removed, and the sutures are tied. (Courtesy R-Med, Inc., Oregon, Ohio.)

Suturing is only as secure as the knots used. Following are general principles that must be observed when tying knots, regardless of the suture material (Ethicon, 1991):

- Extra ties are not needed to secure a properly tied knot. They merely add to the bulk of the knot.
- The completed knot must be secure so that slipping does not occur. Usually the simplest knot for the suture material being used is the most desirable, as long as the knot is tied securely.
- Excessive tension is not needed during knot tying because the extra force could break the suture or cut the tissue.
- When tying a knot, friction or sawing of the suture lengths must be avoided because this could weaken the integrity of the suture.
- The knot should be as small as possible and the ends cut as short as possible. If the suture is absorbable, a smaller knot will prevent excessive tissue reaction. If the suture is nonabsorbable, the foreign body reaction will be minimized.
- Avoid damaging the suture material when handling it. Refrain from excessive crimping or crushing of the suture material with grasping or clamping instruments.

Endoscopic clip applier

Endoscopic clip appliers are used to apply clips to tissue to achieve hemostasis or occlude structures (Fig. 7-102). Usually U-shaped clips made of titanium are used for this purpose and can safely and quickly occlude small vessels and structures. To avoid injury, however, both prongs of the clip must be visible before insertion. Right-angled clip appliers are also available, and these provide easy access to structures so that the clip can be properly placed (Figs. 7-103 and 7-104). Multiple-load or single-load disposable clip appliers are also now available (Fig. 7-105).

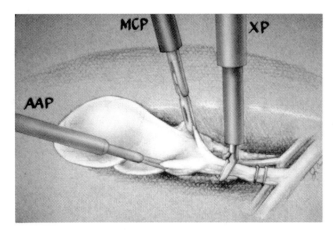

Fig. 7-102 An endoscopic clip applier is being used on the cystic duct. (Courtesy Jack Lomano, MD, Sanibel, Fla.)

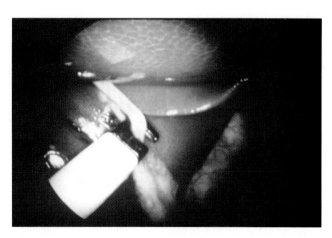

Fig. 7-104 A right-angled clip applier, which can facilitate tissue placement into the apex of the clip. (Courtesy Origin Medsystems, Menlo Park, Calif.)

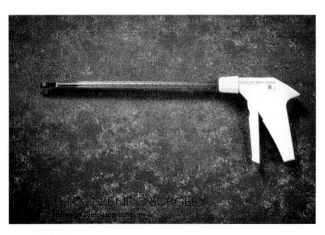

Fig. 7-103 A right-angled clip applier which can gain access to hard-to-reach areas. (Courtesy Ethicon Endo-Surgery Inc., Cincinnati, Ohio.)

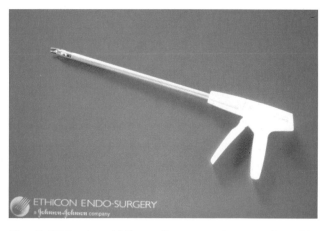

Fig. 7-105 A multiclip applier can apply many clips without the need to reload. (Courtesy Ethicon Endo-Surgery Inc., Cincinnati, Ohio.)

A disadvantage of reusable clip appliers is that the instrument must be removed from the surgical site for reloading, because often they accommodate only one clip at a time. This continual movement of the instrument in and out through the access port may cause a loss of the pneumoperitoneum. It also takes time and causes frustration, especially if the clip is not loaded properly and is dislodged upon reinsertion.

Endoscopic staplers

Endoscopic staplers have been developed to decrease the surgical time needed to repair and suture tissue. Stapling devices have been designed to staple the mesh in place during hernia repairs performed laparoscopically (Fig. 7-106). With their use it takes less time to suture the mesh, thus reducing the surgical time tremendously.

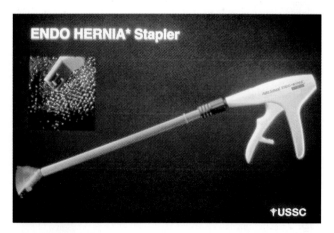

Fig. 7-106 Endoscopic hernia stapler. (Courtesy United States Surgical Corp., Norwalk, Conn.)

Endoscopic linear cutters

Endoscopic linear cutters grasp the tissue, deliver two rows of staples, and then cut the tissue (Fig. 7-107). These devices provide safe dissection and stapling through the endoscope thereby decreasing the need for an open approach to accomplish the same end. With the advent of this technology it is possible to perform a lung resection through the thoracoscope (Fig. 7-108).

Retractors

Retractors are used to hold tissue and expose the operative site.

Endoscopic retractors

Retractors are used during endoscopic (laparoscopic) procedures to maintain optimal visualization by retracting structures, such as the bowel (Fig. 7-109). Retractors can be traumatic to some structures, such as the liver, so they must be used with caution. New retractors, such as the balloon retractor, have been designed that do not cause injury. Small delicate structures can be retracted with a mini-retractor (Fig. 7-110). Other endoscopic retractors have been developed to gently retract tissue. For example, there is a fan-shaped endoscopic retractor that collapses during insertion and then fans out to provide retraction over a larger area (Fig. 7-111).

Abdominal wall–lifting devices

Various abdominal wall–lifting systems have been designed to provide intraperitoneal retraction without the need for gas insufflation (Fig. 7-112). This tool is inserted through the trocar site and then expanded to lift the abdomen (Fig. 7-113). The lifting device is connected to a stabilizing arm that is attached to the surgical table (Fig. 7-114). The stabilizing arm is draped to keep the field sterile (Fig. 7-115).

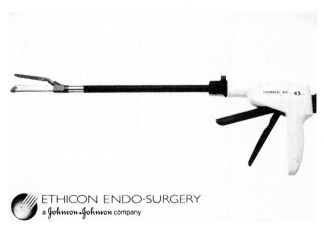

Fig. 7-108 Thoracoscopic linear cutter. (Courtesy Ethicon Endo-Surgery Inc., Cincinnati, Ohio.)

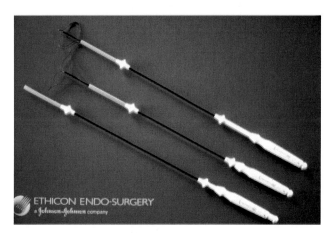

Fig. 7-109 This retractor's working end can be enlarged and changed by moving the handle control. (Courtesy Ethicon Endo-Surgery Inc., Cincinnati, Ohio.)

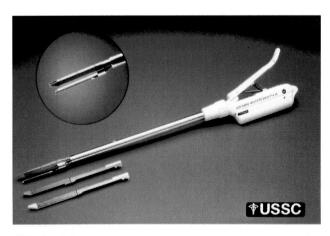

Fig. 7-107 Endoscopic tissue stapler that can be used for stapling and cutting. (Courtesy United States Surgical Corp. Norwalk, Conn.)

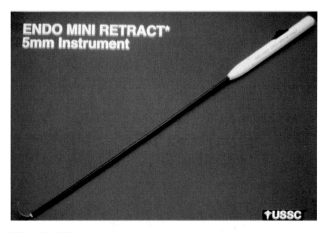

Fig. 7-110 Endoscopic mini-retractor. (Courtesy United States Surgical Corp., Norwalk, Conn.)

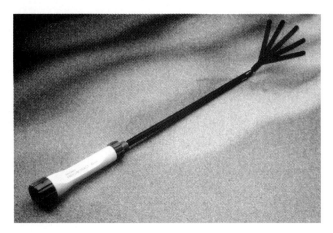

Fig. 7-111 Endoscopic fan retractor with five fingers. (Courtesy United States Surgical Corp., Norwalk, Conn.)

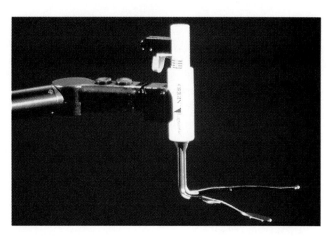

Fig. 7-114 This lifting device is connected to a stabilizing arm attached to the surgical table. (Courtesy Origin Medsystem, Menlo Park, Calif.)

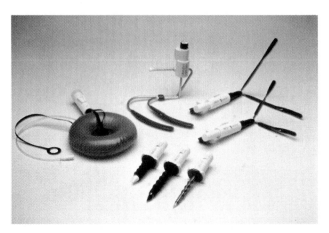

Fig. 7-112 Abdominal wall–lifting systems for gasless laparoscopy. (Courtesy Origin Medsystem, Menlo Park, Calif.)

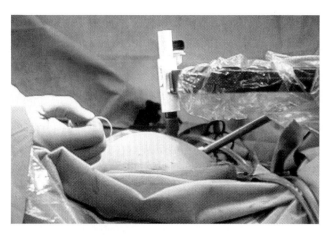

Fig. 7-115 Stabilizing arm draped with a sterile cover. (Courtesy Origin Medsystem, Menlo Park, Calif.)

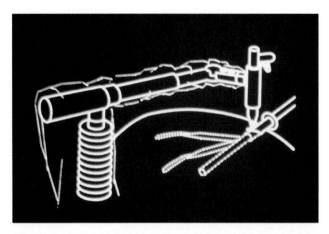

Fig. 7-113 This abdominal wall–lifting system is inserted through the trocar site and expanded to lift the abdomen. (Courtesy Origin Medsystem, Menlo Park, Calif.)

Abdominal wall–lifting systems were not designed, however, to replace gas insufflation and the establishment of a pneumoperitoneum but can be used in select patients who cannot endure the possible trauma resulting from abdominal distention. Such gasless lifting systems are mostly utilized for laparoscopic procedures of the lower abdomen (pelvic area) and are not as effective for procedures of the upper abdomen because of the limited visibility of this area they afford. The abdominal wall–lifting device also may not be used successfully in patients with thick or heavy abdominal walls, because it would be very cumbersome and difficult to lift the abdomen in such circumstances.

Advancements in the wall-lifting system have led to the development of an atraumatic doughnut-shaped lifter that provides a consistent force to elevate the abdominal wall (Fig. 7-116). This system attaches to the surgical table in the same way as the others do.

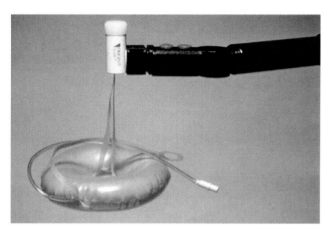

Fig. 7-116 An atraumatic doughnut-shaped lifting device. This provides a consistent force to elevate the abdominal wall. (Courtesy Origin Medsystem, Menlo Park, Calif.)

The development and refinement of this gasless abdominal wall–lifting system may have the benefit of encouraging an increased use of local anesthesia because abdominal insufflation is not needed. More research and product refinement are needed, however, before this device can be used extensively in patients under local anesthesia.

Patients with certain conditions, such as pregnancy, may benefit from the abdominal wall–lifting device. Laparoscopy performed with insufflation is not always recommended for pregnant women because, as noted in an earlier chapter, CO_2 insufflation can cause acid-base changes in the fetus. Insufflation is also not widely used for patients with severe cardiopulmonary disease, because the traditional pneumoperitoneum exerts a significant uplift on the diaphragm and this can compromise the patient's cardiac and respiratory status.

There is continued controversy, however, about the advantages and disadvantages of this lifting tool. Studies are needed that examine the incidence of the postoperative pain caused by the lifting device applying pressure to one area, as opposed to the spreading of pressure over the entire abdominal wall that occurs with insufflation. The amount of exposure and visualization of the internal structures afforded by the two methods also need to be compared, because there have been complaints that the lifting device provides less lateral exposure than insufflation does. The gasless system also sometimes does not adequately compress the intestines, with the result that they obscure the surgical team's vision. This is not the case for gas insufflation, which exerts a uniform pressure throughout the abdomen and adequately compresses the bowel. A steeper Trendelenburg position may be used in patients to help compensate for this problem.

Besides these concerns, the main lifting device that attaches to the surgical bed plus the cost of the sterile disposable item that is introduced into the patient need to be compared with the expense of providing the insufflator equipment and the gas.

An abdominal wall–lifting method that is popular in Japan involves the threading of a cable through the abdominal wall, which is then lifted up like a tent. This is called the *cable-lifting method*.

There are many advantages to using an abdominal wall–lifting method instead of gas insufflation, some of which are listed below:

- Traditional instruments that are longer can be used through a small incision without the worry of gas escaping and instrument seals being inadequate.
- Standard needle drivers can be used, making suturing easier.
- More than one instrument can be used through a port, so fewer trocar sites may be needed.
- High-speed suction devices can be used continually to evacuate smoke, blood, or irrigation solutions because there is no pneumoperitoneum.
- The surgeon's tactile sensation is restored because organs can be manipulated manually to look for abdominal pathology.
- There is less pressure on the blood vessels and other organs posteriorly.
- Patients experience less temperature loss that occurs during longer procedures as a result of the constant flow of the cool insufflation gas.
- There is no pneumoperitoneal pressure to be continually monitored.
- There is less referred shoulder pain postoperatively, which is caused by CO_2 insufflation.
- There is no backspray of tissue debris and fluids, caused by the pressurization, when the cannula ports are released.

Accessory Instruments

The many accessory instruments now available have been designed for the purpose of enhancing the use of basic endoscopic instrumentation.

Probes

Probes are used to manipulate tissue. They should be blunt to avoid causing trauma to tissue and organs. Some probes are marked with centimeter gradations so that structures can be measured. Because many endoscopic lenses magnify, this ability to measure allows for more accurate estimation of the structure size.

Irrigation/aspirator probes

Irrigation/aspirator probes serve the dual function of irrigating and suctioning to enhance visualization of the internal structures (Fig. 7-117). (Irrigation/aspiration systems are discussed in more detail in Chapter 9.)

Electrosurgical probes

Many different kinds of electrosurgical probes are now available that can conduct electrical current to the tissue during endoscopy (Figs. 7-118 and 7-119). The nurse must thoroughly inspect such instruments before use to make sure that the insulation is intact. (Electrosurgery is discussed in greater detail in Chapter 11.) Needle electrodes have been developed for precision cutting (Figs. 7-120 and 7-121). Some disposable laparoscopic needle electrodes have a retractable sheath that can be locked into place for needle protection during insertion. When the sheath is extended and the needle retracted, the instrument can also be used as a blunt dissector. When the needle is extended, it can be used for precision cutting and coagulation.

Endoscopic surgical needles

Endoscopic surgical needles have been developed that infuse solutions or medications during endoscopy. These needles can also be used to withdraw fluids from tissue and organs for pathologic examination. They come in different lengths.

Endoscopic specimen bags

Endoscopic specimen bags can be used to contain a specimen (Fig. 7-122). By securing the specimen within the bag, removal is facilitated and cross-contamination is minimized. For example, an infected appendix can be placed in the specimen bag to prevent spillage of the contents into the abdomen. One specimen removal device on the market has a flexible braided container that can be expanded to collect the specimen and then collapsed for removal of the specimen through the cannula. The container can also be replaced during the procedure (Fig. 7-123).

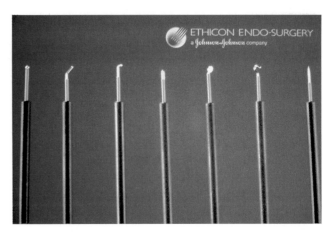

Fig. 7-118 Endoscopic electrosurgical probes and tips. (Courtesy Ethicon Endo-Surgery Inc., Cincinnati, Ohio.)

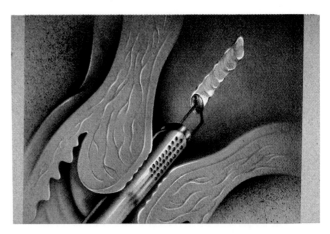

Fig. 7-119 Ablation of the endometrial lining performed using an electrosurgical rollerball probe. (Courtesy Circon Corp., Santa Barbara, Calif.)

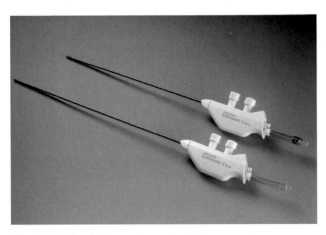

Fig. 7-117 Endoscopic suction irrigators. (Courtesy United States Surgical Corp., Norwalk, Conn.)

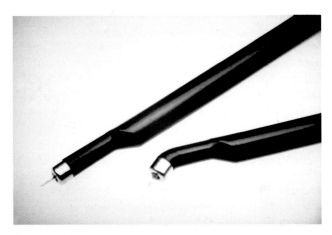

Fig. 7-120 Endoscopic needle electrodes. (Courtesy Erbe USA, Inc., Marietta, Ga.)

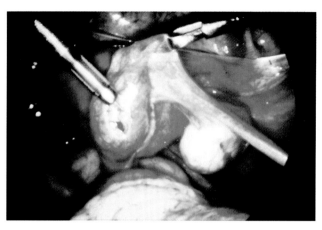

Fig. 7-121 A needle electrode. This device can cut precisely with minimal thermal damage. (Courtesy Erbe USA, Inc., Marietta, Ga.)

Percutaneous cholangiography catheters

Cholangiography is often performed during a laparoscopic cholecystectomy to detect stones in the common bile duct or the cystic duct. To do this, first an introducer sheath is inserted into the abdomen under laparoscopic visualization to function as a percutaneous access port for a catheter. The introducer usually has a 13- or 14-gauge diameter with an internal seal to prevent loss of the pneumoperitoneum. The semirigid catheter is then inserted through the introducer and positioned for transcystic duct cholangiography or transcholecystic cholangiography. After the catheter is in place, a small balloon or atraumatic retention cone is inflated, thereby eliminating the need to suture or clip the catheter in place (Figs. 7-124 and 7-125). Cholangiography is then performed. After this the balloon or cone is deflated and withdrawn and the wound dressed appropriately.

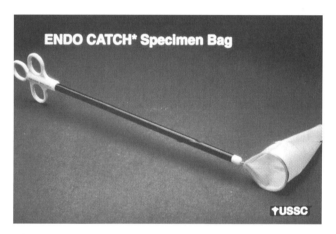

Fig. 7-122 Endoscopic specimen bag instrument. (Courtesy United States Surgical Corp., Norwalk, Conn.)

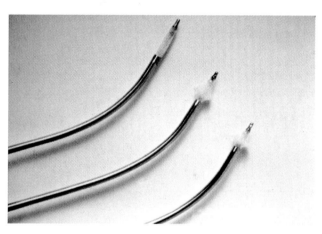

Fig. 7-124 Percutaneous cholangiography catheter with retention cone. (Courtesy Origin Medsystems, Inc., Menlo Park, Calif.)

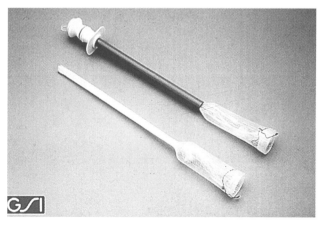

Fig. 7-123 The container of this specimen removal device can be changed during the procedure. (Courtesy General Surgical Innovations, Inc., Palo Alto, Calif.)

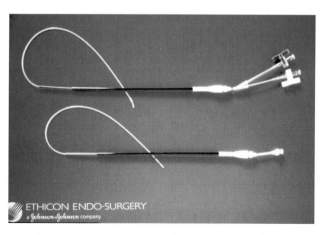

Fig. 7-125 Percutaneous cholangiography catheter with balloon. (Courtesy Ethicon Endo-Surgery Inc., Cincinnati, Ohio.)

INSTRUMENT COUNTS

The counting of instruments for endoscopic procedures has become a very controversial topic for perioperative nurses. Because endoscopy is minimally invasive, many professionals maintain that counting instruments is not necessary, but perioperative nurses are now reexamining this issue. Some nurses contend that making sure each instrument is intact is more important than counting them. Part of this concern stems from the malpractice case involving a $1.6 million award to a patient who underwent laparoscopic tubal ligation and had the sheath of a Veress needle left in her. The sheath was located and removed from the patient one year later (*Laparosc Surg Update*, 1994).

The Association of Operating Room Nurses (AORN) recommends that "an initial instrument count should be taken on all surgical procedures" and that "subsequent instrument counts should be taken before closure of a cavity or incision that might contain an instrument" (AORN, 1995). Some nurses interpret this to mean that endoscopic instruments should be counted before the procedure and then after the procedure only if the incision might contain an instrument. Of course, if the endoscopic approach is converted to an open procedure, all instruments must then be accounted for. The reason for the preoperative count of laparoscopic instruments is that, during conversion to an open procedure, someone could grab an instrument from the endoscopy setup that could get lost in the incision.

The AORN suggests that hospitals develop their own policies regarding instrument counts for endoscopic procedures. The AORN also recommends that "standardization of instrument sets with the minimum types and numbers of instruments in the set should be established" (AORN, 1995). If instrument counts are required, standardization helps to facilitate this and keep track of the instruments used (Fig. 7-126). The use of prepackaged instrument sets also helps to simplify this procedure.

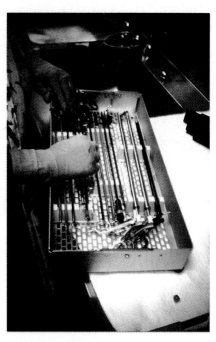

Fig. 7-126   Standardized endoscopic instrument sets. The use of such sets helps the surgical team members keep track of instruments and facilitates instrument counts.

REFERENCES

Association of Operating Room Nurses: *Standards and recommended practices*, Denver, 1995, AORN, p 263.

Ethicon: *Endoscopic suturing and knot tying manual*, Cincinnati, 1991, Ethicon Inc.

Laparosc Surg Update: Should you count instruments after laparoscopic surgery? 2(7):73, 1994.

Laparosc Surg Update: Tips for detecting, avoiding adhesions from prior laparotomy, 3(2):22, 1995a.

Laparosc Surg Update: Avoiding injury without trocar safety shields, 3(3):31, 1995b.

White RA, Klein SR: *Endoscopic surgery*, St. Louis, 1991, Mosby, p 17.

8

Care and Maintenance of Instruments

CARE OF ENDOSCOPIC INSTRUMENTATION

Staff Education

Importance of training

The most critical element in the reprocessing of reusable endoscopic instrumentation and devices is well-trained staff members. Education is the means by which they achieve an appropriate skill level to ensure the proper and safe reprocessing of endoscopic instruments and devices. When reprocessing is delegated to qualified and trained personnel many advantages can be noted, including the following:

- Effective use of resources is fostered
- Cost-efficiency is promoted
- Cross-contamination of pathogens is minimized
- The need for instrument repairs is reduced
- A more consistent outcome from the endoscopic procedures is provided
  Training programs should include information on:
- Instrument design and function
- Cleaning methods and techniques
- Cleaning supplies and equipment
- Disinfection and sterilization methods
- Quality control monitoring
- Protection measures (e.g., proper attire and use of gloves)
- Hazards identification

After workers attend a training program, their competency in the reprocessing of surgical instruments must be verified and documented. Return demonstrations are valuable to document workers' skill level, competency, and ability to perform particular tasks. A com-

petency checklist can be designed to facilitate this process. After workers have achieved competency, then their performance should be checked periodically to make sure they are adhering to standards and facility policies.

Collaborative relationships are essential to provide open communication between the surgical team and the staff members who are responsible for reprocessing endoscopic instruments. The most important goal for all involved is to provide a standardized protocol for infection prevention that has been proved effective and that can be consistently performed over and over again.

In today's health care environment, many infections may go undetected, especially postoperative infections caused by contaminated instruments or faulty technique. This may be due to a variety of different reasons.

- Inadequate surveillance methods.
- Patients who are infected may be asymptomatic.
- Prolonged incubation periods of the infection, such that the infection is not traced back to the actual cause.
- The discouragement of appropriate reporting because of the medicolegal ramifications stemming from publicizing infection incidences.

Pathogen transmission

The staff must thoroughly understand the risks and hazards involved in the reprocessing of endoscopic instruments and devices from the standpoint of the transmission of infection to patients. An additional concern, however, is the transmission of infection to health care workers who come in contact with contaminated or inadequately processed equipment or with infected patients. Decreasing the risk of transmitting bloodborne pathogens, such as human immunodeficiency virus (HIV) and hepatitis B, must become a central concern as protocols for reprocessing are developed.

The incidence of HIV infection continues to grow in the United States, and the infection has now been declared a major health priority throughout the world. The number of persons in the United States who are infected with HIV has been estimated to be well over one million (American Nurses Association, 1992), meaning that now approximately one out of every 250 to 260 people in the United States is HIV positive.

Prevalence studies from 1995 have shown that one out of every 92 American men aged 27 to 39 years is HIV positive. Of the African-American men in this age group, one out of every 33 is HIV positive; of the Hispanic men in this age group, one out of every 60 is HIV positive. Of American women aged 27 to 38 years, one out of every 1667 is HIV positive. Of African-American and Hispanic women, one out of every 98 and 222, respectively, is HIV positive. This ranks HIV infection as the number one killer of people 25 to 44 years of age. In addition, it is predicted that 80 million people worldwide will be infected with HIV by the year 2000, with 13,000 people becoming infected each day (*Columbus Dispatch*, 1995).

Health care statistics from December 1994 have revealed that 42 health care workers have contracted HIV infection as the result of workplace exposure, and approximately 91 more are infected as the result of possible job-related exposure. Of the confirmed workplace exposures, 38 occurred through blood transmission, 37 as the result of percutaneous needle sticks with hollow-bore needles and one as the result of a contaminated scalpel (Bell, 1995). Often, however, health care staff do not even know if a patient is HIV positive, which not only makes the tracking of the source of infection difficult but also makes them more vulnerable to contracting infection because they may not then exercise the proper safety controls. The breakdown of confirmed exposures by health care professional is as follows:

15 phlebotomists
13 nurses
6 physicians
1 respiratory therapist
2 surgical technologists (one got stuck with a biopsy needle)
5 others

It has been postulated that exposure to HIV-infected blood could occur during the release of the pneumoperitoneum during laparoscopy procedures. A closed-suction system can be employed to eliminate this hazard.

There are a few reports of patients being infected with HIV from dirty instruments or contaminated needles. Proper reprocessing is therefore critical to prevent

Box 8-1	*Recent History of Tuberculosis*

1974—decline of TB
1980—Stopped tracking; no federal money available to do so
1986—begin to see increase in incidence
1990—20,000 new cases
1992—52,000 cases
1993 and 1994—slight decrease in incidence

such transmission. One study showed that HIV could survive in the lubricant of endoscopes not adequately removed during cleaning (*Laparosc Surg Update*, 1995a).

Another pathogen of concern to health care workers from the standpoint of transmission to both them and patients is the hepatitis B virus. Approximately 12,000 to 18,000 health care workers in the United States per year contract hepatitis B through workplace exposure. About 250 of these people die each year as the result of the disease's long-term consequences (Margolis, 1995). One study showed that the prevalence of hepatitis markers in health care workers was directly related to the incidence of their exposure to blood (*Laparosc Focus*, 1993). Therefore, because exposure to blood, tissue, and blood fluids is increased in the members of surgical teams, the incidence of transmission is greater in them. Approximately 1% or more hospitalized patients are carriers of hepatitis B, but often their medical charts do not show this. (*Laparosc Focus*, 1993).

Tuberculosis (TB) is another pathogen of concern to health care workers, especially now with the increased incidence of the disease. The history of this disease is chronicled in Box 8-1. The infective pathogen, *Mycobacterium tuberculosis*, is transmitted by means of airborne droplets of oral secretions from infected patients. It can also be transmitted by body secretions or surgical instruments. Health care workers must therefore be extremely careful when reprocessing instruments and devices used on patients with TB.

With the advent of multi–drug-resistant strains of TB (MDRTB), the disease is now even more deadly and difficult to contain. The incidence of this form of TB is higher in people infected with HIV. Seventeen health care workers in the United States are known to have contracted MDRTB. Six have died, and they were also all HIV positive (Jarvis, 1995).

Delayed diagnosis, delayed treatment, and delayed laboratory investigations have all been contributors to the increase in the incidence of MDRTB. The mortality rate in patients with the disease ranges from 72% to 89%, with the interval from diagnosis to death ranging from 4 to 16 weeks (Jarvis, 1995).

Because of the threat posed to health care workers, surgical suite policies and procedures need to be written to provide guidance in the treatment of patients with

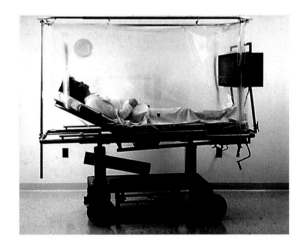

Fig. 8-1   An enclosed cart, designed to control the spread of TB pathogens during transportation of an infected patient.

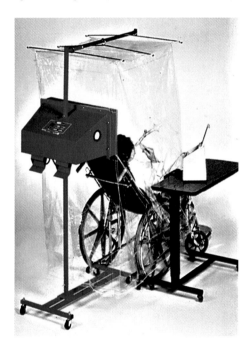

Fig. 8-2   An enclosed wheelchair, used to transport a patient infected with TB.

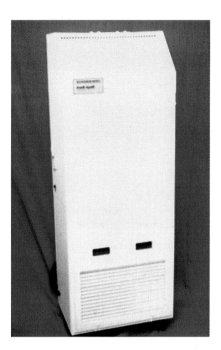

Fig. 8-3   A filtration system, which can be placed in a small room to provide adequate air filtration. (Courtesy of Stackhouse Inc., Palm Springs, Calif.)

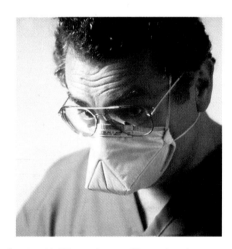

Fig. 8-4   An N-95 respirator filters 1 micron particulate matter at 95% efficiency; worn to protect the health care worker from inhaling air contaminated with TB. (Courtesy Racal Medical, Frederick, Md.)

TB. Some of the key principles that should be followed to minimize the transmission of TB are to:

- Avoid performing elective surgical procedures in patients with active TB. Bronchoscopies in patients with TB should not be performed in the operating room.
- Use new source control devices, such as enclosed carts (Fig. 8-1) and wheelchairs (Fig. 8-2), that have been developed to transport infected patients.
- Construct negative-pressure surgical rooms to decrease the spread of the TB pathogens into other surgical areas.
- Ensure that there are at least 6 to 12 room air exchanges per hour using a high-efficiency particulate air (HEPA) filtration system.

- Air filtration systems for smaller rooms and areas have also been developed (Fig. 8-3).
- Provide isolation postoperative recovery areas for infected patients to prevent transmission of the disease to other patients and health care workers.
- Wear high-filtration masks or respirators that meet OSHA (Occupational Safety and Health Administration) regulations, fit-tested to each health care worker (Fig. 8-4).
- Employ airborne pathogen control measures at all times.

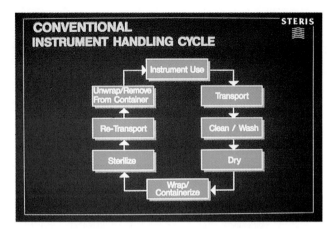

Fig. 8-5 Staff members come in contact with instruments and devices often during the reprocessing cycle. (Courtesy STERIS Corp., Mentor, Ohio.)

- Perform surgery on a patient with active TB at the end of the day's surgical schedule in a room that is not in a high-traffic area. The operating room doors must remain closed as much as possible while the patient is in the room.
- Test and screen the surgical team members for TB at least once a year (ideally every 6 months).

Cleaning

Proper cleaning of endoscopic instruments is vital before disinfection or sterilization is attempted. Cleaning can be accomplished without disinfection or sterilization, but disinfection or sterilization is usually not possible without cleaning. The staff must be taught the proper way to reprocess instruments and other items. Because staff members come in contact with these surgical devices frequently throughout the reprocessing cycle, they must completely understand their roles and responsibilities in the process (Fig. 8-5). Sometimes the technologists responsible for reprocessing should visit the surgical suite to see how the instruments are used and, as a result, note why it is so important to check the integrity of the instrument before it is used again on a patient.

The staff must use universal precautions when dealing with items exposed to bloodborne pathogens (Fig. 8-6). By federal law gloves, gowns, masks, and eye protection must be available. Often shortcuts are taken and reprocessing is hurried when time is limited. For examples, proper protective attire is not always worn (Fig. 8-7). Staff members must completely understand the risks and consequences of not following mandates and hospital protocols.

Reusable instruments must be capable of being disassembled, irrigated, and cleaned. Manufacturers should provide explicit directions for doing this. Instruments must be totally disassembled before cleaning, in-

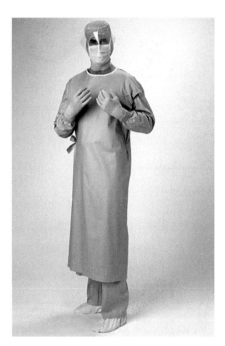

Fig. 8-6 Personal protective attire must be available for staff members to wear while cleaning reusable instruments. (Courtesy Johnson & Johnson Medical Inc., Arlington, Tex.)

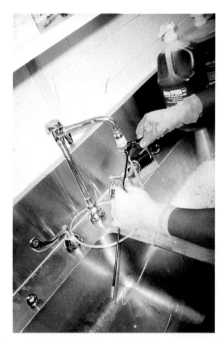

Fig. 8-7 Sometimes staff members try to take shortcuts and do not wear gowns while cleaning contaminated instruments.

cluding the removal of gaskets and other parts (Fig. 8-8). In addition, there must be an adequate supply of instruments so that there is enough time to reprocess them adequately before reuse. Often staff members become rushed because the time between procedures is

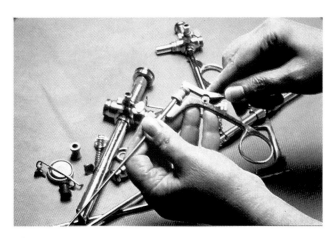

Fig. 8-8 A reusable instrument is disassembled before cleaning.

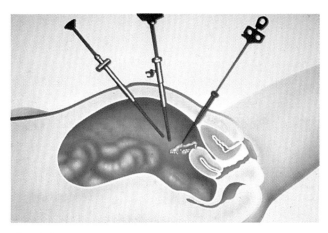

Fig. 8-9 During laparoscopy, instruments are used in a pressurized area, allowing debris to be forced up and into the instruments.

limited and the same instruments must be reprocessed for reuse. Rushing the cleaning process can result in inadequate reprocessing.

There are unique environmental conditions that apply to some endoscopic procedures and that can lead to instrument contamination. For example, during laparoscopy, instruments are used in a pressurized area within the abdomen (Fig. 8-9). This pressurization forces debris and liquid contaminants up into the endoscope and instrument channels, which can solidify during or after the procedure. It is difficult to reverse this process and remove all of the solidified bioburden, so proper techniques must be employed during the endoscopic procedure to keep instrument lumens clean and free from debris.

Instruments should be kept wet and flushed with solutions to prevent bioburden solidification. However, often the handles and not the working parts of endoscopic instruments are submerged in water when the instruments are delivered to the area where cleaning

occurs (Fig. 8-10). This is the opposite of what should be done. The working parts in which debris can collect should be kept moist so solidification does not occur. Soiled instruments also can be placed in a towel saturated with sterile water until they can be cleaned after the case is completed. Contaminated instruments should not be soaked in water for prolonged periods, however, because air bubbles that form on the instruments during soaking in standing liquids can stain the instruments.

Manufacturers' recommendations must be followed closely to ensure thorough cleaning without damaging the instrument. Research has shown that 99% of the bioburden is removed when appropriate cleaning is achieved (Hanson et al, 1990). Appropriate cleaning involves numerous different steps and considerations that should be written into a formal policy. Following are the steps involved in a sample cleaning procedure.

- Completely disassemble the instrument.
- Use an enzymatic cleaner that breaks apart protein bonds and loosens contaminants for thorough cleaning (Fig. 8-11). A detergent with a neutral pH of 7.0 that is low sudsing and produces minimal residue is recommended. A detergent with a higher or lower pH can cause staining and pitting of the instrument. Avoid using abrasives, such as steel wool, that could disrupt the surface of the instrument.
- Never expose instruments to alcohol after use because alcohol binds protein, making cleaning more difficult (*Laparosc Surg Update* 1995b).
- Use appropriate cleaning tools, such as soft-bristle brushes, to adequately clean ports, lumens, serrations, fulcrums, box locks, and crevices (Fig. 8-12). The size of brush must be appropriate for the diameter of the lumen to be cleaned (Fig. 8-13).
- When using brushes, minimize aerosolization to prevent the spread of airborne contaminants (Fig. 8-14).

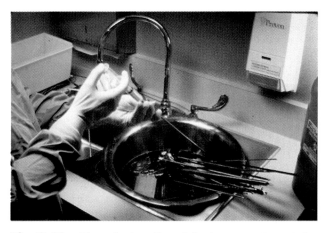

Fig. 8-10 Often the handles of the instruments, not the working ends, are immersed in the solution, allowing debris on the working end to become more solidified and thus more difficult to remove.

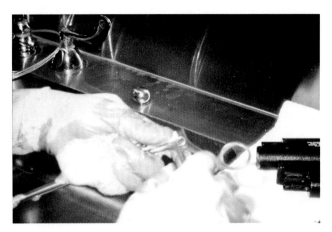

Fig. 8-11 An enzymatic cleaner that breaks apart protein bonds and loosens contaminants should be used for cleaning instrumentation.

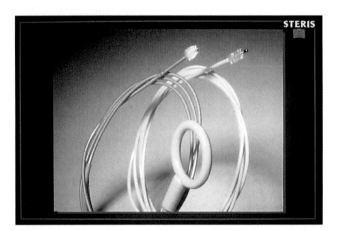

Fig. 8-12 **Cleaning brushes.** (Courtesy STERIS Corp., Mentor, Ohio.)

- Use cleaning devices if available, with port and lumen flusher systems to assist in completely cleaning the device (Figs. 8-15 to 8-17.)
- Use suction devices to help flush the instrument lumen or lumens.
- Use ultrasonic cleaners when appropriate (Fig. 8-18). These cleaners produce sonic waves that form very small bubbles of gas in the cleansing bath. The bubbles expand until they become unstable and implode, thereby disloging debris from the surfaces of the instrument, which is then dissolved in the cleaning solution. Light cables and flexible endoscopes should not be routinely cleaned in an ultrasonic device, however, because the vibration may damage the tiny fiberoptic bundles. There now are special low-vibration cleaners that have been developed to process light cables and flexible endoscopes. When using ultrasonic processing, the gross debris must be rinsed off the instrument first. Any flushing ports should be connected to the ultrasonic machine. The

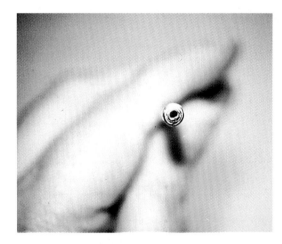

Fig. 8-13 Small brushes should be used to clean instruments with small ports or lumens to ensure adequate cleaning.

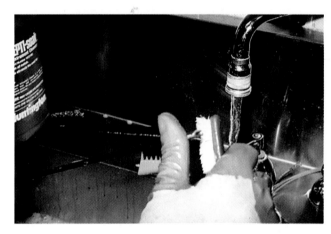

Fig. 8-14 Aerosolization should be minimized during cleaning.

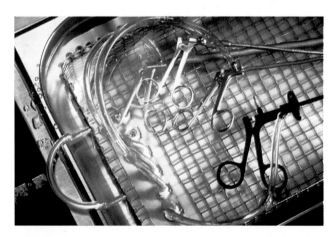

Fig. 8-15 Cleaning systems with automatic port and lumen flusher systems. These systems can help ensure adequate cleaning and rinsing.

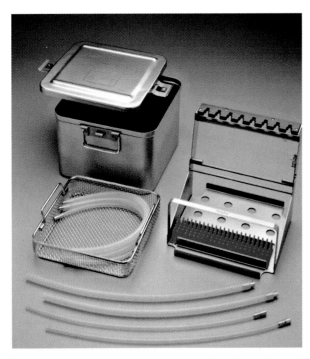

Fig. 8-16 Parts of an automatic cleaning device for endoscopic instruments. (Courtesy Aesculap, Inc., South San Francisco, Calif.)

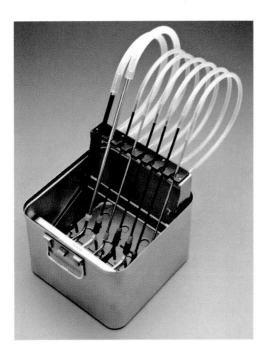

Fig. 8-17 An automatic cleaning device. This device can be used to thoroughly flush the inside lumens and ports. (Courtesy Aesculap, Inc., South San Francisco, Calif.)

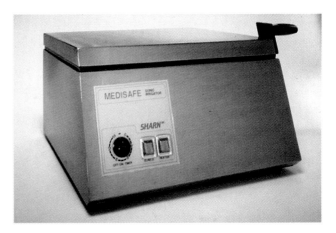

Fig. 8-18 Ultrasonic cleaner. (Courtesy Sharn, Inc., Tampa, Fla.)

vibratory action of the system dislodges debris from the hinges, jaws, and crevices of the instruments. A weakened disinfectant solution is used in some of the ultrasonic machines, but it only cleans and does not disinfect. Ultrasonic cleaners may increase the life expectancy of the instrument because they are more gentle than manual cleaning, which can damage the devices.

- Thoroughly rinse the instrument, especially the internal lumens. Distilled, deionized water should be used because the chemicals and minerals present in most tap water can damage the instrument. If distilled water is unavailable, tap water put through a good water filter can be used.
- Dry the instrument with a soft, lint-free cloth. A blow dryer or a pneumatic air gun can be used to dry internal lumens and the surfaces of delicate instruments. Instruments should not be allowed to drip dry because this can cause spots to develop or minerals to build up on the surface. Lubricants adhere better to dry instruments.
- Reassemble the instrument according to the manufacturer's instructions. (Most instruments should not be reassembled until the disinfection or sterilization process is completed, however.) Lubricate the instrument as recommended. Often instruments are dipped (not soaked) in an antimicrobial, water-soluble instrument lubricant that forms a thin, protective film on the surfaces. This lubricant allows the penetration of steam and gas for sterilization, plus blood and debris cannot coat the surfaces of the instrument as easily.
- Inspect the instruments (Fig. 8-19). Some hospitals periodically involve the manufacturer's sales representatives in the inspection of the instruments to make sure that they are functioning properly. If damage is detected early, expensive repairs or replacement may be avoided. Corrosion on an instrument is caused from the gradual wearing away of a surface as the instrument metal reacts with the chemicals

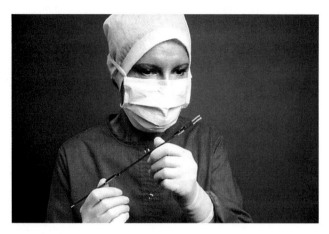

Fig. 8-19 Skilled personnel must inspect instruments and devices during reprocessing. (Courtesy Karl Storz Culver City, Calif.)

and minerals introduced through use and reprocessing. Corrosion may first be noticed on lock boxes or fulcrums, and this form of corrosion usually results from inadequate cleaning. If the corrosion cannot be controlled, then the instrument needs to be repaired by an authorized service company. Pitting occurs if the corrosion becomes extensive.

- Periodically demagnetize stainless steel instruments. Many instruments are made of martensitic steel that can become magnetized during processing and handling. Instruments can also become magnetized as they are touched to magnetic sheets or needle counter boards. This becomes a problem with needle holders or tissue forceps because the needles are then more difficult to manipulate endoscopically. To reduce this problem, a nonmetal cleaning brush and an instrument demagnetizer should be used. Titanium instruments cannot be magnetized because they are made of a nonferrous alloy (Scanlan International, 1995).

If instrument marking is desired for identification or sorting purposes, mechanical engraving should not be done because this will disrupt the rust-resistant chromium oxide skin of the instrument. If an instrument must be permanently marked, then electrochemical or laser etching, done by an experienced service technician, should be performed (Scanlan International, 1995). Instrument banding can also be done using special tape that is steam autoclavable and gas sterilizable. Color-coded instrument tips are available to protect the delicate working ends of endoscopic instruments (Fig. 8-20).

The Association of Operating Room Nurses (AORN) has developed recommended practices to guide the health care worker in the reprocessing of instruments and scopes (AORN, 1995). These practices include the following:

- An instrument should be used only for the specific purpose for which it was designed.
- Instruments should be kept free of gross soil during the surgical procedure.

- Instruments should be decontaminated immediately after completion of the surgical procedure.
- Instruments should be processed in an ultrasonic cleaner after manual or automatic decontamination.
- After every cleaning, instruments with movable parts should be lubricated according to manufacturers' written instructions.
- Instruments should be inspected after cleaning and prepared for storage or sterilization.
- Flexible or rigid endoscopes should be inspected, tested, and processed according to design and type and manufacturer's written instruction.

The use of unclean instruments can easily cause patients to acquire postoperative infections, which can then lead to further complications that could compromise their health. Postoperative infections can also be very expensive. A typical hospital-acquired infection costs the hospital about $14,000 to treat (*Laparosc Surg Update*, 1995a).

A study was conducted in Canada to evaluate the effectiveness of the cleaning process during instrument reprocessing. Three types of instruments (conventional surgical instruments, reusable laparoscopic instruments, and reused disposable laparoscopic instruments) were cleaned using the same process. The 32 instruments studied were visually inspected after cleaning, and all instruments appeared to be clean. However, microscopic examination revealed that there was residual debris on 84% of the instruments, with the most debris on the laparoscopic instruments. These results were startling, because the investigators assumed the cleaning process used was adequate. Further examination of the cleaning process is needed to determine where the inadequacies exist (DesCoteaux et al, 1995).

Another study was conducted to examine the cleanability of hybrid endoscopic instrumentation. The instruments involved were part reusable and part disposable. A consistent cleaning procedure was followed

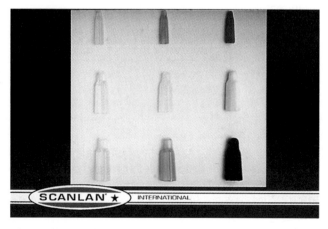

Fig. 8-20 Tip covers are available to protect the working ends of endoscopic instruments. (Courtesy Scanlan International, St. Paul, Minn.)

throughout the study. Visual and microscopic inspection revealed there was no residual debris, showing that all instruments can be adequately cleaned (Marlow and Petruschke, 1995).

Manufacturers must develop a standardized method for validating the efficacy of the cleaning process. Currently different methods are being proposed, but until one method has proved to be successful, the effectiveness of the cleaning process cannot be documented and verified.

Disinfection

The next step in reprocessing is to either disinfect or sterilize the device. The Spaulding classification system has been used to determine the type of reprocessing required for various surgical and medical items. In this system, the degree to which a device is used for purposes that breach the body's immune system determines whether it should be disinfected or sterilized (Rutala, 1990). Following are the classes determined on this basis:

- Critical items—normally used to enter sterile tissue or the vascular system; requires sterilization. An example is a laparoscope.
- Semicritical items—come in contact with mucous membranes or skin that is not intact; requires high-level disinfection. An example is a gastroscope.
- Noncritical items—come in contact with intact skin; requires low-level disinfection. An example is a bedpan.

Disinfection destroys most forms of microorganisms on inanimate objects. High-level disinfection destroys all microorganisms, with the exception of some bacterial spores; therefore, it has been used extensively for devices that come in contact only with mucous membranes. High-level disinfection has also been used to reprocess laparoscopes and laparoscopy instruments, but with the advent of quicker and more effective sterilization processes, sterilization is becoming preferred and recommended for the reprocessing of such equipment.

The effectiveness of a disinfectant is influenced by the following (Rutala, 1996):

- The cleaning of the object
- The organic load present
- The type and number of contaminating microorganisms
- The concentration of the disinfectant
- The exposure time to the disinfectant
- The temperature and pH of the disinfectant
- The type of object to be disinfected

Chemical solutions, such as glutaraldehydes, may be used as disinfectants (Fig. 8-21). Glutaraldehyde can be flushed down the drain with water, unless this is restricted by state or local water and sewer authorities. The sewage microorganisms bioxidize the disinfecting solution, reducing it to glutaric acid and then changing

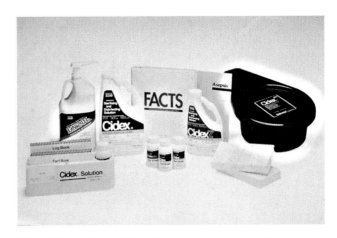

Fig. 8-21 Glutaraldehyde solutions and soaking basin. (Courtesy Johnson & Johnson Medical, Inc., Arlington, Tex.)

it to carbon dioxide and water. Glutaraldehydes achieve effective disinfection, but many concerns about them have been voiced.

Recently the U.S. Food and Drug Administration (FDA) took over the regulation of disinfectants from the Environmental Protection Agency. After assuming this responsibility the FDA demanded more proof of the efficacy of the agents than what the manufacturers had provided in the past. The FDA focused on a study that showed a 45-minute soak time killed 100% of TB pathogens on uncleaned endoscopes. Because of this finding they changed the soaking requirements for achieving high-level disinfection to 45 minutes at 25°C from the previous requirement of 20 minutes at room temperature (Laparosc Surg Update, 1995c).

This has created a dilemma for hospitals because surgical administrators state that they cannot allow 45 minutes for the soaking of devices between procedures. The turnover time must be less than this for the endoscopic surgery schedule to be met. They realize, though, that they must follow the manufacturer's written instructions regarding the reprocessing of the product or have to assume all liability if a lawsuit is filed because a patient suffers a postoperative infection alleged to result from the inadequate reprocessing of instruments. This dilemma places hospitals in a very precarious position.

Some opponents of the new requirement are eager to note that the study the FDA based their decision on involved endoscopes that were not cleaned before immersion in the glutaraldehyde solution. In actual surgical facilities, however, practice guidelines state that a device must be cleaned thoroughly before being disinfected. One study showed that thoroughly cleaned endoscopes soaked in 2% glutaraldehyde for 10 to 20 minutes were safe for reuse in patients (Gerding, 1982).

Researchers and others challenging the FDA requirement state that, if the device is cleaned appropriately, a 20-minutes soak time is sufficient. They also note that no study has shown that the incidence of infection is increased in patients operated on with instruments reprocessed using the 20-minute soaking protocol (*Laparosc Surg Update*, 1995d). Recommendations have been made to the FDA to provide a dual labeling system for the use of glutaraldehydes. One requirement would apply to devices that have not been cleaned; the other would apply to devices that have been thoroughly cleaned (Rutala, 1996).

In another study, endoscopes contaminated with HIV were thoroughly cleaned, which was found to remove 99.9% of the bioburden, and then placed in a glutaraldehyde soak for only 2 minutes. It was found that the endoscopes were completely free of HIV at the end of the processing (Hanson et al, 1990).

Infections documented to stem from endoscopic procedures are known to be caused by breaks in the reprocessing protocols, such as inadequate cleaning, inappropriate use of a disinfecting solution, or inadequate storage of the endoscope.

The value of the new FDA requirement regarding disinfection continues to be debated in the United States. Aside from the fact that the longer soak time is less convenient, it is also more damaging to instruments, plus the warmer solution temperature causes the release of more caustic fumes into the air. Devices are available that can safely heat the glutaraldehyde to 25°C (Fig. 8-22). In the past, health care workers have even used aquarium heaters to safely warm the solution to this temperature.

The maximum recommended exposure level of glutaraldehyde determined by OSHA is a 0.2 parts per million (ppm) (OSHA, 1988, 1989). However, when the solution is being poured or devices are being submerged in it, the level rises to approximately 0.4 ppm, or twice the recommended exposure level (Fig. 8-23). The odor becomes an irritant at only 0.03 ppm, causing tearing, nausea, and other effects. Systems have been

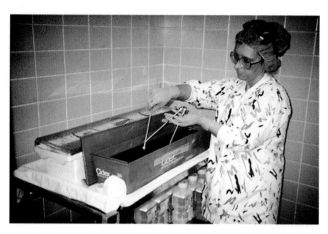

Fig. 8-23 When submerging an instrument into a glutaraldehyde bath, the fumes from the solution increase to 0.4 ppm, or twice the recommended exposure level.

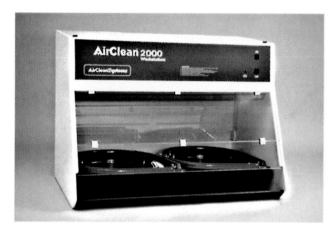

Fig. 8-24 A covered hood system, which can be used to minimize the glutaraldehyde fumes and odor. (Courtesy API Airclean Systems, Raleigh, N.C.)

designed and are now available that can absorb the odor and fumes of the glutaraldehyde solution (Fig. 8-24).

The following guidelines can be used by health care personnel using glutaraldehyde solutions to disinfect instruments and endoscopes:

- The staff members responsible for reprocessing devices must first of all understand the process and the hazards related to use of glutaraldehydes.
- Thorough cleaning before immersion in a disinfecting solution removes the organic debris and pathogenic microorganisms. Research has shown that HIV may survive in lubricants within endoscopes that are reprocessed with a glutaraldehyde solution (*Laparosc Surg Update*, 1995g). Adequate cleaning is therefore critical to remove the bioburden and may also reduce the soaking time necessary to achieve high-level disinfection and eradicate all microbial pathogens, including HIV, hepatitis B virus, and *M. tuberculosis*.

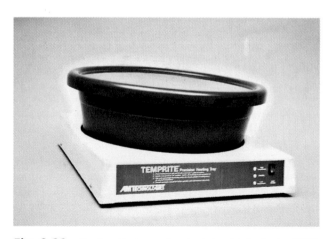

Fig. 8-22 Device that can heat glutaraldehyde to 25°C. (Courtesy API Airclean Systems, Raleigh, N.C.)

- Glutaraldehyde fumes must be kept to a minimum. Devices should be gently immersed in and removed from the glutaraldehyde bath so that the solution is not agitated, thus giving off caustic fumes. OSHA does not require the monitoring of glutaraldehyde fumes but a facility may be fined for high concentrations in the air.
- Glutaradelhyde soaking bins should be located in a central area that is well ventilated (Fig. 8-25). Covers must be used to prevent fumes from escaping.
- Contact lenses can absorb glutaraldehyde fumes, so workers wearing contact lenses should not repeatedly expose themselves to these fumes while wearing them.
- The glutaraldehyde soak pan should adequately accommodate the instrument.
- The placement of wet instruments into a glutaraldehyde bath will cause the soaking solution to become diluted. Instruments should therefore be dry before they are immersed in the solution. Test strips are now available that can detect a glutaraldehyde concentration of 1.5% or less. Any solution with a concentration less than that is too diluted to be effective for disinfection (Rutala, 1996).
- A clock must be available where manual chemical disinfecting is being done so that immersion can be properly timed.
- The glutaraldehyde must be thoroughly rinsed off the device after the soak cycle is complete. In an anecdotal experience, it was noted that some patients who underwent sigmoidoscopy suffered bloody diarrhea afterward. Further investigation revealed that poor rinsing techniques on the part of an inexperienced technician allowed residual glutaraldehyde to become trapped in the endsocope lumens. Glutaraldehyde was then introduced into successive patients, leading to this postoperative complication.

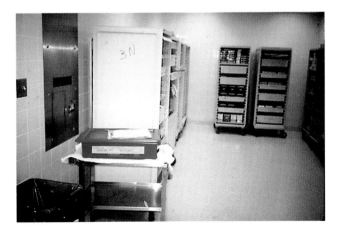

Fig. 8-25 To prevent exposure, the glutaraldehyde solution should be located in a well-ventiliated, centralized area, not on a cart that is wheeled around the surgery suite.

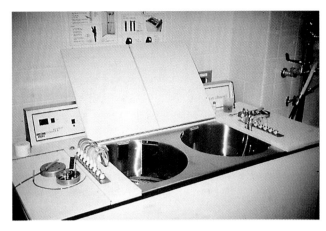

Fig. 8-26 An automatic endoscope washer, which can also disinfect with a glutaraldehyde solution.

- An emergency eye wash station should be readily available so that if glutaraldehyde solution is splashed into a worker's eye, it can be washed out.
- Automatic glutaraldehyde processors are available for some endoscopes (usually flexible) and instruments. Such processors clean the devices and then disinfect them with a glutaraldehyde soak (Fig. 8-26).

Personnel should not wear regular latex surgical or treatment gloves when working with glutaraldehyde because the gloves can start to deteriorate (*Laparosc Surg Update*, 1995e). Such gloves feel sticky with extended contact. Because the breakdown of the latex in gloves can cause the health care worker to be exposed to glutaraldehyde, OSHA has issued citations to people found using latex gloves to work with this disinfecting solution for extended periods of time.

There has been debate over the time it takes for glove materials to deteriorate. Union Carbide tested surgical gloves made of several types of material and found the following (*Laparosc Surg Update*, 1995e).

Latex glove: Glutaraldehyde permeated within 1 hour.

Polyethylene glove: Glutaraldehyde permeated in 4 to 6 hours.

Synthetic surgical glove: Glutaraldehyde permeated in 6 to 8 hours.

Nitrile rubber or butyl rubber gloves: Glutaraldehyde did not permeate during the 8-hour duration test.

Double-gloved latex gloves: Glutaraldehyde permeated in 3 to 4 hours.

Neoprene and polyvinyl chloride gloves: Glutaraldehyde is quickly retained or absorbed by these gloves.

On the basis of these findings, suggestions were made to double glove or change gloves every 10 minutes to minimize the penetration of the glutaraldehyde solution. Because the typical exposure to glutaraldehyde during surgery is less than 10 minutes, latex gloves may be worn during such procedures and will provide adequate protection if rinsed well afterward.

Sterilization

Sterilization completely destroys live organisms and eliminates all microbial viability; this includes the inactivation of bacterial spores. Spores are the most challenging life form to kill since they represent the most resistant microbials.

Often instruments and endoscopes are sterilized at the end of the day and merely disinfected with a chemical solution between procedures. This has provoked discussion about the difference in the level of care delivered to surgical patients. The Joint Commission on the Accreditation of Healthcare Organizations (JCAHO) has stated that this situation should not be construed as the rendering of different levels of care to patients. Even though this situation is not a regulatory concern, many nurses view it as a practice concern. They are not satisfied that sterile instruments are used for the first patient in the day scheduled for surgery and disinfected instruments are used for the rest of the patients. For this reason, quick sterilization methods are rapidly evolving and instruments, endoscopes, cables, and cameras are being developed that can withstand different sterilization methods. Storage trays are also being designed to minimize instrument mishandling or damage (Fig. 8-27).

Steam sterilization

For many years autoclaves have been used to steam sterilize surgical devices (Fig. 8-28). Steam sterilization can be divided into five distinct phases (Meeker and Rothrock, 1995):
1. Loading phase—objects are packaged and placed into the sterilizer.

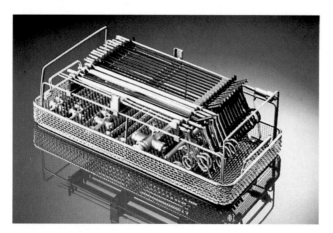

Fig. 8-27 Endoscopic instrument trays. Use of these can help minimize damage to instruments during reprocessing. (Courtesy Aesculap, Inc., South San Francisco, Calif.)

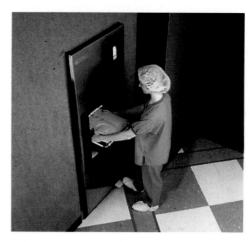

Fig. 8-28 Steam sterilizer. (Courtesy STERRIS Corp. Mentor, Ohio.)

2. Heating phase—steam is generated and surrounds the objects in the chamber.
3. Destroying phase—all live microbes are exposed and killed by the steam; this is also known as the *time-temperature cycle*.
4. Drying and cooling phase—objects are dried and cooled, then removed from the chamber for use or storage.
5. Testing phase—the efficiency of the sterilization process is monitored and validated.

In a gravity-displacement sterilizer, unwrapped metal instruments placed in a perforated tray can be sterilized in 3 minutes at 132°C (270°F) or in 15 minutes at 121°C (250°F). If unwrapped porous instruments are mixed with metal instruments in a perforated tray, they must be exposed to the steam for 10 minutes at 132°C or for 20 minutes at 121°C. Instruments wrapped in four thicknesses of muslin should be exposed to the steam for 15 minutes at 132°C or for 30 minutes at 121°C. If a prevacuum sterilizer is being used, instruments and supplies need to be exposed for 4 minutes after the temperature at the center of the pack has reached at least 132°C (Meeker and Rothrock, 1995).

The disadvantage of steam sterilization is that surgical team members and patients have sustained burns from devices that have not been allowed to adequately cool before reuse. This applies especially to trocars and cannulas because they cool much slower as the result of the bulk of metal in their design.

Surgical team members often wear double gloves when handling instruments that have come directly from the autoclave. This is one source of inadvertent instrument burns because, if double gloving is done, then they may not realize how hot the instrument is. Experiments have shown that when a surgical team member wearing double gloves touches an instrument heated to 195°F for 5 seconds, it only feels like 92°F. An instrument at 195°F touched by a double-gloved hand for 30 seconds feels like 130°F (Adoumi et al, 1994). It has therefore been suggested that surgical managers should develop protocols that require specific cooling times after instruments have been autoclaved.

The AORN and the Association for the Advancement of Medical Instrumentation (AAMI, 1992a) have developed guidelines for steam sterilization, and these should be referred to whenever policies and procedural protocols are being developed. These guidelines include recommendations on such topics as decontamination, packaging, cycle parameters, maintenance, monitoring, and record keeping. Three areas that have aroused the most concern are flash sterilization, frequency of monitoring, and shelf life (Spry, 1995).

Flash sterilization has become a very controversial method. It is now recommended that it be used only in emergencies or in special clinical situations. Institutions have even been penalized for using flash sterilization routinely. To avoid the need to use it, and because longer autoclave cycles are now recommended, many surgical suites are purchasing more instrument sets to have enough available for procedures.

The AAMI standard "Good hospital practice: Flash sterilization–steam sterilization of patient care items for immediate use" has been used as the basis for discouraging flash sterilization. It states that (AAMI, 1992b):

> Flash sterilization may be used when there is an immediate need for an individual item (e.g., a dropped instrument) and there is no alternative. . . . Implantables should never be flash sterilized. . . .
>
> In many health care facilities, flash sterilization has been used as a convenience to compensate for inadequate inventories of instruments. . . . Use of flash sterilization should be restricted to unplanned or emergency situations.

The frequency with which steam sterilizers should be monitored has been a controversial topic over the years. The AORN recommends that steam sterilizers should be monitored daily (AORN, 1995), and the AAMI suggests that monitoring should be done at least once a week, but preferably daily (AAMI, 1994).

The factors that determine the shelf life of instruments also have been the source of much debate among surgical team members. Both the AORN and AAMI contend that the shelf life of a package is event related and not time related. Surgical units using the event-related standards must develop policies that address the criteria used to determine event-related sterility. Following are some recommended ways to optimize event-related conditions, and thereby increase shelf life:

- Rotate the sterile packs and instruments.
- Ensure the storage area is:
   Well ventilated.
   Temperature and humidity controlled.
   Relatively free of traffic.
- Store sterile supplies at least 8 to 10 inches (20 to 25 cm) from floor and 18 inches (45 cm) from the ceiling.
- Not use sterile packs that have been crushed or are wet.
- Keep pack handling to a minimum (each pack should not be handled more than four times before being used on a patient).

Gas sterilization

Ethylene oxide (EO), or gas, sterilization has been used for the sterilization of surgical devices since the 1940s. EO is a colorless gas with an odor similar to that of ether, but its use is associated with an inhalation hazard similar to that of ammonia gas (Fig. 8-29).

EO is also highly explosive and very flammable in its pure state, so other gases are mixed with it to minimize fire and explosion hazards. Mixtures such as 12% EO with 88% chlorofluorocarbon (CFC), known as the *12:88 mixture*, were used as alternatives, but because CFCs damage the ozone layer of the atmosphere that blocks out the harmful ultraviolet light from the sun, this mixture could no longer be used as of the end of 1995 (Spry, 1995).

EO is now being mixed with hydrochlorofluorocarbon (HCFC) and is 50% less damaging to the ozone layer (Spry, 1995), but the use of HCFC is being phased out by the year 2030. Other countries are pressuring their governments to abolish the sale and use of HCFC as early

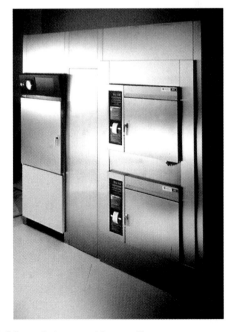

Fig. 8-29 Ethylene oxide sterilizer. (Courtesy STERIS Corp. Mentor, Ohio.)

as 2003, however (United Nations Environment Programme, 1992).

Since pure EO must be stored in explosion-proof cabinets because of its flammability, other mixtures are being used. EO has been successfully combined with carbon dioxide. However, the sterilizing chamber for an EO-CO_2 combination must be able to accommodate increased pressure and a longer exposure time to the gas mixture. The mixture of EO with inert gases does not destroy the sterilization effect of EO; it merely reduces the flammability hazard.

The rate of EO sterilization depends on several factors, including the gas concentration, relative humidity, temperature, and contact time. A relative humidity of at least 35% to 85% is required for sterilization to be effective (AAMI, 1992a). Humidity is necessary to allow the EO to penetrate the cellular membranes.

There have been many theories regarding the way in which EO sterilization affects cellular structures. The most widely accepted one is that EO sterilization destroys the cells as the gas diffuses through the cell walls. This causes chemical interference within the cell, thus inactivating the reproductive process.

Instruments and devices must be dry when placed in the sterilizer, because EO can react with water to form ethylene glycol, which is a toxic chemical similar to antifreeze. This byproduct is not eliminated during aeration.

Aeration after sterilization is mandatory, however, to allow the residual EO gas to escape. EO sterilizers also require special exhaust systems, including abators and aerators, and special venting capabilities. Written policies must be established to ensure that the appropriate aeration cycle is completed to discourage early removal of packs and supplies from the sterilizer.

There are three basic steps in the gas sterilization process: sterilant penetration, biological kill, and sterilant removal (Amsco International, Inc., 1995), and three phases to the EO sterilization process (Joslyn Sterilizer Corporation, 1995):

1. Preconditioning—The items to be sterilized are loaded into the sterilization chamber. After the system is closed, air is removed to enhance heating and allow complete penetration of the humidity and the EO-gas mixture.
2. Exposure—After the air is removed, the EO is released. The pressure of the chamber is increased, and the items are exposed to a combination of EO, humidity, and temperature until sterilization is achieved.
3. Detoxification—After sterilization is completed, the EO is removed from the chamber and from the processed items. When this aeration cycle is completed, the sterilized items can be removed without the risk of residual EO exposure.

EO poses many safety hazards to the health care team, however. Research has shown that EO irritates the eyes, skin, and respiratory systems of workers who are close to the sterilizer (Grant, 1995). EO is also known to be a possible human carcinogen and mutagen and is a reproductive hazard to men and women. In addition, EO can cause skin burns on contact.

To prevent occupational exposure to the EO, the gas sterilizer should be located in a well-ventilated area where at least 10 air exchanges occur per hour (Meeker and Rothrock, 1995). Many states have developed regulations regarding EO emission; therefore hospitals and other surgical facilities must be cognizant of any such local, state, and federal regulations to ensure compliance.

OSHA states that the exposure limit to EO is 1 ppm weighted over an 8-hour period. Because EO is odorless below 700 ppm, environmental monitoring must be conducted (Grant, 1995). Warning devices are available that can detect EO leaks. Facilities must ensure that there is regular medical surveillance and that continuing education is provided to minimize any hazards associated with the use of gas sterilizers.

Liquid chemical immersion sterilization

Liquid chemical immersion sterilization has recently become very popular in the United States because it is a quick way of reprocessing (Fig. 8-30). Instruments and endoscopes can be reprocessed within 30 minutes using this method, thereby helping to minimize surgical scheduling conflicts. Several systems may be placed within the surgical suite so that they can be immediately available. This minimizes the time needed to transport instruments and endoscopes to another area or department for reprocessing. It also minimizes the chances of device damage resulting from the extra handling required during transportation.

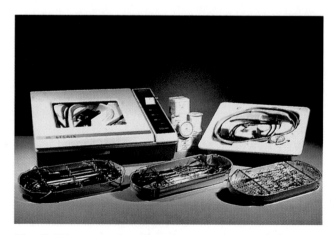

Fig. 8-30 Peracetic acid sterilizer. (Courtesy STERIS Corp., Mentor, Ohio.)

Peracetic acid is the most common agent used for liquid chemical immersion sterilization. It is a highly biocidal oxidizer that sterilizes even in the presence of high levels of organic soil. Peracetic acid consists of acetic acid plus an extra oxygen atom that reacts with most cellular components to cause cell death. The mechanism of action of the sterilizing solution is not truly understood, but it has been theorized that the peracetic acid disrupts the sulfhydryl and sulfur bonds in proteins and enzymes, oxidizes essential enzymes within cells, acts as a protein denaturant, ruptures cell walls, interferes with active transport across membranes, and inactivates catalase, which is known to detoxify caustic hydrogen peroxide (STERIS Corp, 1995).

Because peracetic acid breaks apart protein bonds, debris buildup is prevented. This can be seen by comparing an endoscope lumen that has undergone multiple glutaraldehyde exposures with the same lumen after only two cycles of the peracetic acid process (Fig. 8-31).

To qualify for liquid chemical immersion sterilization, devices must be fully immersible, able to withstand temperatures up to 56°C, and fit into one of the varieties of sterilizing trays and into the chamber of the unit (Fig. 8-32).

The procedure for sterilizing devices using this method is as follows: After a device is completely cleaned, it is placed in the sterilizing system. All instrument or endoscope lumens are attached to the unit with special connectors so that the solution can flow freely through the internal workings of the devices. A single-use container holding the sterilant and buffer is placed in the unit, the lid is closed, and the start button is pushed (Fig. 8-33).

The system combines 35% peracetic acid with water heated to 50° to 56°C. A buffer is automatically added to keep the peracetic acid from corroding the instrument.

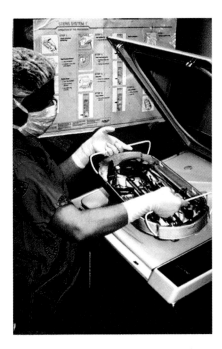

Fig. 8-32 Instruments and endoscopes to be sterilized must fit easily inside the sterilizing tray. (Courtesy STERIS Corp., Mentor, Ohio.)

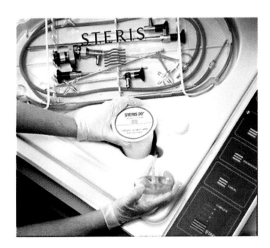

Fig. 8-33 A single-use container holding the sterilant and buffer is placed inside the sterilizing unit. (Courtesy STERIS Corp., Mentor, Ohio.)

As all of these solutions combine, a "use dilution" is formed, lowering the concentration of the peracetic acid to 0.2% with a pH of approximately 6.4.

After the sterilization process is finished, the devices are thoroughly rinsed with sterile water within the automated, enclosed system. The end-products of the process (i.e., acetic acid, water, oxygen) are safely disposed of in the normal sanitary sewer system without environmental concerns.

During the cycle, the system continually monitors the solution concentration, temperature, and exposure

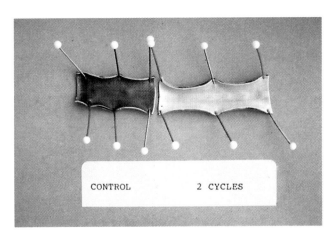

Fig. 8-31 An endoscope lumen processed repeatedly with glutaraldehyde solution and then subjected to two peracetic acid sterilization cycles. (Courtesy STERIS Corp., Mentor, Ohio.)

time to validate sterility. The parameters are documented on paper, which can then be filed or placed on the patient's chart (Fig. 8-34). Chemical and biologic indicators also can be added to the load to validate that conditions for sterilization have been met. Currently, monitoring the sterilization parameters (noting the solution concentration, temperature, and exposure time) is being discussed as a process to validate that sterilization conditions have been met. It may some day replace the need to perform biologic and chemical indicator testing to validate sterile processing conditions have been met.

After the process is completed, the sterilized instruments and endoscopes can be immediately transported to the nearby sterile field for use (Fig. 8-35). A method for sterile storage after the peracetic acid sterilization process is completed needs to be developed, however, so that such sterilized devices can be stored and used at a later date.

Plasma sterilization systems

Plasma sterilization systems are rapidly evolving that may serve as an alternative means of sterilizing wrapped dry instruments and devices, especially those that may be heat or moisture sensitive. Because the instruments must be wrapped, they can be stored for future use after the sterilization process. The instruments must be adequately cleaned, however, or these systems cannot sterilize them.

There are two popular systems; one uses hydrogen peroxide gas plasma that sterilizes within 75 minutes and the other uses peracetic acid vapor and gas plasma that sterilizes within 3 to 4 hours. Both of these systems use and emit nontoxic and nonflammable gases. They also do not produce byproducts that threaten the environment, so they quickly have become acceptable alternatives.

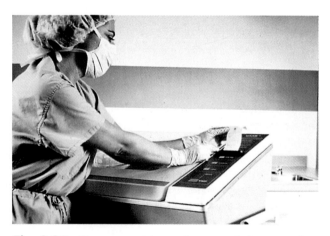

Fig. 8-34 The parametric readings can help to confirm that appropriate sterilization parameters have been met. (Courtesy STERIS Corp., Mentor, Ohio.)

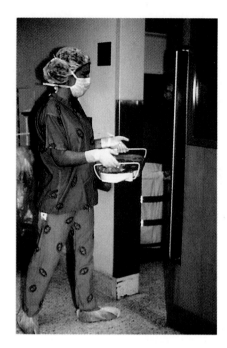

Fig. 8-35 Sterile instruments and endoscopes are transported to the nearby surgical area for use. (Courtesy STERIS Corp., Mentor, Ohio.)

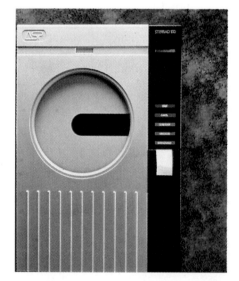

Fig. 8-36 Hydrogen peroxide gas plasma sterilization system. (Courtesy Advanced Sterilization Products, Irvine, Calif.)

Hydrogen peroxide is a well known and recognized germicide. The hydrogen peroxide gas plasma system uses hydrogen peroxide at a 56% concentration (Fig. 8-36). To reprocess devices using this system, cleaned instruments and devices are first placed in nonwoven polypropylene wraps or Tyvek-Mylar pouches. Muslin and cellulose wrappers (such as paper or linen) cannot be used. Instruments and endoscopes with smaller lumens can be processed using a special adapter that allows the plasma to penetrate into the internal workings. Cellulose materials, liquids, or powders cannot be processed using this system.

Following are the steps in the hydrogen peroxide gas plasma sterilization process:

- The items are placed in the chamber, the door is closed, and the system is activated.
- A vacuum is created within the chamber.
- Hydrogen peroxide and water are infused into the chamber and surround the items.
- A radiofrequency-induced electrical field causes plasma to be formed from the hydrogen peroxide gas. The electrons collide with each other within the plasma.
- Free radicals and other collision products in the plasma cloud interact with the cellular membranes, disrupting life functions and thereby destroying the microorganisms.
- At the completion of the cycle, the end-products, vaporized water and oxygen, are formed. Aeration is not necessary because there are no toxic residues or harmful emissions.
- The sterile items can be immediately used or stored for future use.

In the peracetic acid vapor and gas plasma sterilization system, the two gases are alternated during the sterilization process (Fig. 8-37). Instruments and devices can be wrapped in either woven or nonwoven

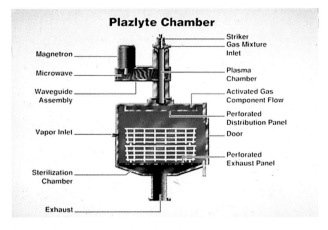

Fig. 8-38   Cross-section showing the chamber configuration of the peracetic acid vapor and gas plasma sterilization system. (Courtesy Abtox Inc., Mundelein, Ill.)

material. The procedure for sterilizing devices using this system is as follows:

- The items are placed in the sterilizing chamber, the door is closed, and the system is activated.
- Peracetic acid vapor is formed by vaporizing a 5% peracetic acid solution into the chamber under vacuum pressure.
- Gas plasma is formed in a separate chamber by flowing a mixture of stable gases (argon, oxygen, and hydrogen) through an electromagnetic field. The items in the sterilizer are not exposed directly to the electromagnetic energy of the charged plasma particles.
- A plasma consisting of electrons, ions, atoms, and free radicals is formed in the separate chamber as the gas molecules are excited.
- The highly charged ions and electrons remain in the separate chamber while the uncharged atoms, molecules, and free radicals are introduced into the sterilization chamber (Fig. 8-38).
- In a repetitive sequence, the peracetic acid vapor and the gas plasma surround and diffuse through the wrappers to sterilize the contents.
- The sterilizing effects are bactericidal, sporicidal, virucidal, tuberculocidal, and fungicidal as the cellular protein structures and bonds are destroyed.
- The gas plasma is evacuated from the system, and the reactive components are combined to form water, oxygen, and hydrogen, which are safely discharged into the environment. The cycle also includes an aeration period to remove any odor. No special exhaust system is required.
- No residues are left on sterilized items, so they can be used immediately after the 4-hour cycle is completed.

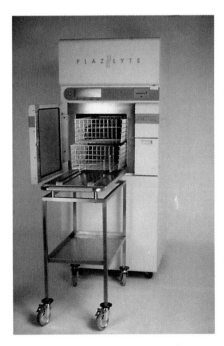

Fig. 8-37   Peracetic acid vapor and gas plasma sterilization system. (Courtesy Abtox Inc., Mundelein, Ill.)

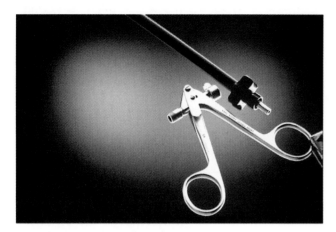

Fig. 8-39 Reassembly of the device.

Reassembly

After the device has been sterilized or disinfected, it must be reassembled for use (Fig. 8-39). Often this is done at the sterile surgical field, so the nurse and other team members must know how to properly reassemble a reusable item quickly, while at the same time making sure that it works safely and appropriately.

Quality Checks

Inadequate processing puts the patient, surgical team, and reprocessing staff at risk. Improper processing can result in broken valves, inadequate lubrication, insulation breaks, leaky gaskets, clogged ports and lumens, missing parts, and cracked fiberoptics. The staff members responsible for reprocessing must therefore be able to check the instrument or device to ascertain its integrity and proper function. If, however, the staff member is not experienced, the instrument may be reassembled incorrectly. In addition, if the staff member does not understand how the instrument is used or how to check the device, then faulty instruments may be placed back into service. Currently there are not many reliable methods for checking reusable devices during reprocessing. The use of magnification to examine an instrument can help in checking the integrity, but this does not ensure that the instrument will function properly (Fig. 8-40). Trocars need to be sharpened regularly, but there are no standards that pertain to the frequency with which tips should be sharpened. There appear to be no consistent guidelines for inspecting instruments before reuse.

Unfortunately, it is the patient who is often the quality check point for reusable devices. In many instances, the only way a nurse knows that instruments, such as reusable scissors, are not sharp enough is when the surgeon complains that they are not cutting the tissue easily. If a malfunctioning instrument is identified during a surgical procedure, the delay incurred while a replacement instrument is procured puts the patient at risk and also increases the expense of the surgery. A disposable instrument, on the other hand, must pass rigorous quality checks at the manufacturing site before being packaged, so the user can be assured that it will function adequately.

Instruments and devices that have not been adequately cleaned are sometimes placed back into service after reprocessing (Figs. 8-41 to 8-43). The FDA conducted a study of 26 health care centers involving 71 gastrointestinal endoscopes that had been cleaned and disinfected. A significant bacteria count was found on 24% of the endoscopes. Problems noted to be responsible for the inadequate reprocessing of the endoscopes included failure to time the disinfection period, to clean all channels, to flush all channels with the disinfectant, and to fully submerge the endoscope in the disinfectant

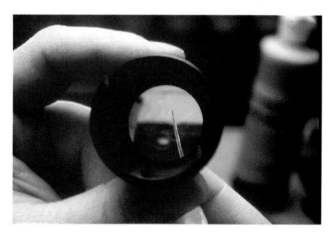

Fig. 8-40 The tip of a reusable laser fiber is checked using magnification.

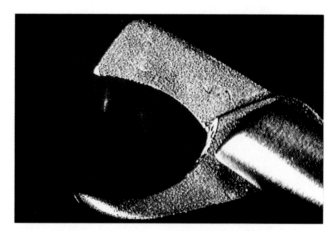

Fig. 8-41 Sterile laparoscopic scissors contaminated with debris from a previous use. (Courtesy United States Surgical Corp., Norwalk, Conn.)

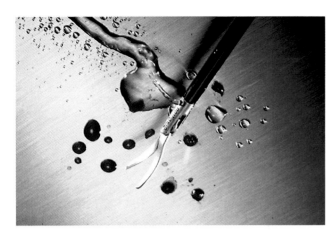

Fig. 8-42 A laparoscopic irrigation suction device ready for patient use contains blood that was not removed during cleaning (Courtesy United States Surgical Corp., Norwalk, Conn.)

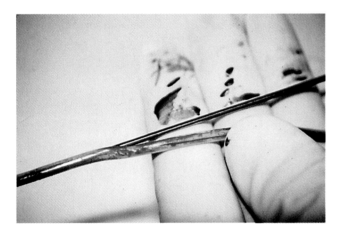

Fig. 8-43 An instrument ready for patient use that has been dissected. The lumen is found to be contaminated. (Courtesy United States Surgical Corp., Norwalk, Conn.)

solution. This study demonstrates the importance of having a quality-management program wherever reprocessing is performed (Kaczmarek et al, 1992). As noted earlier in this chapter, the cost of treating a hospital-acquired infection is usually about $14,000 (*Laparoscopic Surgery Update*, 1995a) and this points up the importance of adequate reprocessing. It is hard to calculate the actual incidence of postoperative infections, however, because in the United States many physicians use prophylactic antibiotics.

Some consider the bioburden on reprocessed instruments or endoscopes to be sterile dirt. However, even though the contaminant may be sterile after processing, sterile dirt can cause adhesion formation and can cause the immune response to be increased postoperatively.

A study was conducted to determine the knowledge of hospital administrators and other professionals regarding infection control practices. These people were asked whether a policy and procedure existed at their facility for the cleaning, sterilization, and inspection of instruments before surgery. All of the hospital administrators stated their hospitals had policies in place, but only 41% of the hospital staff said that such a policy actually existed (United States Surgical Corp., 1993).

There is a big difference today between recommendations that everyone understands and those actually put into practice. This gap between recommendations and actual practice must be closed. To help achieve this, it is mandatory for staff members to understand the steps involved in the reprocessing of instruments and devices and to comply with policies regarding reprocessing.

Instrument discoloration and staining are often noticed when instruments are inspected. The following may be observed on stainless steel instruments (Scanlan International 1995):

- Light brown veneer—may especially form on satin-finished instruments. It usually denotes the formation of a chromium oxide layer, which actually offers more protection for the instrument.
- Brown/orange stain—indicates a chemical stain, usually from phosphates or rust. May result from the use of inferior water, the use of highly alkaline detergents or sterilant solutions with a high pH, inadequate cleaning, or the use of surgical wrapping material that has residual phosphate detergents.
- Black stain—usually results from an acid reaction with the stainless steel. May be caused by a low-pH detergent.
- Bluish gray stain—usually occurs when instruments made of dissimilar metals, such as stainless steel and aluminum, are placed together in an ultrasonic bath or autoclave. Chemical sterilizing or disinfecting solutions may also stain instruments this color.
- Multicolor stain—usually results from exposure to excessive heat.
- Water spot discolorations—usually caused by inadequate drying.
- Purplish black stain—usually caused by detergents or solutions containing ammonia or amines. To minimize this problem, autoclaves and steam lines should be routinely cleaned to remove any detergent residues.

It is not as common for titanium instruments to become stained because these instruments have an oxide layer that protects against this. However, because oxides are sensitive to halogens, such as fluorine and chlorine, exposure of instruments to these elements can cause them to degrade and become stained.

If instruments or endoscopes need to be repaired, a qualified service organization that can provide experienced and skilled services needs to be contacted. This organization can be the original equipment manufacturer or an independent service agency. The following criteria need to be considered when contracting with organizations to repair instruments and endoscopes:

- The reputation of the company
- The quality of repair services
- The timeliness of service and return of devices
- Loaner capabilities
- The cost of services
- The warranty period
- Technician skill, experience, and knowledge
- The ability to return instrument to original equipment specifications
- The type of replacement parts used (i.e., new versus refurbished)
- Other materials used for repair (i.e., are the glues compatible with sterilizing processes?)
- The range of devices repaired (i.e., does the company service both instruments and endoscopes)
- The response time to answer the initial call for service
- The process used to ensure device integrity after repair

REUSABLE, SINGLE-USE, AND REPOSABLE INSTRUMENTS

During the past decade there has been a tremendous increase in the number of minimally invasive surgeries performed, which is attributable to the technological advancements made during this time. Endoscopy performed on an outpatient basis has almost become a universal standard of care. Because patients are sent home much sooner after surgery, it is a challenge for the nurse to provide consistent follow-up and to evaluate the perioperative care delivered (Fig. 8-44). Determining whether a postoperative infection has resulted from the use of a contaminated instrument or whether a complication has resulted from the use of a malfunctioning device can be very arduous. Quality and appropriate instrumentation must be provided that will ensure safe care is delivered. Nurses have joined the team of professionals who determine which instruments are most suitable. Knowledge and experience form the foundation on which these decisions are made.

Definitions

There are three categories of instruments from which to choose—reusable, single use, and reposable—and these are defined and discussed in the following sections.

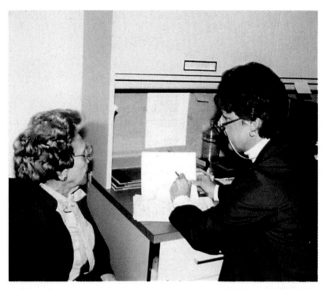

Fig. 8-44 Because patients are sent home quickly after surgery, it is often a challenge for the perioperative nurse to provide consistent postoperative follow-up and to evaluate the perioperative care delivered.

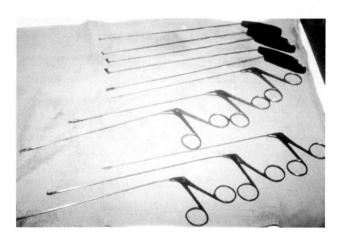

Fig. 8-45 Reusable instruments can be used over and over.

Reusable instruments

Reusable instruments are ones that can be used over and over (Fig. 8-45). They must therefore be designed so that they can be adequately cleaned, and they must be made of materials that can withstand reprocessing. The reusable instrument must also be easy to disassemble and reassemble and ideally should have component parts that can be replaced if broken or missing. The manufacturer should provide literature that describes how to reprocess and maintain the instrument. Usually

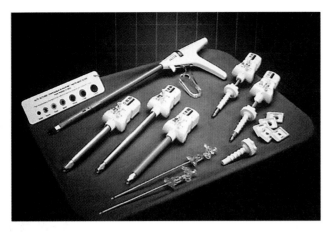

Fig. 8-46 Single-use instruments are warranted for use only one time. (Courtesy United States Surgical corp., Norwalk, Conn.)

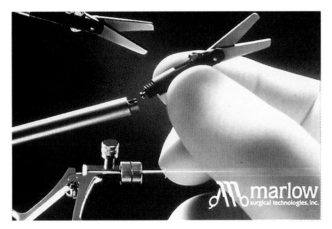

Fig. 8-47 Reposable instrument with a single-use and a reusable component. (Courtesy Marlow Surgical Technologies, Willoughby, Ohio.)

manufacturers do not state the number of times an instrument can be used because this differs from institution to institution, depending on how they are cared for. Because reusable instruments are made of materials that must withstand continual reprocessing and use, they typically cost more. If the cost of the instrument is high, planning for the purchase appears in the capital budget.

Single-use instruments

A single-use instrument is one that is used only once and then discarded (Fig. 8-46). These instruments are often called disposable, but some object to use of the term in this sense because even reusable instruments can be "disposable" if they cannot be repaired. Single-use instruments usually cost less because they are made of materials intended to last for only one use. Usually the cost of such

instruments appears on the operating budget. Because more of these instruments are needed, single-use items may appear to be a major expense for the surgical unit. Single-use instruments are often used to solve the problems with reusables, such as the need to continually sharpen some instruments. Because the manufacturer performs stringent quality cheeks before packaging, single-use instruments may be more reliable.

Reposable instruments

Reposable is a term that was coined to refer to instruments with both reusable and disposable components (Fig. 8-47). These devices can be compared to razors that have a reusable handle but blades that are discarded with each use or after a few uses (Fig. 8-48). There are different instruments, such as scissors, that have a disposable working end but a reusable shaft.

Debate

Today there is a big debate going on throughout the world as to whether to use reusable, single-use, or reposable instruments. All of the players are adamant about their views, though there is one common thread: Everyone is convinced that their view is the only logical one.

Cost is the major issue in the debate. At one end of the cost spectrum are high-cost items, such as endoscopes and fiberoptics, that are usually reusable. At the other end are the low-cost items, such as blades and sponges, that are usually single-use items. The debate, however, is focused on instruments in the mid–cost range. This is the combat zone, and it is here that debate rages over whether it is best to use reusable, single-use, or reposable devices, or a combination of devices.

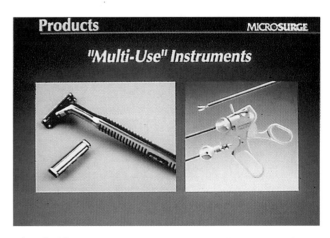

Fig. 8-48 A reposable instrument can be compared to a razor that has a reusable and a single-use or limited-use component. (Courtesy Microsurge, Needham, Mass.)

Deciding Factors

Although cost is an important consideration in the selection of instruments, it is not the only factor that should be considered. There are many other factors that must also be considered, and these, plus the financial considerations, are discussed in the following text.

Financial considerations

The financial advantages and disadvantages of reusable, single-use, and reposable instruments sometimes obscure the other important deciding factors. Unfortunately, often decisions are made more on the basis of economics than science, especially if unrealistic monetary comparisons are presented.

There is no financial formula for conclusively showing which type of instrument is most appropriate for all surgical environments. There are too many other variables that can affect the dollar amount. For example, the overall cost to reprocess a reusable item at a large metropolitan hospital with an extensive central service department would probably be less than that for a small rural hospital with only one person who reprocesses the instruments. A smaller hospital performing less than 250 procedures per year may find that using single-use instruments for laparoscopy is more economical because it avoids the high overhead costs of reprocessing and maintaining reusable instruments. The expense of single-use items is very visible in an operating budget, whereas the costs of reusables are not as noticeable because they are hidden in the staffing, equipment, and supply costs needed for reprocessing. The cost of reusable items may even appear only in the capital budget because they are usually more expensive than disposables. There are a variety of costs that can be considered and compared when examining the expense of using reusable or single-use items. When considering the use of reposables, combinations of each grouping can be used. Factors to be considered in evaluating the cost of using reusables may include:

- Individual instrument cost
- The life expectancy of the instrument
- The number of instruments needed
- The number of backup instruments needed
- The cost of repairs
- The frequency of repairs
- The cost of reprocessing (staff wages, personal protective equipment, processing supplies, processing equipment)
- The cost of educating the staff responsible for reprocessing
- Instrument maintenance and quality checks

Factors that apply to single-use instruments may include:

- Individual instrument cost
- The number of instruments needed
- The cost of staff time involved in ordering instruments

- The cost of staff time in maintaining inventory
- The expense of extra storage area
- The disposal cost of instruments and packing materials

There are many other variables that can be factored into the equation, such as the cost to treat a postoperative infection caused by an instrument that was improperly prepared, the cost to treat an employee who has been injured by a sharp instrument during reprocessing, and the revenue loss incurred while waiting for instruments to be reprocessed.

Because each surgical facility has unique circumstances that must be considered, one financial model is not appropriate for all. The focus should also not be on the numbers shown by any particular study but on the process used to determine the differences. Other deciding factors, such as instrument reliability and physician preference, should also be considered in the final decision. However, quality and safety must never be compromised in favor of what may appear to be a lower cost.

Other financial concerns need to be explored whenever the economic impact of reusables versus single-use is being examined. These include the cost of the procedure, the patient charge, and the reimbursement expected.

In considering the cost of a procedure, both the direct expenses, such as the cost of the device, plus the indirect expenses, such as the cost of reprocessing the device, must be included. As previously noted, the indirect costs associated with the use of reusables include the cost of cleaning, sterilizing, sharpening, repairing, staffing, and repackaging. The costs for single-use items include the expense of purchasing the instruments, maintaining the inventory, and disposing of used instruments.

Physicians are also becoming more involved with the financial aspects of endoscopy. Some hospitals provide quarterly records of the costs incurred for different endoscopic procedures performed by surgeons. This causes physicians to compete with each other to control the expenses of each procedure. If this practice is used, however, then both the indirect and direct expenses must be reported.

Many facilities have discovered that standardizing instrumentation has had a great impact on the cost of procedures. Purchasing instruments in kits has also helped to defray extra expenses. For example, if single-use items are desired, kits that contain one trocar and several cannulas can be purchased instead of multiple packages of trocar/cannula sets, which ultimately are more expensive. The medical instrument industry has been very appreciative of and responsive to the need to offer cost-effective alternatives to help control endoscopic expenses.

With the expansion of capitation, the patient charge has not become as critical an issue. In capitation environments the patient pays for health care before receiving it

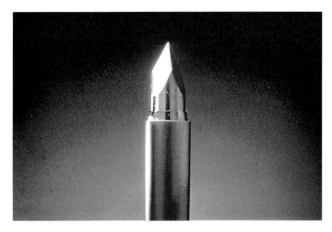

Fig. 8-49 The reliability of a reusable trocar's sharpness has been questioned, but it is almost guaranteed for single-use instruments.

and the income is fixed. Therefore, the surgical unit must control expenditures to ensure that expenses do not exceed the predetermined income.

For facilities still offering fee-for-service care, patient charge remains very important. In the United States, the patient may be charged directly for a single-use device, but the patient charge may be double or triple the cost of the item to the hospital. If patients complain to their physicians or to the hospital about excessive surgical fees, this causes the cost of single-use items to be explored again. The cost of a single-use item may be more evident on the patient's bill than the cost of reusable items, but, in fact, once all the costs are analyzed and compared, the overall cost of the single-use item may prove to actually be less than that of the reusable.

Because reimbursement has become very limited in the United States, decision-makers are faced with trying to choose the most cost-effective type of instrument. By realistically exploring as many financial variables as possible in the context of the other deciding factors, they can make a pragmatic decision.

Financial concerns continue to be a major influence in determining whether to purchase reusable, single-use, or reposable instrumentation. Most surgical units are discovering that a combination of such instruments is the best approach to realizing cost control and savings. As the medical instrument industry continues to lower the costs of single-use and reposable instruments, however, the financial impact will continue to be difficult to analyze.

Reprocessing

The need to reprocess reusable instruments is a major consideration in the decision regarding the type of instruments to use. This factor was discussed in detail at the beginning of this chapter. The effectiveness of the processing of reusable instruments has a direct impact on product integrity and the safety of the staff and patient.

If the process is sound and is being performed by skilled personnel, then costs and risks are controllable. If the process is inconsistent and ineffective, then the costs and risks increase appreciably.

Reliability

The reliability of an instrument must also be carefully considered when deciding whether to use reusable, single-use, or reposable instruments. For example, a reusable trocar may not be consistently as sharp as a single-use trocar, whose sharpness can almost be guaranteed (Fig. 8-49).

Reliability needs to be monitored using a consistent process that checks the integrity and function of an instrument after each use. The difficulty is making sure the process is followed with each reprocessing of the instrument and that the proper tools are available to test the instruments. Single-use instruments are often preferred if reliability is in question because they go through such rigorous checks for reliability before being packaged. However, if a reposable or single-use instrument malfunctions during a procedure, then the reliability of these instruments must also be challenged.

Life expectancy

The life expectancy of an instrument is similar to its reliability. The number of uses is difficult to determine, however, because the life expectancy of an instrument varies tremendously with each surgery suite. For example, the life expectancy of reusable instruments used in teaching hospitals tends to be less because the residents, nursing students, and other novices who use them may not fully understand the appropriate care and handling required. Differences in surgical practices also have a bearing on the life expectancy of instruments.

The number of times a reusable instrument can be used safely is critical. Usually instrument manufacturers cannot determine this because of the differences among surgical practices just noted. However, in one attempt to eliminate this problem, a manufacturer of reposable instruments has designed a limited-use instrument working end that has a heat-sensitive dot that changes color with multiple uses (Fig. 8-50). When the dot becomes black, this indicates that the instrument working end should be discarded. Companies are trying to develop other methods to determine usage for limited-use instruments.

Another concern pertaining to reusable instruments is that sometimes they malfunction while being used on a patient, thus becoming a patient safety issue. For liability reasons, the patient must not continue to be the quality check point for validating instrument integrity.

When trying to determine the life expectancy of an instrument, many factors should be considered, such as the number of uses per year, the technique and expertise of the operator, the quality of the reprocessing, and

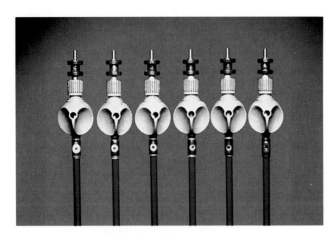

Fig. 8-50 The heat-sensitive dot on the limited-use instrument changes color after it has been subjected to multiple steam autoclave sterilizations. (Courtesy Microsurge, Needham, Mass.)

the care and handling of the instrument. Once life expectancy has been estimated, the number of instruments needed can be calculated.

Liability

Liability always needs to be considered whenever a decision is being made regarding the type of instruments to purchase. Decision-makers involved in examining the sources of patient complications stemming from endoscopic procedures look to determine if faulty instrumentation is implicated. For example, if a patient suffers a postoperative infection and an endoscopic instrument used in the patient is found to have been contaminated before its use in the patient, then the reprocessing of reusable instruments would need to be examined. If the problem continues to surface, consideration may need to be given to the use of single-use instruments instead.

Because manufacturers include care and handling information with each product, reprocessing should become more consistent, thus minimizing the incidence of patient and staff injuries.

Availability

Instruments need to be readily available whenever surgery is being performed. However, there are three problems that tend to be encountered in this regard:
1. Having enough instruments so that delays do not occur
2. Having the appropriate instruments available when procedures are performed on off-shift hours
3. Having enough storage for instruments (especially single-use instruments)

There should be enough instruments so that delays are not caused by their reprocessing between procedures. A shortage of instruments could also cause instru-

ment preparation to be rushed, with the result that mistakes are made and the processing may not be adequate. This in turn increases liability because the likelihood of patient or staff injury or infection escalates. If reusable laparoscopic instrument sets are used, then there should be at least four sets for every 300 procedures performed annually.

Another concern is having the appropriate instruments available 24 hours a day. Sometimes instruments are sent to another department for processing at the end of the day with the result that the endoscopic instruments may not be available should the on-call staff come in to perform an emergency procedure. Therefore, enough instruments, supplies, endoscopes, and other devices must be available in the surgical suite at all times. Often physicians and nurses store favorite instruments in their lockers so they are available for the cases they are involved with. This, of course, means that if others are trying to find these instruments for use in a procedure, they would be unavailable. This practice must also be stopped

Storage is always a problem for surgical departments (Fig. 8-51). If single-use instruments are used, careful planning must be done so that there is enough storage space for the extra packages of these instruments. To help remedy this problem, many instrument companies have resorted to providing a "just in time" inventory. This involves the continual delivery of instruments so that the surgical suite has a comfortable supply but overstocking and the need for expansive stock rooms are eliminated

The space needed for the storage of disposed single-use instruments can also be a problem. Because many endoscopic procedures may be conducted during a day, used single-use instruments can rapidly accumulate. Space therefore needs to be allocated for this waste, and regular removal is critical.

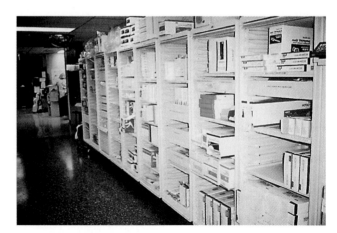

Fig. 8-51 Storage space for the variety of single-use instruments needed for endoscopic procedures must be adequate.

Environmental concerns

In the United States, regulated medical waste or infectious waste must be made unrecognizable and decontaminated before being placed in a landfill (AORN, 1995). Single-use sharp instruments, such as trocars and scissors, are considered regulated medical waste and must be disposed of as such. Because it costs much more to dispose of regulated medical waste than regular waste, the use of single-use instruments has compounded this problem and increased the cost of the hospital waste stream.

The medical instrument industry has helped solve environmental concerns by constructing instruments made of more environmentally friendly material. The amount of packing materials used has also been decreased to lessen the amount of environmental waste. In another approach to solving this problem, the peanuts used for packing can be made out of dissolvable materials (Fig. 8-52).

One company has developed a piece of equipment that simultaneously grinds and decontaminates regulated medical waste, rendering it safe and unrecognizable in less than 15 minutes (Fig. 8-53). The regulated medical waste is placed directly into a portable processing chamber (Fig. 8-54). When full, the processing chamber is transported to the central system in a special mobile caddie (Fig. 8-55). The chamber is then placed in the processor for automatic grinding and decontamination. The end-products can then be treated as clean refuse and placed directly in a landfill without extra costs. This piece of equipment offers tremendous cost savings to the hospital and surgical suite in the disposal of single-use instruments.

Product development

New endoscopic techniques are continually evolving in today's fast-paced surgical environment. Advancements

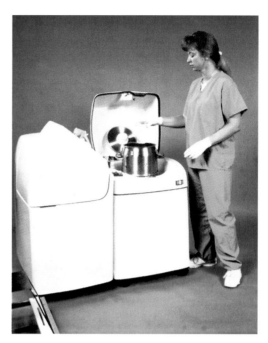

Fig. 8-53 Device that grinds and decontaminates regulated medical (infectious) waste so that it can be safely discarded with noninfectious waste. (Courtesy STERIS Corp., Mentor, Ohio.)

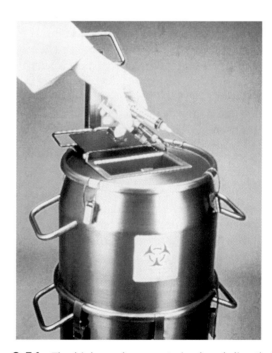

Fig. 8-54 The biohazardous waste is placed directly into the portable processing chamber. (Courtesy STERIS Corp., Mentor, Ohio.)

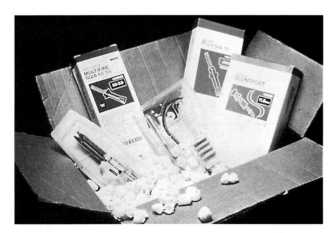

Fig. 8-52 Packing peanuts used for the packaging of single-use instruments can be made out of dissolvable materials to help minimize environmental problems with the disposal of packing materials. (Courtesy United States Surgical Corp., Norwalk, Conn.)

in instrumentation have made it possible for complex procedures to be performed successfully using an endoscope. Often single-use instruments are introduced as the prototypes for new instruments, because it's easier to change the design of these instruments as refinements are made. Obsolescence is usually not a concern

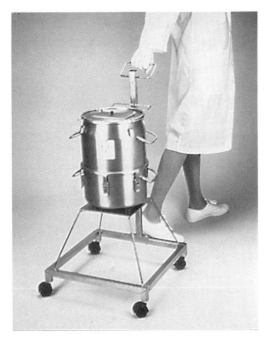

Fig. 8-55 A special caddie, used to transport the full chamber to the processor. (Courtesy STERIS Corp., Mentor, Ohio.)

with single-use items. Sometimes surgeons prefer to use single-use instruments for the performance of newly introduced procedures because reusables cost more and they want to see whether the procedure is scheduled as often as expected. As a procedure becomes more accepted and the caseload increases, then it may be more cost-effective to purchase the reusable version of the instrument.

Physician preference

Physician preference is also a critical factor in determining whether to use reusable, single-use, or reposable instruments. If a surgeon attends a training program on endoscopic procedures sponsored by a company that manufactures single-use devices, then the surgeon will be more inclined to prefer the single-use instruments. As a surgeon becomes comfortable with one instrument design, then his or her decision will be based more on the comfort level experienced. The surgeon's opinion about an instrument is critical and must always be considered in purchasing decisions. Such standardization may be more difficult, however, for surgical suites staffed by many surgeons.

Reuse of Single-use Items

Reusing single-use items has become a very controversial topic in the United States, even though this practice has become widely accepted in other countries. For example, many facilities in Canada are reprocessing single-use items and believe that they can do this with-

out posing harm to their patients (English, 1996). So far there have not been reports of significant increases in the infection rates at these institutions.

In the United States, administrators and risk managers sometimes are adamantly against this practice because of the threat of lawsuits should a reprocessed device fail or cause infection (*Laparosc Surg Update*, 1995f). If a single-use instrument is reprocessed within the facility and problems occur, then the hospital or surgical suite assumes the liability for this.

As managed care organizations and capitation gain an even stronger hold on the health care market, more pressure will be brought to bear on surgical administrators to explore new avenues to lower costs. In addition, as health care dollars become increasingly limited, the practice of reprocessing single-use items will resurface as a potential cost-savings measure.

Currently some hospitals are successfully reprocessing single-use laser fibers (Fig. 8-56). The protocol for studying the validity of reprocessing laser fibers shown in Box 8-2 may be used as a model for the reprocessing of other single-use items. As long as a device can be adequately cleaned and reprocessed and its integrity is not destroyed, then reuse of single-use items may be justified.

Before 1996, there was a Joint Commission on the Accreditation of Health Care Organization (JCAHO) standard stating that single-use products should not be reprocessed by the hospital unless the original manufacturer provided written instructions for doing so. This standard prevented many hospitals from even contracting with an outsourcing service for reprocessing. As a result, this standard was eliminated in the "1996 JACHO Surveillance, Prevention and Control of Infection Standard IC.4," which states that, "the hospital [should take] action to prevent or reduce the risk of nosocomial infections in patients, employees and visitors." For implementation the standard requires that

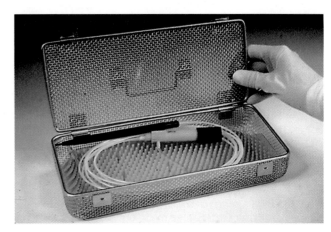

Fig. 8-56 Some facilities reprocess single-use laser fibers.

| Box 8-2 | *Reprocessing of Single-use Laser Fibers* |

1. Obtain approval for the study from the laser committee and the risk manager.
2. Conduct a survey of other hospitals and ambulatory surgery centers to determine if they are reprocessing single-use laser fibers.
3. Develop criteria for single-use laser fibers that may be reprocessed.
   Example:
   - The fibers must be able to be cleaned adequately.
   - The fiber can be resterilized.
   - The fiber's physical characteristics or quality will not be changed by the reprocessing.
   - The fiber remains safe and effective for its intended use.
4. Contact manufacturers for their recommendations on how the fibers should be reprocessed. If they cannot give any recommendations, then ask the company to document what materials are used in the manufacture of the fiber so that appropriate sterilization methods can be chosen. Also ask the manufacturers for free product to use during the research.
5. Collaborate with Central Processing Services to develop a reprocessing protocol for the laser fibers.
   Example:
   - Clean the fiber.
   - Inspect the fiber using magnification.
   - Place the fiber in a sterilizing container.
   - Label the container.
   - Gas-sterilize the container (other sterilization methods may be used)
6. Conduct a cost analysis of the reprocessing expense for comparison with the cost of using a new single-use fiber for every procedure.
7. Test the integrity of the reprocessed fiber before the next procedure by calibrating the fiber to determine the transmission of the laser energy. If the transmission is less then 75%, the fiber should be discarded.
8. Evaluate the results of the cost comparison and the fiber integrity testing.
9. Report the results to the laser committee and risk manager. Get approval to reprocess single-use laser fibers if results warrant this action.
10. Communicate the results to the laser team and other surgical staff.
11. Pass the cost savings onto the patients.

"processes [be] designed to provide for the continued sterility of hospital-sterilized and commercially prepared items through appropriate packaging, storage and other methods to provide for package integrity" (JCAHO, 1996). With the advent of this less restrictive standard, hospitals feel more comfortable about using outsourcing services for the reprocessing of single-use items. Such companies provide reprocessing services for single-use items that have been used in patients or the outer package may have been opened but the item itself was not used. These companies assume the liability for the reprocessed item's sterility and integrity and warrant the item for another use.

Because specific standards for reprocessing single-use items are still being developed, hospitals wanting to use a service company for reprocessing should address this issue in a policy that reflects actual hospital practice. The hospital needs to (Orris, 1996):
1. Revise the old hospital policy to read "single-use items will not be reprocessed at the hospital but may be reprocessed by any FDA-registered remanufacturing facility with appropriate liability insurance."
2. Have the certificate of insurance on file to show that the service company assumes the liability for the performance of the product.
3. Ensure that the reprocessing company validates their sterilization processes with an independent laboratory.

There are three areas of concern to consider whenever a decision is being made to reprocess single-use items (*AORN J*, 1995).
1. The function and safety of the device after reprocessing
2. The legal and ethical issues associated with reprocessing
3. Economic concerns with reprocessing

Usually low-risk devices can easily be reprocessed if they can be adequately cleaned and sterilized, but patient safety should continue to be the primary concern. If the device's effectiveness, safety, and integrity can be ensured, then reprocessing of single-use items may be a solution to help control health care expenditures.

SUMMARY

The decision to use reusables, disposables, or reposables will continue to be a challenge for health care professionals. Probably the best approach is to use a combination of all three while the pros and cons of each system and the resources of the hospital are being considered. Perioperative nurses must continue to be involved in this decision because of its impact on nursing practice and patient care.

Benefits of reusable instruments:
- Environmental waste is not a concern, except for the supplies and agents used for reprocessing.
- Sometimes appear to cost less than single-use items.
- Costs of the instruments are not easily observed in the operating budget.
- Less storage space is required.
- May have more of a high-quality feel for the surgeon.
- Greater life expectancy.

Benefits of single-use instruments:

- Reliable performance with every use.
- Always available if in stock.
- No disassembly or reassembly is needed.
- No need for sharpening or repair; therefore, instrument documentation logs are not needed.
- Some disposable instruments are designed with safety parts that protect the patient and the surgical team (e.g., trocars with safety shields).
- No need for cleaning or lubrication, thus reducing the risk of malfunctioning instruments and the risk of pathogen transmission to the health care team and possibly to other patients.
- No indirect costs to reprocess or repair the instruments, including labor costs, equipment, and supply expenses.

Benefits of reposable instruments:

- Replaces single-use and reusable instruments.
- Economically priced.
- Increased reliability with single-use working end.
- Fewer repairs because the part that needs repair is usually the working end.
- Reusable component is easily cleaned and reprocessed.
- Minimal extra storage space needed.
- No major economical concerns because only the working end is discarded.

REFERENCES

Adoumi R, Smith B, Chiu RCJ, et al: Double gloving might predispose to injury by blunting temperature perception, *Surg Laparosc Endosc* 4(4):284, 1994.

American Nurses Association: *Compendium of HIV/AIDS positions, policies, and documents,* Washington DC, 1992, ANA.

Amsco International, Inc: Ethylene oxide sterilization and alternative methods, *Surg Serv Management* 1(2):16, July 1995.

AORN J: Clinical issues, 61(3):581, 1995.

Association for the Advancement of Medical Instrumentation: *American National Standard: good hospital practice: steam sterilization and sterility assurance,* Arlingotn, VA, 1992a, AAMI.

Association for the Advancement of Medical Instrumentation: *American National Standard: good hospital practice: flash sterilization–steam sterilization of patient care items for immediate use,* Arlington, VA, 1992b, AAMI.

Association for the Advancement of Medical Instrumentation: *American national standard, good hospital practice: steam sterilization and sterility assurance,* Arlington, Va, 1994 16, AAMI.

Association of Operating Room Nurses: *1995 standards and recommended practices,* Denver, 1995, AORN.

Bell DM: Healthcare related HIV—can exposure be avoided?, Presented at Association of Operating Room Nurses First Annual Conference on Infectious Diseases, May 1995, Atlanta, Ga.

Columbus Dispatch: p A1 1:92 young men have HIV, Nov 24, 1995, (Based on article by Rosenberg PS, in *Science,* 270:1372, 1995).

DesCoteaux JG, Poulin EC, Julien M, Guidoin R: Residual organic debris on processed surgical instruments, *AORN J* 62(1):23, 1995.

English, Nancy: Reprocessing disposables: one strategy to balance cost reduction and quality patient care, *Today's Surg Nurse* 18(4):23, July/Aug. 1996.

Gerding DN, Peterson LR, Vennes JA: Cleaning and disinfection of equipment for gastrointestinal flexible endoscopy: evaluation of glutaraldehyde exposure time and forced-air drying, *Gastroenterology* 83:613, 1982.

Grant M: EtO monitoring compliance requirements, *Infect Control Steril Technol* May 1995, p 28.

Hanson PJV, Gor D, Jeffries DJ, et al: Elimination of high titre HIV from fiberoptic endoscopes, Gut: 31:657, 1990.

Jarvis WR: Tuberculosis: an old disease—new threat, Presented at the Association of Operating Room Nurses First Annual Conference on Infectious Diseases, May, 1995, Atlanta, Ga.

Joint Commission on the Accreditation of Healthcare Organizations: Surveillance, prevention and control of infection standards, In *Standards, scoring guidelines and aggregation rules,* Chicago 1996, JCAHO, p 453.

Joslyn Sterilizer Corporation: Ethylene oxide sterilization, *Surg Serv Management,* 1(2):14, 1995.

Kaczmarek RG, Moore RM, McCrohan J, et al: Multi-state investigation of the actual disinfection/sterilization of endoscopes in health care facilities, *Am J Med* 92: March 1992.

Klacik ST: Cleaning endoscopes: the basics, *Infect Control Steril Technol* June 1995, p 24.

Laparosc Focus, Laparoscopic instrumentation, 1(1):7, 1993.

Laparosc Surg Update: What to do when equipment techs won't clean properly? (3(5):59, 1995a.

Laparosc Surg Update: Tips on reprocessing instruments, 3(6):70, 1995b.

Laparosc Surg Update: Change in Cidex label causes confusion, could increase OR costs, 3(6):61, 1995c.

Laparosc Surg Update: Special section: laparoscopic reprocessing, 3(8):88, 1995d.

Laparosc Surg Update: Letter from OSHA clearly says latex gloves not okay with Cidex, 3(8):90, 1995e.

Laparosc Surg Update: "Disposables commonly used outside US, Why not here?, 3(9):97, 1995f.

Laparosc Surg Update: Scope lubricants may shield HIV from high level disinfection, 3(11):123, 1995g.

Margolis HS: Hepatitis: are you aware of the dangers? Presented at the Association of Operating Room Nurses First Annual Conference on Infectious Diseases, May 1995, Atlanta, Ga.

Marlow SC, Petruschke HK: Cleanability of hybrid laparoscopic instruments, *AORN J,* 62:32, 1995.

Meeker MH, Rothrock JC: *Alexander's care of the patient in surgery,* ed 10, St. Louis, 1995, Mosby.

Occupational Safety and Health Administration: Air contaminants, *Federal Register* 54:2464, 1989.

Occupational Safety and Health Administration: Occupational exposure to ethylene oxide, Final standard (29 CFR Part 1910), *Federal Register* 53:11413, 1988

Orris, *Operating room recycling and instrument service,* Houston, TX, 1996.

Reichert M: GI flexible endoscopes cleaning and disinfection effectiveness, *Infect Control Steril Technol* June 1995, p 20.

Rutala WA: APIC guideline for selection and use of disinfectants, *Am J Infect Control* 18:101, April, 1990.

Rutala WA: New sterilization technology and high level disinfection, Lecture sponsored by the Cleveland Clinic and STERIS Corp., 1996, Cleveland, Ohio.

Scanlan International: Making the most of your surgical instrumentation investment, St. Paul, 1995, Scanlan International.

Spry CC: Sterilization regulations—who's in charge here? *Surg Serv Management* 1(2):56, July 1995.

STERIS Corp.: Peracetic acid sterilization, *Surg Serv Management,* 1(2):30, July 1995.

United Nations Environment Programme: *Report of the fourth meeting of the parties to the Montreal protocol on substances that deplete the ozone layer,* Nov 1992.

United States Surgical Corp: Single-use instruments for safety and cost-effectiveness, Norwalk, Conn., 1993, USSC.

9

Basic Endoscopic Equipment

As the trend toward less invasive surgery is encouraged, more endoscopic procedures have been introduced, thus requiring the development of more sophisticated equipment. The nurse working in this field must be knowledgeable about the variety of different endoscopic systems and devices available today and experienced in their use. This includes an understanding of equipment operation, troubleshooting protocols, safety measures, and how to set up the room to provide a safe traffic pattern.

ENDOSCOPES

Type of Endoscopes

An endoscope is a tube that is inserted into a natural body orifice or through a tiny incision to access internal organs or structures. Endoscopes are used for either diagnostic or operative purposes. The development of endoscopy began with the need to provide minimally invasive diagnostic methods. Endoscopes used for diagnostic applications do not have channels and are used only for observation. Sometimes such diagnostic endoscopes have superior imaging capabilities because of the absence of an operating channel. With the advances made in endoscopes, light sources, and instrumentation, however, it became possible for operative procedures to be performed through the endoscope. Operative endoscopes therefore have ports or lumens that are used for irrigation, suctioning, biopsying, and inserting instruments. Because of the addition of the operating channel in the endoscope, the number of fiberoptic bundles had to be reduced and often the lens system had to be made smaller, with the result that the lighting may not be as defined as that possible with a diagnostic en-

doscope. Attempts are being made to improve lighting and optical technology to address this problem.

Endoscopes can have a rigid, semirigid, or flexible viewing sheath, and the diameter and length of this sheath depend on the location of the structure being visualized. Rigid endoscopes include laparoscopes, bronchoscopes, hysteroscopes, cystoscopes, and sinuscopes. Flexible endoscopes include colonoscopes, gastroscopes, hysteroscopes, and bronchoscopes. Many scopes come in either a rigid or flexible form. Semirigid endoscopes have a rigid section and a flexible section. An example of the latter is a ureteroscope, which has a shaft that is fairly rigid but does allow some movement.

Endoscopes have a lens system that can magnify or enhance the image. This system may consist of a single eyepiece or a series of sophisticated telescopic lenses.

A rigid endoscope has a lens structure that conducts the light through a quartz rod system (Fig. 9-1). The light is also conducted through an objective lens and an eyepiece mechanism to visualize the image. The older traditional lens systems contained a series of small lenses placed at certain intervals within the rigid endoscope shaft with air spaces between the lenses. In the newer rod lens systems, special long glass rods are placed at intervals within the endoscope shaft. The newer lens systems interchanged the amount of air with lenses (Fig. 9-2). The rod lens system allows for the endoscope shaft to be smaller while the viewing angle is large and the imaging bright. The type and placement of the lens determine the endoscope angle of vision, field of view, and resolution.

The angle of view is determined by the lenses within the endoscope (Fig. 9-3). The optical capabilities through a rigid endoscope can be direct or angled to

111

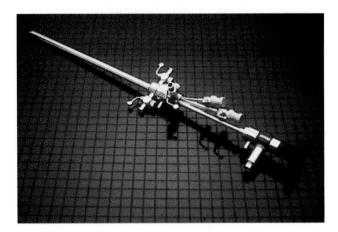

Fig. 9-1 Rigid endoscope.

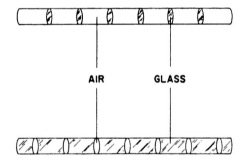

Fig. 9-2 The lens system within a rigid endoscope. The newer Hopkins lens system interchanges the air spaces and glass lenses, resulting in better imaging. (White RA, Klein SR: *Endoscopic surgery*, St. Louis, 1991, Mosby.)

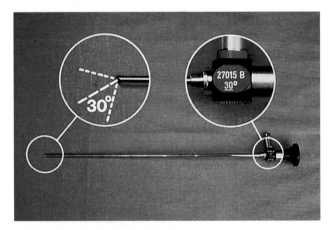

Fig. 9-3 The lenses inside the endoscope determine the anlge of view. (Courtesy Karl Storz, Culver City, Calif.)

better visualize internal structures. A 0-degree lens is usually the easiest lens to use because it provides a straight forward view. However, sometimes a structure cannot be viewed easily with a 0-degree lens, so an angled lens is needed. Following are the angles some lenses come in and the view afforded (Fig. 9-4).

- 30-degree angle—forward oblique
- 70-degree angle—lateral
- 90-degree angle—lateral
- 120-degree angle—retrospective

Many rigid endoscopes are used in fluid environments, and some of these endoscopes therefore have irrigation ports built right into the distal end of the scope shaft to provide rapid delivery of solution (Fig. 9-5).

A flexible scope can be bent in different directions, with some limitation, to reach hard-to-reach areas and to facilitate insertion into curved structures such as the lower colon (Fig. 9-6). Flexible endoscopes have complex systems consisting of optical fibers and internal lumens (Fig. 9-7). Light is carried via the fiberoptics to illuminate a structure. A panoramic view can be obtained merely by moving the end of the scope to different positions using a control near the eyepiece. These endoscopes have suction and irrigation ports to remove liquids and plume and provide irrigation solution. The design of a flexible endoscope is very complex, because many different components are compressed into a small control head and a flexible shaft (Fig. 9-8).

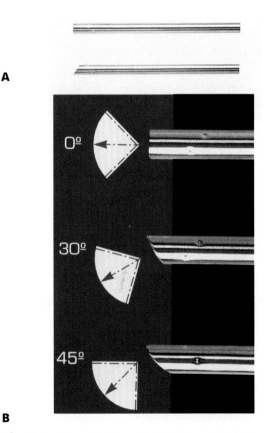

Fig. 9-4 A and B, Examples of some rigid endoscope lens angles. (Courtesy Devmed Group. Inc., Palm Beach Gardens, Fla.)

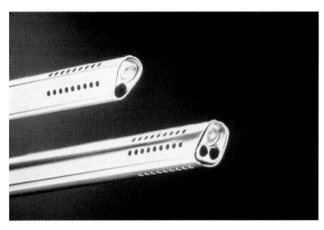

Fig. 9-5   Distal ends of continuous-flow operative hysteroscopes. (Courtesy Circon Corp., Santa Barbara, Calif.)

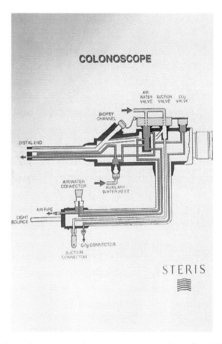

Fig. 9-8   The internal components of a flexible colonoscope. (Courtesy STERIS Corp., Mentor, Ohio.)

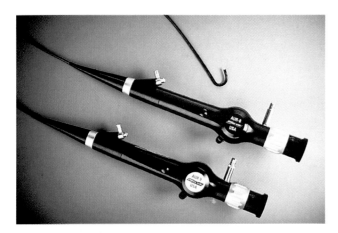

Fig. 9-6   Flexible endoscopes. (Courtesy Circon Corp., Santa Barbara, Calif.)

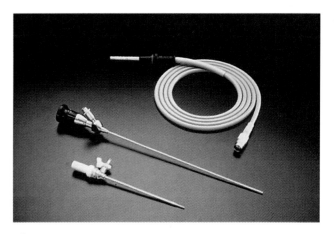

Fig. 9-9   Microlaparoscope. (Courtesy Olympus America, Inc., Melville, N.Y.)

Very small rigid endoscopes, such as microlaparoscopes, have been developed that are approximately 2 mm in diameter (Fig. 9-9). Because of their smallness, laparoscopy can be performed in a physician's office with the patient under local anesthesia. Image clarity is not compromised, however, because advanced fused-image–fiber technology has been incorporated into the design of the endoscope. This technology affords exceptionally high resolution and sharpness. Microinstruments have also been developed for use with this endoscope. The abdomen is entered after the Veress needle is used for insufflation. Trocar/cannula insertion is not necessary because the access port for the endoscope is so small.

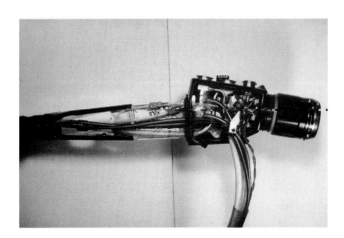

Fig. 9-7   A dissected flexible endoscope, showing the complexity of the internal structure and design. (Courtesy STERIS Corp., Mentor, Ohio.)

A study was conducted to compare the results from laparoscopy using a 2-mm scope and a traditional 10-mm scope. In this study a series of patients underwent laparoscopy, first with the small scope and then immediately with the larger scope. All of the cases were videotaped. It was found that the images yielded by the 2-mm laparoscope were sufficient to permit accurate diagnosis, as shown by the fact that no pathology was missed. Minor procedures can also be performed through the microlaparoscope (Molloy, 1995). Other small-lumen flexible and rigid endoscopes are being developed to access body structures using less invasive techniques (Figs. 9-10 to 9-12).

Rigid endoscopes, such as laparoscopes, are being designed that are reusable, but only for a limited number of procedures (Fig. 9-13). They are discarded either after a certain number of uses or when repair is needed. They have the advantage of being less expensive, first because they are less expensive to make and second because the repair expense is eliminated.

Care of the Endoscope

All endoscopes must be handled, cleaned, disinfected or sterilized, and stored according to the manufacturer's recommendations. Endoscopes should be prepared in the same manner for every patient. If the first patient of the day gets a sterile endoscope, then the rest of the patients undergoing surgery during that day deserve a sterile endoscope. Reprocessing policies should ensure consistency within the endoscopic program.

Appropriate supplies must be available to allow for adequate cleaning of an endoscope (Fig. 9-14). The endoscope should be disassembled for cleaning immediately after use while organic debris is still moist (Fig. 9-15). If allowed to dry, mucus, debris, and other contaminants become extremely difficult to adequately remove.

Endoscopes should be washed in warm water with a mild, nonabrasive detergent that does not leave a residue (Fig. 9-16). Before immersion in the cleaning solution, however, flexible endoscopes should first be tested for leaks, to make sure the internal lumens are intact. Brushes and other tools must be used to thoroughly clean the ports and lumens of the endoscope (Fig. 9-17). These instruments should not be cleaned using ultrasonic cleaning devices, however, because the high-frequency motion causes the glass fibers to vibrate, which could damage them. New low frequency ultrasonic devices specifically made for endoscope cleaning are now available.

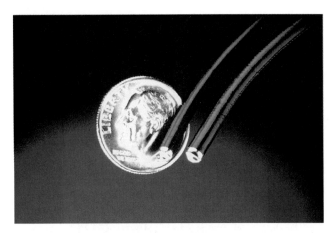

Fig. 9-11   Distal ends of small flexible ureteropyeloscopes. (Courtesy Circon Corp., Santa Barbara, Calif.)

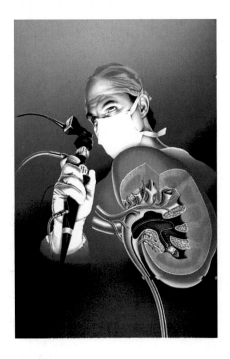

Fig. 9-12   A small flexible ureteroscope is being used to examine the kidney. (Courtesy Circon Corp., Santa Barbara, Calif.)

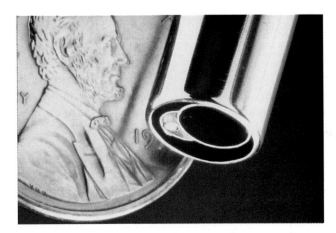

Fig. 9-10   The distal end of a small rigid percutaneous nephroscope. (Courtesy Circon Corp., Santa Barbara, Calif.)

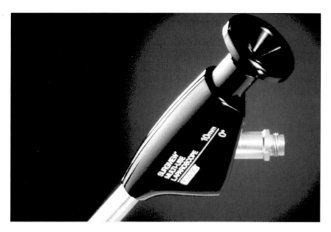

Fig. 9-13 Limited-use laparoscope. (Courtesy United States Surgical Corp. Norwalk, Conn.)

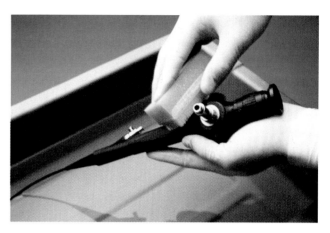

Fig. 9-16 The endoscope shaft is washed with a soft-bristle brush and a mild, nonabrasive detergent. (Courtesy Karl Storz, Culver City, Calif.)

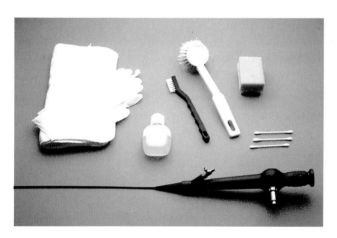

Fig. 9-14 Supplies that may be used to clean an endoscope. (Courtesy Karl Storz, Culver City, Calif.)

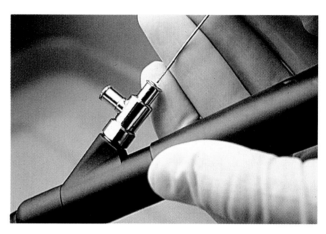

Fig. 9-17 The endscope port is thoroughly cleaned with a brush. (Courtesy Karl Storz, Culver City, Calif.)

After thorough cleaning, the endoscope is rinsed with demineralized water to prevent the formation of water spots and endoscope discolorization (Fig. 9-18). Complete drying is then necessary to prevent bacterial growth and corrosion of the metal surfaces (Fig. 9-19). Lumens can be dried by attaching a suction line or a compressed-air line. A water-base lubricant should be applied to all movable parts to prevent sticking and immobility.

The endoscope is then disinfected or sterilized according to the manufacturer's recommendations. Flexible endoscopes are currently made from flexible elastomeric materials that would be destroyed during steam sterilizing, but rigid endoscopes are now being designed that can withstand the steam autoclaving used to sterilize the rest of the instruments (Fig. 9-20).

Special endoscope processors are also available. Some processors, such as the peracetic acid sterilizer, require that the endoscope be cleaned before being

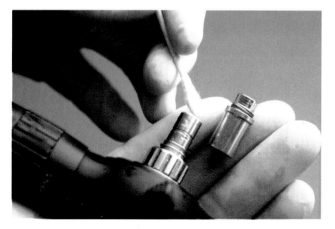

Fig. 9-15 Removable parts of the endoscope are disassembled for cleaning. (Courtesy Karl Storz, Culver City, Calif.)

placed in the unit (Fig. 9-21). Other processors clean the endoscope and then soak it in a disinfectant (Fig. 9-22) (see Chapter 8). Endoscopes should never be soaked for more than 30 minutes in any solution, however, including sterile water.

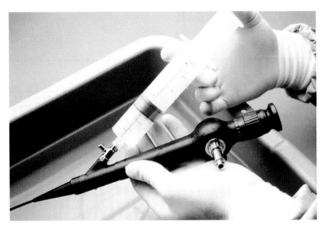

Fig. 9-18 The endoscope port is rinsed with demineralized water. (Courtesy Karl Storz, Culver City, Calif.)

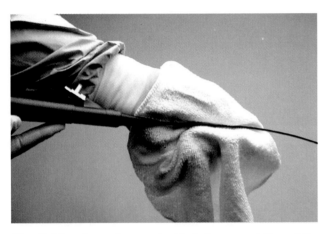

Fig. 9-19 The endoscope is dried after completion of the cleaning process. (Courtesy Karl Storz, Culver City, Calif.)

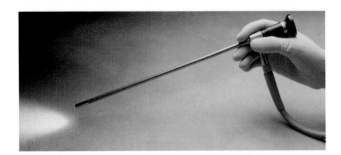

Fig. 9-20 Some rigid endoscopes have been designed for steam sterilization. (Courtesy Aesculap, Inc., South San Francisco, Calif.)

Endoscopes should always be stored dry in a protected case or in a specially designed storage area or cabinet (Fig. 9-23). Flexible endoscope cabinets are also available in which the scopes can be stored vertically so the sheath is not kinked (Fig. 9-24).

Endoscopes should be inspected before each use to assess their functional integrity. The eyepiece should be examined to evaluate the clarity of the image from the reflected light against the ocular and objective lenses (Fig. 9-25). Any scratches or fingerprints on the surface will be obvious.

A study was conducted in which the working and suction channels of 241 flexible endoscopes were examined using 1.4-mm and 2.4-mm inspection endoscopes. Of the 80 facilities in the study, at least one endoscope with encrusted debris in the channels was found at 38 of the facilities. Twenty-six of the 241 scopes were found to have severely scratched channels that could easily harbor debris. At only 56 of the 80 facilities were attempts made to dry the endoscopes after processing; an effective drying method was noted to be used at only three of these 56 sites (5.4%). This study showed that flexible endoscope reprocessing is not being performed adequately and that small-lumen inspection endoscopes can be used effectively to examine the lumens to validate the cleaning process (McCracken, 1995).

Endoscope Fogging

Endoscopes have a tendency to fog upon insertion, because the endoscope is usually cooler than the warm environment of the body. Following are some tips for preventing this problem:

- Use sterile antifogging solutions to coat the lens to provide defogging.
- Heat the scope near the temperature of the body.

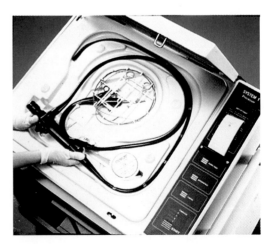

Fig. 9-21 A flexible endoscope that has been cleaned is placed in the peracetic acid sterilization system for processing. (Courtesy STERIS Corp., Mentor, Ohio.)

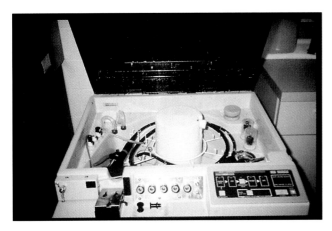

Fig. 9-22 Some automatic endoscope processors can clean and disinfect the endoscope.

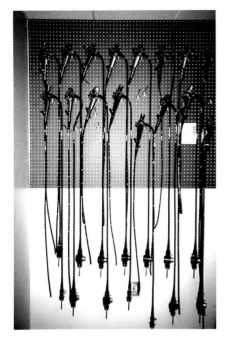

Fig. 9-23 Endoscopes should be dry before being stored in a designated area.

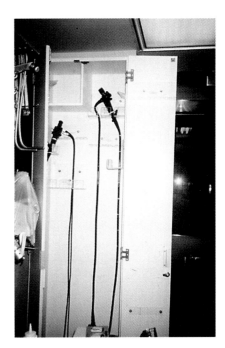

Fig. 9-24 Flexible endoscopes can be hung vertically in a cabinet for storage.

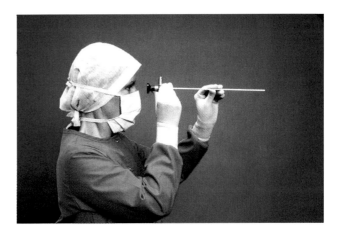

Fig. 9-25 The endoscope lens should be inspected to assess the clarity of an image from reflected light. (Courtesy Karl Storz, Culver City, Calif.)

- If using a cold chemical-disinfection process, warm the final rinsing solution.
- Use an endoscope warmer.
- Warm the irrigation solution.
- Avoid touching the scope to tissue upon insertion or when positioning the scope close to the tissue. If the scope is cooler than the tissue, fogging will occur.
- Replace faulty or leaking O-ring seals.
- During laparoscopy, do not provide insufflation through the endoscope port because unheated insufflation gas flowing across the scope will cause fogging. Ideally the insufflation gas should be warmed.

A laparoscope-washing device is available that flushes the lens system to clean it of fog, fat, and blood during the procedure without the need to remove the endoscope from the surgical site (Fig. 9-26). The protective irrigating sheath can be sterilized by autoclave, ethylene oxide, or other sterilization methods. The sheath can also be soaked in a glutaraldehyde solution if disinfection is desired. To clean the sheath, the cap and the O-ring are separated from the sheath (Fig. 9-27). A rigid 10-mm laparoscope is placed through the cap and O-ring and then inserted into the sheath (Fig. 9-28), which comes in different lengths and can accommodate

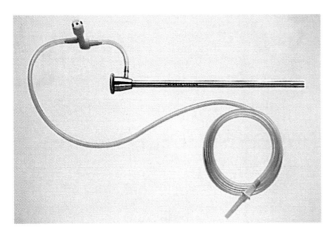

Fig. 9-26 An intraoperative lens-washing system. (Courtesy Devmed Group, Inc., Palm Beach Gardens, Fla.)

0-, 30-, and 45-degree angled scopes. The cap is then tightened to seal the endoscope into the protective sheath (Fig. 9-29). The sterile tubing with a standard bag spike is inserted into the solution bag. The tubing has an in-line trumpet valve that allows both washer and irrigation functions to be controlled with a single push-button action. The distal lens of the endoscope is protected from tissue and blood contact that could obscure the endoscopic image (Fig. 9-30).

LIGHT SOURCES

The first crude light sources utilized incandescent light bulbs, but these generated a lot of heat and it was unsafe to use them for long periods. Fiberoptics not only

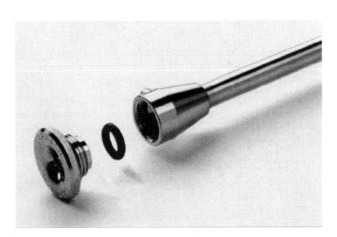

Fig. 9-27 The cap, O-ring, and sheath are separated before the laparoscope is inserted. (Courtesy Devmed Group, Inc., Palm Beach Gardens, fla.)

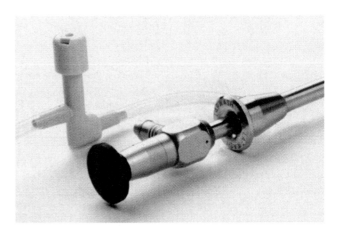

Fig. 9-29 The cap is tightened to seal the laparoscope within the protective sheath. (Courtesy Devmed Group, Inc., Palm Beach Gardens, Fla.)

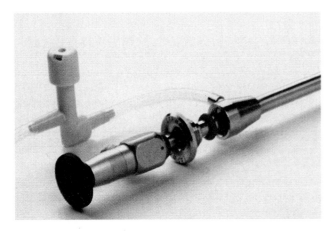

Fig. 9-28 The laparoscope is placed through the cap and O-ring and inserted into the protective sheath of the washing system. (Courtesy Devmed Group, Inc., Palm Beach Gardens, Fla.)

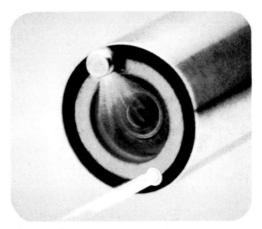

Fig. 9-30 The distal lens of the laparoscope is protected from tissue and blood contact. (Courtesy Circon Corp., Santa Barbara, Calif.)

provided better illumination and did not produce a lot of heat, but the intensity could be controlled at the light source.

Heat from a light source is not transmitted through the scope and thus cannot injure the tissue, but intense heat can be emitted from the end of the fiberoptic cable if it is disconnected from the scope. A disconnected cable with the light still on must therefore be protected from coming in contact with dry combustible drapes or sponges. Either the end of the cable should be placed on a moist towel to prevent fires or burns or the light source should be turned off (Meeker and Rothrock, 1995).

Light Source Types

The most popular types of light sources available today are the xenon, metal halide, and halogen light sources (Fig. 9-31), and the bulbs most commonly come in 300, 270, and 150 watts, respectively (Frantzides, 1995). The heat generated by the high-wattage bulbs is attenuated by high-speed fans within the light source.

Xenon light bulbs cost about twice as much as halide ones but last twice as long. The xenon light can be focused down to a small area, so this is the preferred light source for smaller-lumen endoscopes. Xenon is the preferred light source for video endoscopy because of the higher-wattage bulb that is available and the more consistent light intensity generated. If the light does not come on when ignited, then re-ignition should be attempted. If the light goes out during a procedure, usually the bulb has burned out and needs to be replaced.

Metal halide bulbs are less expensive but have a shorter life span than xenon bulbs. These bulbs are also easy to handle and replace and do not require large fans to cool them.

Halogen light sources are popular in physicians' offices but do not offer the light intensity usually needed for endoscopy and some video requirements. They are generally not preferred for video endoscopy, because they produce a yellow cast and they have only a 150-watt capacity (Spellman, 1995).

Light bulbs should be changed by an experienced person according to the manufacturer's instructions; this is to prevent an electrical shock, avoid damage to the bulb, and minimize the risk of finger burns. Most light bulbs are located in light assembly drawers, making them readily accessible. It is usually necessary to use a cloth or a 4 × 4 sponge to both remove the burned out bulb and replace it with the new one; this protects against burns from the hot bulb being replaced and keeps oils from rubbing off one's hands onto the glass of the new bulb, thus extending its life. If a newly replaced bulb still does not work, then the problem may be in the light source itself.

A light source ideally should have a lamp life status monitor and adjustable brightness modes. An automatic brightness mode that adjusts the brightness according to the video image eliminates the need for continual adjustments. As already indicated, the light source should be easily accessible to facilitate bulb changing.

Because different light sources produce different colors, the camera must be white-balanced so that the signals between the light source and camera are communicated properly. After white-balancing is performed on the camera, then the camera can properly identify all primary colors. (See Chapter 10 for more information on white-balancing.)

Light Source Cables

The light source cable must be adaptable to different endoscopic systems. Universal light cable adapters are available on many light sources, which enhances their utility and versatility (Fig. 9-32). There are interchangeable light source adapters and endoscope adapters available for other cables.

Light cables are liquid filled or fiberoptic, but both are fragile and should not be dropped, kinked, or wound tightly (Fig. 9-33). Liquid-filled light cables are usually more durable than fiberoptic cables and produce more light. However, they are also more expensive and produce more heat at the endoscope. They are usually only available in the standard 6-foot (1.8-meter) lengths (Nezhat, et al, 1995).

Inside fiberoptic light cables are hundreds of glass fibers that transmit light (Fig. 9-34). These fibers can be broken if the cable is dropped or bent at extreme angles. Cables should therefore be checked before each use. Broken fibers can be noted by holding one end of the cable toward a bright light while looking at the other end (Fig. 9-35). Any fibers that appear as black dots

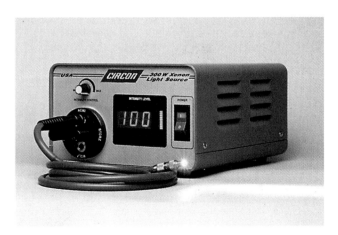

Fig. 9-31 300-Watt xenon light source. (Courtesy Circon Corp., Santa Barbara, Calif.)

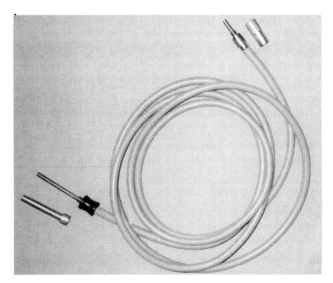

Fig. 9-32 Universal light cable adapters allow the light cable to be connected to many different light sources and endoscopes. (From Meeker MH, Rothrock JC: *Alexander's care of the patient in surgery,* ed 10, St. Louis, Mosby.)

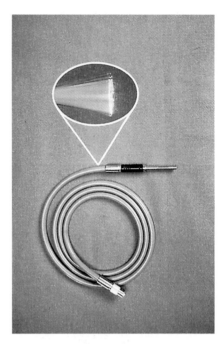

Fig. 9-34 Inside the light cable are hundreds of glass fibers that transmit light. (Courtesy Karl Storz, Culver City, Calif.)

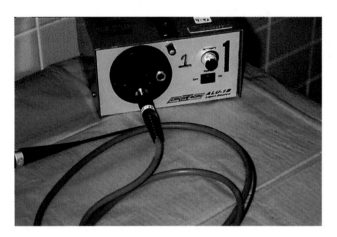

Fig. 9-33 The light cable should be wound loosely to prevent damage.

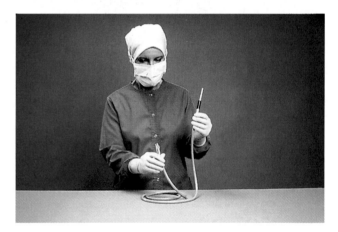

Fig. 9-35 The light cable can be checked for broken fibers by holding one end toward a bright light while looking at the other end. (Courtesy Karl Storz, Culver City, CA)

(peppering) are broken. This cannot be done with the cable hooked into the light source, however, because the light would then be too bright. If 18% to 20% of the cables are broken, the fiberoptic should be replaced because not enough light will be transmitted to perform the endoscopy (Fig. 9-36) (Meeker and Rothrock, 1995).

The light cable is usually 4 to 5 mm in diameter, with the light efficiency increasing with increases in the cable diameter, until the fiberglass bundle exceeds the diameter of the bundle within the endoscope (Soderstrom, 1986). Fiberoptic light cables usually come in 6-, 8-, and 10-foot (1.8-, 2.4-, and 3-meter) lengths (Nezhat, et al, 1995).

Transluminal illumination systems have been introduced that consist of light carriers which can be attached to traditional light cables. These light carriers can be

inserted into the esophagus, rectum, ureters, and other organs to improve visibility and enhance identification of structures during laparoscopic and thoracoscopic procedures. For example, an illuminated bougie that is sheathed in biocompatible silicone elastomer and has a soft, clear, flexible tip has been introduced (Fig. 9-37). Light is transmitted through the clear tip, creating a glow that can be seen through the walls of the organ or structure. Because anatomic parts are then easily identified, endoscopic surgery is facilitated. The illuminated bougie has been used for laparoscopic Nissen fundoplications in the treatment of gastroesophageal reflux. During the procedure, the illuminated bougie is inserted to identify esophageal structures and esophageal patency, and to ensure that the gastric wrap is not too loose or too tight (Stengel and Dirado, 1995).

Care of Light Cables

Following are tips regarding the care and maintenance of fiberoptic light cables that can be incorporated into written policies and procedures:

- Avoid squeezing, stretching, or sharply bending the cable.
- Grasp the connector piece when inserting or removing the light cord from the light source (Fig. 9-38). Never pull the cable when disconnecting it from the light source.

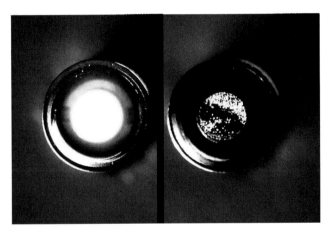

Fig. 9-36 The light cable should not be used if more than 20% of the fibers are broken. (Courtesy Karl Storz, Culver City, Calif.)

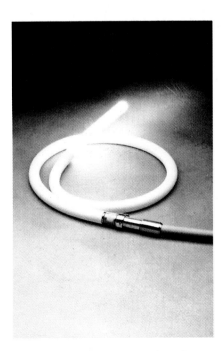

Fig. 9-37 Transluminal illumination bougie. (Courtesy BioEnterics Corp., Carpinteria, Calif.)

- Secure the cable to the surgical drape by placing it in a pocket created in the draping material (Fig. 9-39). Avoid puncturing the cable with towel clips or squeezing the cable between forceps jaws when securing it to the drape.
- Do not turn the light source on before connecting the cable to the endoscope, because the end of the cable gets hot and could ignite dry combustibles.
- Inspect the cable for broken fibers before each use.
- Inspect the ends of the cable to ensure each end has a clean, reflective, polished surface.
- Use a mild detergent solution to remove foreign matter from the cable. Oil, debris, or fingerprints on the cable ends can act as a local heat source, thus reducing the light output and leading to premature failure of the cable.
- Use a cotton-tipped applicator moistened with 70% isopropyl alcohol to clean the cable ends (Fig. 9-40).

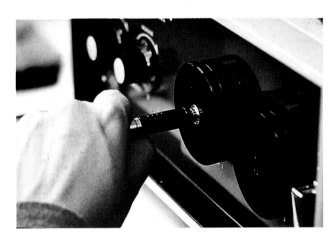

Fig. 9-38 The connector piece is held during insertion or removal of the light cable from the light source.

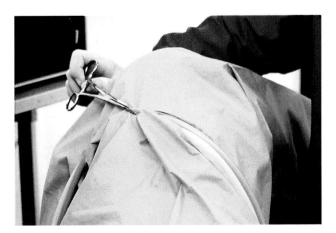

Fig. 9-39 The light cable can be secured to the surgical drape by placing it in a pocket created in the draping material.

- Do not subject the fiberoptic cables to usual ultrasonic cleaning, because the vibratory motion can destroy the tiny fiber bundles. Special low-frequency ultrasonic cleaning devices are now available for fiberoptics.
- Thoroughly rinse and dry the cable.
- Store the cable loosely coiled.
- Sterilize or disinfect the cable according to the manufacturer's instructions.
- Fiberoptic cables may be placed in a peel pack for ethylene oxide sterilization (Fig. 9-41).

Review of Most Frequently Occurring Accidents

Endoscopes, light cables, and other accessories can easily be damaged during procedures. Figures 9-42 to 9-51 illustrate some of the most frequent ways in which endoscopic equipment is damaged.

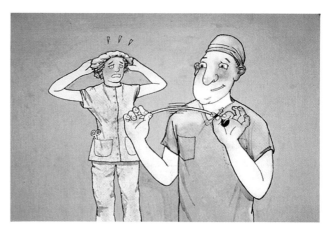

Fig. 9-42 Rigid endoscopes should not be bent during handling. (Courtesy Karl Storz, Culver City, Calif.)

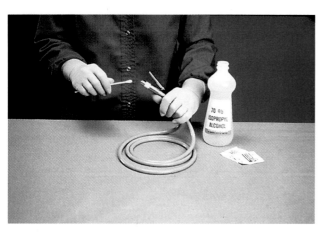

Fig. 9-40 A cotton-tipped applicator moistened with 70% isopropyl alcohol can be used to clean the cable ends.

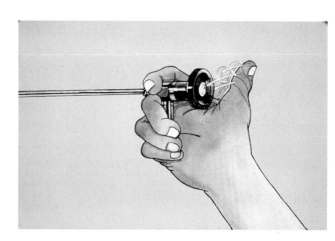

Fig. 9-43 Thumb and finger prints on an endoscope lens will distort the image. (Courtesy Karl Storz, Culver City, Calif.)

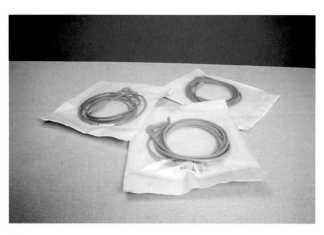

Fig. 9-41 Light cables packaged in peel packs for ethylene oxide sterilization. (Courtesy Karl Storz, Culver City, Calif.)

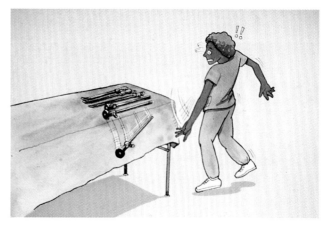

Fig. 9-44 The endoscope and other instruments should not be placed near the edge of the surgical table. (Courtesy Karl Storz, Culver City, Calif.)

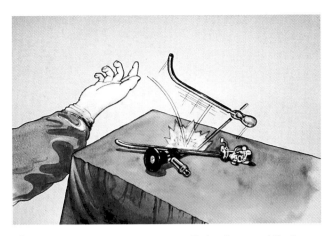

Fig. 9-45   An endoscope can easily be damaged if a heavy instrument is accidentally thrown on top of it. (Courtesy Karl Storz, Culver City, Calif.)

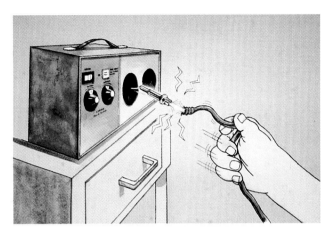

Fig. 9-48   The light cable connector should be grasped when disconnecting it from the light source. (Courtesy Karl Storz, Culver City, Calif.)

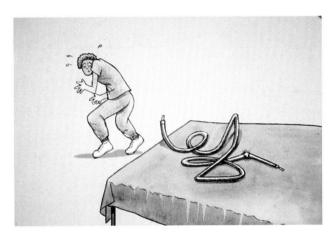

Fig. 9-46   The light cable should not be kinked or twisted. (Courtesy Karl Storz, Culver City, Calif.)

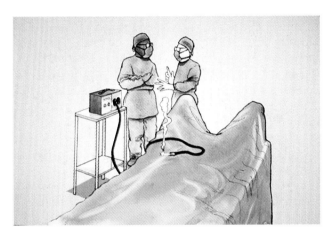

Fig. 9-49   To prevent a surgical drape fire, the light source should not be turned on unless the light cable is attached to the endoscope. (Courtesy Karl Storz, Culver City, Calif.)

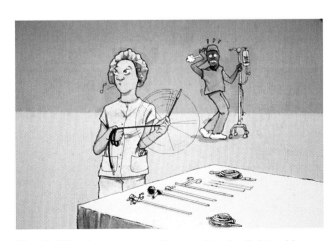

Fig. 9-47   The tiny glass fibers inside the light cable can easily be damaged. (Courtesy Karl Storz, Culver City, Calif.)

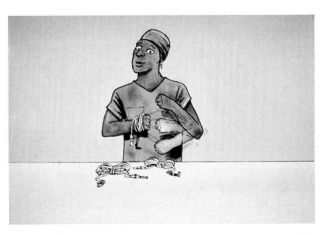

Fig. 9-50   To prevent damage, an electrosurgical cable should not be wound tightly. (Courtesy Karl Storz, Culver City, Calif.)

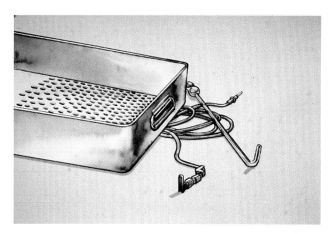

Fig. 9-51 Placing an instrument tray or instruments on top of an electrosurgery cable can cause damage to the cable. (Courtesy Karl Storz, Culver City, Calif.

INSUFFLATORS

Insufflation is usually performed to establish a pneumoperitoneum, which improves visualization by separating the intracavitational organs from the body wall. Insufflation originally was achieved by injecting room air by hand into the peritoneal cavity (White and Klein, 1991). Today an insufflator is used to provide a flow of gas to distend the body cavity so that internal organs and structures can be visualized and surgery can be performed safely (Fig. 9-52). There are two routes used: the transabdominal approach, which is the route more commonly used, and the posterior vaginal fornix approach.

Insufflator Controls and Safety Measures

The insufflator printouts or panel must be easily identifiable and read by the surgical team at all times. The importance of this is pointed up by one case in which a patient died of a CO_2 embolism as a result of the insufflation gas being instilled into a blood vessel during a laparoscopic procedure. A $1.6 million settlement was awarded. When the physician was shown a picture of the insufflator and was asked to point to the gauge he was watching before the patient died, he responded by pointing to the wrong gauge (*Laparosc Surg Update*, 1993). To prevent such accidents and ensure adequate insufflation, the following variables must be monitored and displayed on the control panel:

- Rate of flow
- Volume delivered
- Intraabdominal pressure

The rate of flow should be low initially to allow time to determine that the Veress needle is correctly placed and that insufflation is proceeding safely. A separate switch is

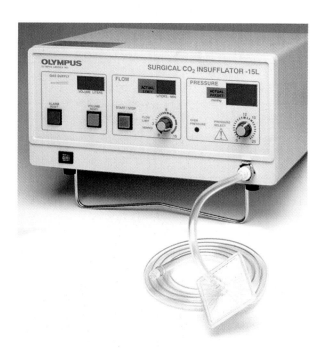

Fig. 9-52 Laparoscopic insufflator with a gas filter. (Courtesy Olympus America, Melville, N.Y.)

used to deliver the gas from the tank into the storage gas cylinder within the insufflator device. An indicator is therefore needed to show how much gas is available in the insufflator and ensure that an adequate amount is provided for the procedure.

The volume delivered must be monitored to determine the amount of gas that has actually been used to develop the pneumoperitoneum. Usually more gas is needed for larger adults and less for smaller patients. As more ports are established for access, more leakage can occur and more gas is needed.

The intraabdominal pressure monitoring system is necessary to determine the pressure of the gas at the end of the Veress needle. This reading can show whether the gas is flowing appropriately or whether clogging or overinsufflation has occurred. Monitors warn the operative team if overpressurization is occurring or other insufflation variables are not being met. An audible alarm also sounds, alerting the team to a potential problem that must be handled immediately. This control feature is extremely important in pediatric laparoscopy and in procedures being performed in patients in critical or compromised conditions.

A continual low-pressure reading may indicate that there is a leak in the line, the gas tank is empty, or the connections are not secure.

Some insufflators have an automatic mechanism that causes any gas that leaks out during the procedure to be continually replaced. However, proper functioning of this control must be monitored closely so that overpressurization does not occur. In addition, two older insufflator units should not be used in a patient in the hope of providing faster insufflation, because the pressure readings cannot accurately reflect the amount of intraabdominal pressure achieved. Insufflators are also not designed to work in tandem. The solution to this problem is to invest in a later-model high-flow insufflator.

Shutoff valves are recommended as a safety measure to immediately shut off the gas. Other shutoff valves that can interrupt the flow of gas are located on the Veress needle and on the trocar/cannula (Fig. 9-53). These controls permit the surgeon to regulate the flow throughout the endoscopic procedure. Most insufflators are designed to stop the flow of gas automatically when a predetermined pressure limit has been met or exceeded.

Because hypothermia can become a problem, especially during prolonged laparoscopic procedures, heating of the insufflation gas is recommended. This is essential for pediatric and debilitated patients. Special heating units can be used for this purpose.

Insufflation Gases

CO_2 is the most commonly used insufflation gas. The signs and symptoms of CO_2 toxicity must be recognized early to prevent untoward effects. Intraoperative blood gas levels should be checked, especially during prolonged laparoscopic procedures, because the incidence of CO_2 toxicity is greatest in patients undergoing these procedures. Following are the signs and symptoms of CO_2 toxicity:

- Respiratory acidosis
- Acid-base imbalances
- Hypertension or hypotension
- Gastric distention

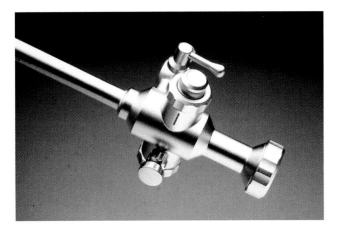

Fig. 9-53 A shutoff valve on the side of the trocar/cannula interrupts the flow of gas during insufflation. (Courtesy Aesculap, Inc., South San Francisco, Calif.)

- Confusion
- Irritability
- Electrolyte imbalances
- Nausea and vomiting

It is important to interpret the blood gas results, recognize the signs and symptoms of acid-base imbalance, and make sure the staff is aware of the potential for CO_2 toxicity, especially during long procedures. Some of nursing measures used to treat these symptoms include:

- Assisting the patient with ventilation
- Elevating the patient's head
- Instructing the patient to deep breathe and cough to improve ventilation
- Assisting the anesthesia provider with treatment measures

Insufflation during laparoscopy may introduce foreign matter or pathogens into the sterile site, but these usually do not originate with the gas but with the gas cylinder that holds the CO_2. CO_2 gas has been shown to be contaminated with iron, copper, metal filings, rust particles, molybdenum, and chromium (Ott, 1991). Particle matter contamination is not a problem when stainless steel tanks are used because rust cannot form on them.

Bacterial colonization has also been discovered in the insufflator itself (Ott, 1991). Organisms such as *Klebsiella, Pseudomonas,* and *Staphylococcus aureus* can be introduced into the patient in this way (Meeker and Rothrock, 1995).

A single-use hydrophobic filter that is impervious to fluids should be used to prevent insufflation gas contamination (see Fig. 9-52). The filter should be changed before each procedure because contamination on the filter cannot be visually assessed. Changing filters not only ensures proper filtering of the gas but also prevents cross-contamination between patients.

Sometimes substitute gases are considered if a CO_2 cylinder becomes empty during a procedure. Because oxygen is readily available in the operating room, it may appear to be a convenient alternative. However, oxygen should never be used as an insufflation gas because it readily supports combustion. The use of an electrosurgical device or laser during laparoscopy would then place the patient at very high risk. The use of oxygen or room air also increases the risk of embolism formation.

In the past, nitrous oxide was used successfully as an insufflation medium. It is inexpensive and rapidly absorbed and eliminated. However, its use for insufflation has also been discouraged lately, because a nitrous oxide pneumoperitoneum is combustible if a significant level of hydrogen or methane is present. Advocates of the use of nitrous oxide maintain that the likelihood of the two gases combining and causing combustion is very remote. It would take an additional 125 liters of 100% hydrogen or methane to make combustion possible in the

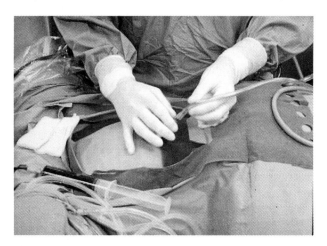

Fig. 9-54 After proper insertion and placement of the Veress needle, the insufflation gas tubing is connected to the port. (Courtesy InnerDyne, Inc., Sunnyvale, Calif.)

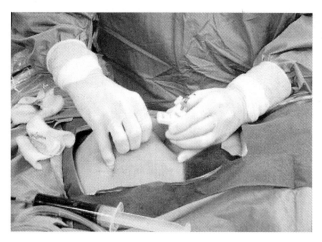

Fig. 9-55 The abdominal wall can be grasped on each side of the Veress needle to facilitate insufflation. (Courtesy InnerDyne, Inc., Sunnyvale, Calif.)

presence of a typical 3-liter pneumoperitoneum. Improperly prepared bowels can release significant amounts of hydrogen during surgery, but it is not known whether this would be enough to support combustion.

Opponents of the use of nitrous oxide as an insufflation gas state that postoperative pain is greater in patients in whom it is used. Sometimes this postoperative pain is caused by the residual gas as it dissolves. There is also concern that the embolism risk may be higher in patients who receive nitrous oxide than in those who receive CO_2 (*Laparosc Surg Update*, 1995b).

Because the use of nitrous oxide has been discouraged due to its proposed combustibility, an animal study was conducted to determine whether an ultrasonic scalpel could be used in a nitrous oxide environment instead of the laser or electrocautery. It was found that the ultrasonic scalpel generated temperatures of less than 100°C, meaning that the scalpel is less likely than the other tools to cause combustion. It was concluded from this that nitrous oxide can be used safely in conjunction with the ultrasonic scalpel (*Laparosc Surg Update*, 1994e).

Even argon gas has been tried as an insufflation gas. A study in which this gas was used to distend the abdominal cavity showed that discomfort was minimal postoperatively. Other advantages to using argon gas are that it can be used with existing insufflators, it is not flammable, it does not cool the body tissues as CO_2 or nitrous oxide do, it is inexpensive, and it can be obtained easily (*Laparosc Surg Update*, 1994a). More studies need to be done, however, to validate the benefits from using argon gas for insufflation.

Art of Insufflation

After the Veress needle is inserted and its proper position has been determined, the insufflation tubing is at-

tached to the needle's port (Fig. 9-54). (See also Chapter 7 for detailed information about needle placement.) A flow rate of 1 L/min is used initially to establish the pneumoperitoneum and then this is increased to more than 9 L/min to maintain the distention. The slow initial flow rate is used to allow time to determine proper needle placement and to identify any subcutaneous emphysema or respiratory problems that could become serious. A high initial flow rate could rapidly aggravate any ensuing problems. Once the flow of insufflation gas is proceeding, a high-pressure reading may be encountered, which may be caused by a kink in the tubing or a blocked valve. Sometimes this problem can be eliminated by gently shaking the patient's abdomen from side to side, which moves the needle tip away from a structure it is abutting against and that is causing the gas flow to be restricted. If this technique fails, then the abdominal wall on either side of the Veress needle can be grasped using towel clips or the operator's fingers and then elevated to allow the viscera to fall away from the wall (Fig. 9-55). If this measure fails also, then the needle should be withdrawn and inserted elsewhere.

After initial insufflation has been achieved, the Veress needle is removed (Fig. 9-56) and the trocar is inserted. Sometimes a surgeon temporarily increases the pressure in the lower abdomen by gently pressing on the epigastrium. This increased pressure pushes the peritoneum tightly against the abdominal wall, making it rigid and thus easier to puncture and allowing for safer insertion of the trocar. The increased pressure also may cause the bowel to be compressed, thus reducing the risk of bowel injury during insertion.

After placement, the deflation valve should be depressed to ensure that the gas can flow freely through the trocar. If blood or intestinal contents come out the

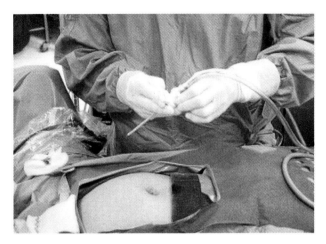

Fig. 9-56 The Veress needle is removed after a pneumoperitoneum has been achieved. (Courtesy InnerDyne, Inc., Sunnyvale, Calif.)

trocar/cannula site or no rush of gas is heard, this indicates a possible problem with trocar placement.

As already mentioned, a flow rate of 9 L/min is usually required to maintain the pneumoperitoneum, but because multiple ports are often needed for the performance of today's laparoscopic procedures, the flow rate may be increased to 15 to 20 L/min to maintain insufflation (Fig. 9-57).

The insufflation pressure for an adult is usually 14 to 16 mm Hg (Meeker and Rothrock, 1995). Intraabdominal pressures of more than 16 mm Hg should be avoided to minimize complications, such as hypocapnia, increased pulmonary pressure, cardiac arrhythmias, increased peritoneal stretching, decreased venous return or bradycardia, vagal collapse, and even cardiac arrest. The surgical team should therefore be aware of

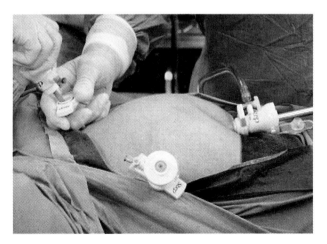

Fig. 9-57 The insufflation flow rate may have to be increased when multiple ports are used during laparoscopy. (Courtesy InnerDyne, Inc., Sunnyvale, Calif.)

and watch for the cardiovascular and respiratory changes that can occur with insufflation.

Overpressurization during the procedure can become hazardous to the patient. For example, excess pressure can force the CO_2 into the patient's bloodstream, causing hypercapnia. This can be detected through end-tidal CO_2 monitoring. Excess pressure can also increase pressure on the diaphragm, which could result in regurgitation and even aspiration of the stomach contents. In addition, it can affect the respiratory effort and cardiac output. If an injury occurs during the laparoscopic procedure and, as a result, gas is being instilled into the bowel or stomach, then flatulence or eructation may occur. If the CO_2 is accidentally introduced into the liver or vena cava, then an unusual heart murmur may be noticed. This problem must be dealt with immediately because it could lead to the formation of an embolism that could be fatal.

If the pneumoperitoneum is difficult to maintain during the procedure, then the connections, fittings, reducers, and trocar valves should be checked to make sure all are functioning properly. If, on the other hand, high pressure is noted during the procedure, then this may be due to the fact that the patient is starting to wake up. The anesthesiologist or nurse anesthetist can easily rectify this problem.

At the completion of the laparoscopic procedure, the CO_2 must be expelled from the abdomen. Ideally this should be done with a low-flow evacuator to provide a closed system. Otherwise pathologic contamination, such as with HIV-contaminated blood, could occur as the result of exposure to the aerosol or splatter released. To begin with, the main trocar is left in place with the valve open to expel as much gas as possible. The trocar is then grasped with one hand and pointed toward the pelvis while the lower abdominal wall is pulled up, drawing in room air to dilute the CO_2. Then the abdomen is gently depressed downward to expel more gas. This is done several times to try to dilute and expel the CO_2. This technique often causes postoperative pain to be reduced, especially the shoulder and neck pain that is so common after laparoscopic procedures and that results from the CO_2 irritating the phrenic nerve.

At the end of the laparoscopic procedure, while the pneumoperitoneum is being decreased, male patients should be assessed to determine if there is any testicular swelling. If swelling is noted, then gentle pressure should be applied on the testes to prevent any further gas escape into this area. Testicular swelling after laparoscopy will slowly disappear without treatment, but it often is very alarming to the patient and family.

Some professionals advocate using a less expensive system similar to the peritoneal lavage technique to develop the pneumoperitoneum instead of using the

Veress needle technique. This involves inserting a small-gauge needle with a catheter sheath to carry the gas. Insufflation can be accomplished with this method. Because the needle is smaller, the risk of injury is less, making this a valuable method for trauma patients. If blood is detected, then peritoneal lavage can be performed employing the same needle/catheter system used to introduce the gas for laparoscopy. This setup is more difficult to use in obese patients, however. Many surgeons do not use this technique because they are not familiar with it.

It has become a matter of debate whether to perform laparoscopy on patients with abdominal organ or tissue cancer. One study showed that laparoscopy should be avoided in patients with colon cancer until more is known about the proper procedure and about the status of tumor growth at the trocar site in the particular patient. One animal study showed that the pneumoperitoneum caused tumor implantation at the trocar site to be increased by three times (*Laparosc Surg Update*, 1995a).

Troubleshooting Insufflation Problems

Insufflators are not very complex, so problems with them can usually be readily assessed and remedied. Some of the typical problems are given in Box 9-1, along with questions to be answered that can lead to the solution (*Laparosc Surg Update*, 1994c).

IRRIGATION/ASPIRATION SYSTEMS

Irrigation/aspiration systems are used to administer irrigation solution and aspirate fluids and surgical smoke. There are many different systems available today that are versatile and have added features to meet the irrigation-suction needs that arise during endoscopic procedures.

Irrigation is extremely important to enhance visualization during endoscopy, because it is not easy to directly swab the tissue as it is in open procedures. Irrigation is accomplished by means of irrigation channels built into endoscopes, irrigation instruments inserted through the endoscope operating channel, or an irrigation probe inserted into a secondary trocar site.

Irrigation solution can be delivered manually during the endoscopy via a syringe hooked to the irrigation port. An irrigation bag attached to the port with irrigation tubing can also be used to deliver irrigation fluid.

The flow of the irrigant is achieved through gravitational pull, or the fluid can be delivered using a pressure bag to increase the flow. An external irrigation pump may also be used to provide high-flow irrigation, the pressure controlled by an adjustment switch (Figs. 9-58

Box 9-1	*Troubleshooting problems with insufflation*

PROBLEM: The insufflation gas is not flowing.
- Has the flow rate been set?
- Is the insufflation tubing kinked or twisted?
- Is the stopcock open on the Veress needle?
- After switching the tubing to the cannula, is the Luer lock partially closed?
- Has the tubing been obstructed with a clip used to secure it onto the drapes?
- Is the CO_2 gas tank turned on?
- Is the CO_2 tank empty? (At least two full tanks should be available before a laparoscopic procedure is started.)
- Is the insufflator turned on?
- If using a separate tube to monitor the pressure, is it connected correctly?

PROBLEM: The gas was flowing and then stopped.
- Has the insufflator been set to automatically disable the output flow in order to maintain a certain pressure?

PROBLEM: The insufflator alarm is sounding.
- Has overpressurization occurred? Is the patient exhibiting signs of overpressurization (i.e., difficulty breathing, heart arrhythmias):
- Is the tubing kinked or twisted, cutting off the gas flow? (A backflow would cause the overpressurization alarm to sound.)

PROBLEM: The insufflator stops working during the procedure.
- Is the gas tank upright?
- Has the power cord been disconnected?

---

and 9-59). The desired flow rate can vary from a constant drip to one that would permit hydrodissection (Fig. 9-60). The irrigation solution may also be delivered in pulsations or in a continual stream.

Irrigation systems are available that are controlled by a CO_2-powered pump or an electrical pump, which creates the force for the flow by inflating a pressure bag. If CO_2 is used, however, the appropriate wrench to open the tank valve must be readily accessible. The tank pressure must also be monitored to ensure that there is enough gas in the tank for the entire endoscopic procedure. In some systems employing an electrical pump, the desired amount of pressure can be set. These systems have bladders that inflate and exert pressure on the solution bag, thus controlling the flow of the irrigant (Fig 9-61).

The normal pressure needed for irrigation is approximately 300 mm Hg. Hydrodissection, used to separate tissue and divide planes, can be accomplished with a pressure of approximately 750 mm Hg. The pressure provided is directly related to the size of the tubing and

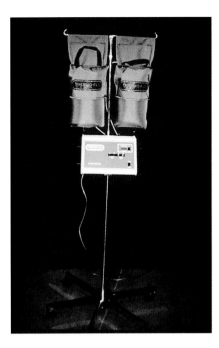

Fig. 9-58 Irrigation pump. (Courtesy Sanese Medical Corp., Columbus, Ohio.)

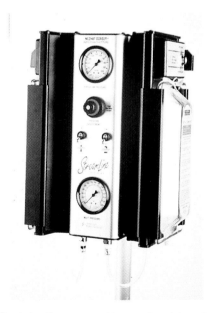

Fig. 9-59 Irrigation pump. (Courtesy Davol, Inc., Cranston, R.I.)

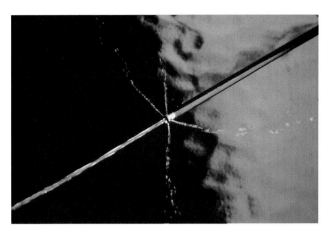

Fig. 9-60 The rate of irrigation flow can vary from a constant drip to one that would permit hydrodissection.

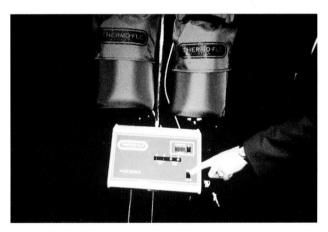

Fig. 9-61 The flow of the solution is controlled by adjusting the pressure in the bags. (Courtesy Sanese Medical Corp., Columbus, Ohio.)

the probe. An irrigation probe is usually 5 mm in diameter. The smaller the diameter of the probe, the more increased is the pressure of the solution flow.

High-flow irrigation systems should have a mechanism that switches from an empty solution bottle or bag to a full bottle or bag without an interruption of flow. Disposable tubing is used to connect the irrigation solution to the irrigation delivery system. Connections must be made using sterile technique so that the inner tubing is not contaminated when the irrigant bag or bottle is punctured. Usually there is a clamp on the tubing, and this should be closed to prevent leakage or spillage while connections are being made. After the system is completely connected, the clamp can be opened to allow irrigant flow.

The distal tubing connects to the irrigation probe or delivery system. The probe can be disposable or reusable and can have different tip configurations (Fig. 9-62). If a reusable probe is used, it must be one that can be easily disassembled for thorough cleaning and reprocessing. The irrigation probe may be used as a suction probe, too.

A trumpet valve may be incorporated into the probe, which allows for both irrigation and suctioning to occur (Fig. 9-63). There are also trumpet valves that attach to existing instrumentation. Following are some of the important features of trumpet valves used for this purpose (Nezhat, et al, 1995).

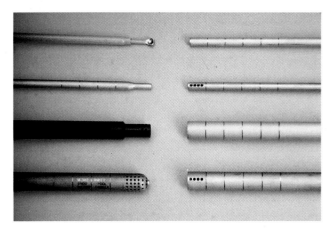

Fig. 9-62 Probe tips are available in different configurations. (Courtesy Davol, Inc., Cranston, R.I.)

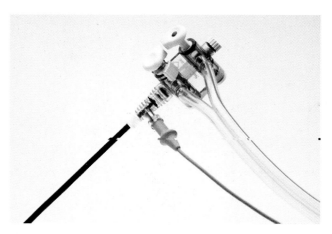

Fig. 9-63 A trumpet valve controls irrigation and suction. (Courtesy Davol, Inc., Cranston, R.I.)

- The valve must be easy to activate and constantly control the flow of irrigation fluid and the suction.
- The valve must have a large enough lumen to accommodate the passage of fluid, blood, and debris and to maintain constant irrigation flow.
- Reusable trumpet valves must be easy to disassemble, clean, and sterilize or disinfect.

Some irrigation systems have monitoring devices that show the amount of solution administered. This helps in determining the amount of fluid absorbed which is done by subtracting the amount of fluid removed from the operative area from the amount delivered.

Irrigation pumps used for arthroscopic procedures may be controlled with a foot switch, which is very convenient for the surgical team because of the large amount of irrigation usually needed during arthroscopies.

Saline is the most popular irrigant, but there are other irrigants that can be used. The decision to use them depends on the surgeon's preferences, the patient's condition, the reason for the irrigation, the surgical tools to be used, the bleeding anticipated, and the cost of the solution.

Many concerns have been raised about the use of conductive irrigation solutions with electrosurgery devices. The passage of electrical current through a conductive irrigant, such as saline, during endoscopy disperses the current over a wide area. Although the current is then being delivered to untargeted tissue, hazards are minimized because the current is dispersed over such a large area. However, this also has the effect of diminishing the surgical effect of the electrosurgical device, thus requiring an increase in the power from the electrosurgical unit to restore the surgical effect. If this problem is perceived to be significant, one of the more expensive nonconductive irrigants available can be used. However, if a nonconductive irrigant is used,

then resistance between the electrodes may occur, also necessitating the use of more energy.

It is recommended that warmed irrigation solution be used to prevent patient hypothermia and endoscope fogging. Solutions may be prewarmed to about 100°F (37.7°C) and maintained at this temperature by the irrigation system. Some systems do this while the solution is in the irrigation bag; other systems heat the solution while it is in the tubing. However, a disadvantage to the later system is that it may not perform as well should rapid flow of the solution be needed.

SMOKE EVACUATION EQUIPMENT

Smoke evacuation is needed for all endoscopic procedures that produce surgical smoke. Multiple studies have shown that the plume generated by electrosurgery devices is just as hazardous as a laser plume (*Clin Laser Monthly*, 1993). Any surgical smoke must therefore be evacuated adequately to minimize hazards to the surgical team and the patient. In one new advancement, a smoke evacuator system has been combined with an insufflator. (See Chapter 11 for more details on smoke evacuation.)

Smoke Evacuation Methods

An inline suction filter is used to evacuate small amounts of surgical smoke, such as that produced during some laparoscopic procedures. The filter is placed in the suction line between the wall outlet and the suction canister (Fig. 9-64), which collects any fluids as the filter purifies the air. The filter can be used without the canister if solutions are not to be suctioned. If the filter gets wet, however, it will not function effectively.

A smoke evacuator, capable of filtering particulate matter that is larger than 0.1 μm in diameter, is used to remove larger amounts of plume (Fig. 9-65). Usually

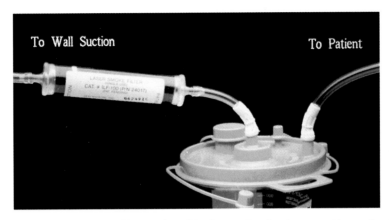

Fig. 9-64 An inline suction filter is placed in the suction line between the wall outlet and the suction canister. (Courtesy Stackhouse Inc., Palm Springs, Calif.)

smoke evacuators have a three-step filtering process involving a prefilter that captures large particles and fluid, an ultra–low penetration air (ULPA) filter, and a charcoal filter (Fig. 9-66).

The smoke evacuator should have a ULPA filter that can capture 0.1-μm particulate matter at a flow rate of 30 cubic feet per minute and that is 99.9999% efficient. High-efficiency particulate air (HEPA) filters that are sometimes found in smoke evacuators have a filter rating of 0.3 μm and an efficiency rating of 99.97% (Ball, 1995).

ULPA or HEPA filters are usually made of a maze of glass or thermal plastic fibers. This medium forms a tortuous path that entangles particulate matter within the mesh (Fig. 9-67). Filtering occurs in three different ways as the particles come in contact with the mesh (Ball, 1995):
1. Direct interception: Particles larger than 1 μm are captured by the filtering media (Fig. 9-68).
2. Inertial impaction: Particles that are 0.5 to 1.0 μm collide with the fibers and are held at the point of collision (Fig. 9-69).
3. Diffusional interception: Particles that are less than 0.5 microns are captured through the effects of brownian motion or random thermal motion (Fig. 9-70).

Particulate matter that is 0.12 μm is the most difficult to capture because it can slip through the filtering mesh and is not small enough to exhibit brownian motion. This particle matter is known as the *most penetrating particle* (MPP) (Stackhouse, 1992).

Charcoal filters made from activated virgin coconut shells have been found to be the most effective for removing the offensive odor caused by toxic gases in the surgical smoke (Stackhouse, 1992), because coconut-based charcoal has more absorptive capabilities than wood-based charcoal.

Special chemicals are used in some smoke evacuators to treat the plume as it moves through the filtering system. It has been theorized that this can help reduce the carcinogenic and mutagenic elements in laser and electrosurgical smoke.

Smoke evacuator filters must be changed according to the manufacturer's recommendations. Some smoke evacuator systems have an indicator light that is activated when a filter needs to be changed. Once a filter is contaminated, it should never be left on the smoke evacuator for later changing because the odor from a contaminated filter can travel into the smoke evacuator, causing the internal components of the unit to absorb the offensive smell. Gloves should be worn while the filter is changed to minimize the risk to the health care worker. The contaminated filter should then be placed

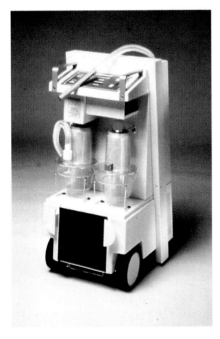

Fig. 9-65 A smoke evacuator should be used if a plume is visible. (Courtesy Stackhouse Inc., Palm Springs, Calif.)

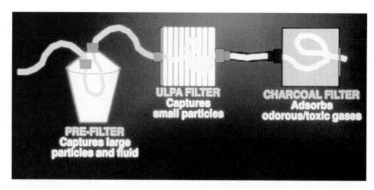

Fig. 9-66 Smoke evacuation may involve a three-step process. (Courtesy Stackhouse Inc., Palm Springs, Calif.)

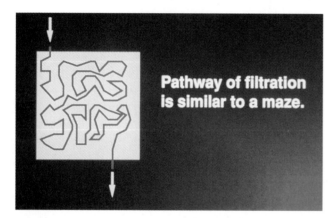

Fig. 9-67 The medium in a smoke evacuator filter forms a tortuous path that entangles particulate matter within the mesh. (Courtesy Stackhouse Inc., Palm Springs, Calif.)

in a plastic bag and discarded in the general hospital waste. Research has not conclusively shown that there is a need to treat a contaminated filter as infectious or regulated medical waste.

Selecting a Smoke Evacuator

Several factors should be taken into consideration when selecting a smoke evacuator, including (Ball, 1995):
- Filtering capacity
- Size
- Noise level
- Portability
- Air movement or suction capability
- Reliability and ease of use
- Cost
- Maintenance requirements
- Cost of supplies

The rate of air movement, or flow rate, produced by the smoke evacuator is very important, because it often determines the effectiveness of the unit. Using a wall vacuum, fluid can be aspirated through ¼-inch (0.6-cm) tubing at a rate of approximately 2 cubic feet per minute, whereas a smoke evacuator can move plume through ⅞-inch (2.2-cm) tubing at about 50 cubic feet per minute. This illustrates the importance of using wall suction with an inline filter to evacuate only small amounts of surgical smoke.

Surgical Team Responsibilities

The surgical team has many different responsibilities with regard to ensuring that surgical smoke is eliminated. Proper positioning of the smoke wand, the appropriate use of high-filtration surgical masks, and ensuring that the plume is removed during endoscopic procedures are some of these obligations.

To be effective, the smoke evacuation suction tip or probe must be held as close as possible to the site where the plume is being generated. Research has shown that, as the smoke evacuation wand is moved away from the site of origin, more plume is allowed to escape into the air. Approximately 98% of the smoke is removed if the wand is held within 1 cm of the plume generation site. If the wand is held 2 cm from the site, the efficiency of smoke evacuation is decreased to 51% (Mihashi, et al, 1975).

Surgical masks should never be worn in lieu of using a smoke evacuator, though high-flow surgical masks can be worn to protect against unevacuated plume that may not have been captured by the evacuator.

Smoke poisoning may occur if smoke evacuation is not adequate during endoscopic procedures. Dr. Doug Ott conducted research into the effects of laser and electrosurgical smoke released during laparoscopic procedures and found that intraabdominal smoke caused an increase in the patient's levels of methemoglobin and carboxyhemoglobin (resulting from the smoke's carbon monoxide content). Anesthesia monitoring devices such as pulse oximeters did not detect this increase, but intraoperative blood gas results showed changes in the patient's oxygen saturation. This study also showed that the problems stemming from exposure to an unevacuated plume were similar to those experienced by people who smoke eight to nine cigarettes within 90 minutes to

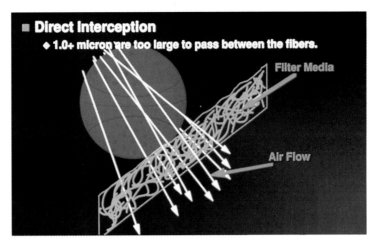

Fig. 9-68   Direct interception. (Courtesy Stackhouse Inc., Palm Springs, Calif.)

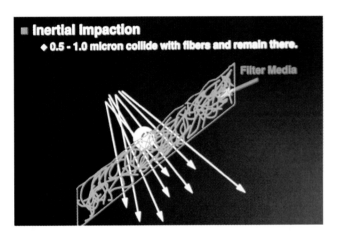

Fig. 9-69   Inertial impaction. (Courtesy Stackhouse Inc., Palm Springs, Calif.)

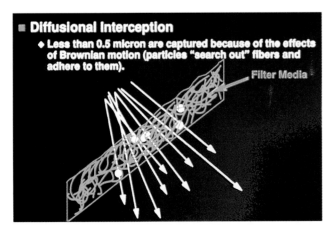

Fig. 9-70   Diffusional interception. (Courtesy Stackhouse Inc., Palm Springs, Calif.)

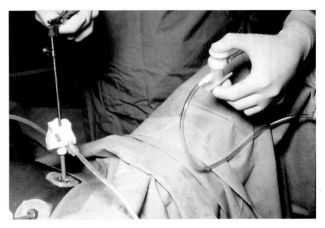

Fig. 9-71   A low-pressure suction valve can be used to provide gentle movement of the insufflation gas to remove the surgical smoke.

2 hours. Ott theorized that postoperative complications such as nausea and headaches may result from acute smoke poisoning. He also stated that proper evacuation during laparoscopy can remove 98% of the plume and should be performed to minimize patient complications (*Laparosc Surg Update*, 1994d).

The intraabdominal smoke produced during laparoscopy can be evacuated using a low-pressure suction valve that gently removes the plume without destroying the pneumoperitoneum (Fig. 9-71). A high-flow, "on demand" insufflator should also be available to replace the insufflation gas as it is evacuated.

OTHER EQUIPMENT

Other equipment that may be used during endoscopic procedures include the laser, electrosurgery unit, argon-enhanced electrosurgical equipment, ultrasonic devices, cryosurgery units, and diagnositc equipment.

These devices produce energies that may be used in the performance of either operative or diagnostic procedures. They are discussed in detail in Chapter 11.

ROOM SETUP

A surgical room must be selected that can accommodate all of the endoscopic equipment and provide enough space to deliver safe patient care. A study showed that laparoscopic procedures involve the use of 17% more furniture, 40% more equipment, and 35% more cables or tubes than open procedures (*Laparosc Surg Update*, 1994b). Because the presence of these devices can impair the movement of the surgical team, clutter needs to be reduced. Preplanning is therefore vital to ensure that equipment and devices are properly arranged. The perioperative nurse may even draw a schematic for use as a guide (Fig. 9-72).

An electric operating table is most desirable so that the patient can be placed in the different positions required for visualization, patient comfort, and safety. Foot controls that move the table facilitate positioning and are more convenient for the surgical team.

Because most endoscopic physicians use video technology to perform sophisticated techniques, usually two monitors are preferred. Regardless of the number of monitors used, they must all be strategically placed to ensure that the entire surgical team can view the procedure and better anticipate the surgical needs (Fig. 9-73).

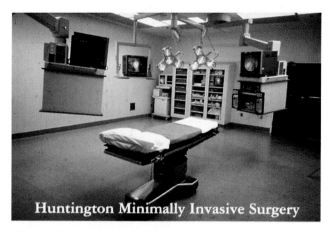

Fig. 9-73 Three monitors are strategically placed so that the entire surgical team can see the video image. (Courtesy Dr. David Lourie and Huntington Minimally Invasive Surgery, Pasadena, Calif.)

Advocates of using only one monitor often describe their setup as being more simplistic and easy to arrange.

Often the single-monitor setup is all that is available to the surgical team. If a single-monitor setup is used, the monitor may be placed over the patient's head for upper abdominal procedures or near the patient's feet for lower abdominal procedures. The team is then positioned according to where the monitor is placed and the anesthesia provider is sitting. The monitor can be placed on a cart or suspended from the ceiling. If a cart is used, then there must be enough room for the anesthesia provider to operate safely and monitor the patient easily.

The monitor is placed at eye level or just slightly higher so that the image can be easily seen (Fig. 9-74). If only one monitor is used, extra-long cords are needed so that the monitor can be moved to allow members of the team to have access to the patient's head or feet areas.

If two monitors are used, then usually a monitor is placed on either side of the patient. Ideally the monitors should be similar so that the surgical team sees the same-quality image as they look from one monitor to the other while changing positions during the procedure. In either a one- or two-monitor setup, there should be a backup monitor should a monitor fail.

Storage cabinets are used to keep video and endoscopic equipment within limited spaces. Locking cabinets are also being designed to prevent the theft of expensive video equipment. Multiple devices are housed in one mobile cart so that the cart can be easily moved from one place to another so endoscopy is not confined to one area or room (Fig. 9-75).

Cabinetry design so the stacking of video and needed endoscopic equipment minimizes the number of cords and cables seen, because the system is configured to allow for easy connection and operation.

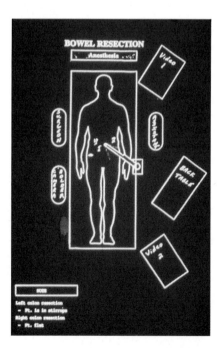

Fig. 9-72 A schematic drawing can be made to determine the proper positioning of the endoscopic team members and the equipment. (Courtesy Origin Medsystems, Menlo Park, Calif.)

Power strips are used to plug in the various equipment pieces so that only one connection must be made to power the entire system. Nurses must remember to turn the power switch on for all the equipment to work, however.

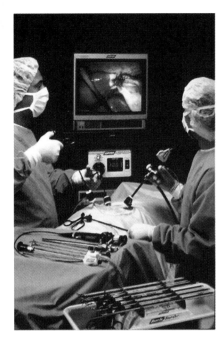

Fig. 9-74   The monitor is placed at eye level or just slightly higher so that the image can be easily seen. (Courtesy Circon Corp., Santa Barbara, Calif.)

Articulating arms can also be used to suspended monitors and other equipment from the ceiling (Fig. 9-76). This eliminates the number of power cords and cables on the floor and also allows more direct access to the patient than that afforded by a cart that takes up floor space. Suspension arms should be able to be moved or swiveled easily for proper viewing of the monitor. However, the surgical team must be very aware of the articulating arms to avoid injuring themselves. The corners of the overhead suspension devices can be padded to prevent such injuries.

Once the monitors and other devices are in place, the proper connections between the equipment must be made to ensure that all systems work. The connections between the main pieces of equipment are usually already done, so reconnection is not necessary for each procedure. The basic wiring configuration can be diagrammed for reference by the surgical team members.

ROOM DESIGN

New endoscopy suites are being designed that consist of at least 24 × 24 feet (7 × 7 meters) of floor space to ensure the accommodation of continually advancing equipment. There also should be a 15- to 16-foot (4.5- to 5-meter) ceiling height to allow for construction of a dropped ceiling to accommodate electrical wiring, video cables, and suspension arms. The electrical cords should

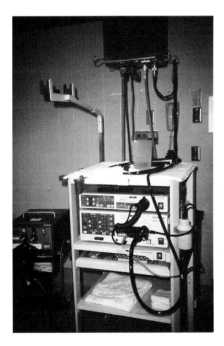

Fig. 9-75   Storage cart for video equipment.

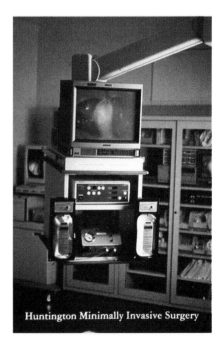

Fig. 9-76   A monitor can be suspended from the ceiling so that the monitor does not have to be placed on a cart. (Courtesy Dr. David Lourie and Huntington Minimally Invasive Surgery, Pasadena, Calif.)

drop from the ceilings to prevent physical hazards for the endoscopic team (Gruendemann and Fernsebner, 1995). The electrical system in each endoscopy suite also should be isolated so interference from other rooms is prevented. Multiple electrical outlets must be provided to accommodate the large number of electrical devices needed in this high-tech environment. If lasers are to be used, then the appropriate electrical connections must be installed. If it is anticipated that radiographic examinations will be performed during endoscopic procedures, then the appropriate high-voltage connections must be placed and the walls of the room lead lined.

A rheostat should be installed to the overhead lights so they can be dimmed during the endoscopic procedure. There must be adequate lighting for the anesthesia personnel when the lights are dimmed.

Endoscopy rooms should each be provided with their own temperature control panel so that each can be made warmer or cooler depending on the patient's and endoscopy team's needs. Usually the endoscopy room should be maintained at 70° to 75°F (21.1° to 23.9°C) to provide comfort and reduce the metabolic demands on the patients (Meeker and Rothrock, 1995). It must also be possible to control the humidity. The relative humidity should be between 50% and 60% to suppress static electricity and reduce bacterial and other pathogen growth (Meeker and Rothrock, 1995).

The doors to the endoscopy room must be wide enough to accommodate the patient and equipment. If a minimally invasive suite for the performance of simple endoscopic procedures is being planned, even though most patients are expected to be able to walk into the room, the doorway must still be wide enough to accommodate those brought in by wheelchair or those on a transportation cart. For example a patient from a nursing home may be transported to the endoscopy suite on a cart, or a patient may experience complications that require him or her be hospitalized and a transportation cart is needed to move the patient out of the endoscopy room.

If state law permits drains in surgical areas, then a drain may be desirable for rooms where cystoscopy or arthroscopy is to be performed. Any overflow or excess solutions can then be directed to this drain to prevent spillage on the floors. The drain should be cleaned regularly and covered when not being used.

Any storage rooms must have enough space for large pieces of equipment that may not be used during every procedure. The doorway to this room must be wide and high enough to accommodate these larger pieces of equipment, such as lasers. Electrical outlets also should be installed in the storage area so battery-operated devices can be recharged during storage.

ROBOTICS

New advancements in endoscopic equipment are continually changing the way in which procedures are performed. Robotics constitutes one of these areas, and robotic devices are being introduced to minimize some of the more common problems experienced during endoscopic procedures, such as laparoscopy.

One new robotic device used for laparoscopy, called *AESOP* (automated endoscopic system for optimal positioning), has received a lot of attention lately (Fig. 9-77). AESOP was developed to help minimize problems with shaky video images, miscommunication between the surgeon and the assistant, and fogged or dirty scope lenses resulting from inadvertent contact with tissue (*Minimally Invasive Surg Nurs*, 1994). This device is designed to hold and manipulate the laparoscope under the physician's direct control. The robot's movement can be controlled by foot pedals (Fig. 9-78), a hand-held control (Fig. 9-79), or voice activation.

This robotic device was not created to replace staff members, however, but to free up surgical team members to perform other roles and responsibilities. AESOP was designed to facilitate the laparoscopic procedure, promote safety, and minimize the time needed to perform the procedure.

AESOP, which has been approved by the FDA, consists of several components. The chassis houses the power system and the control computer (Fig. 9-80). The

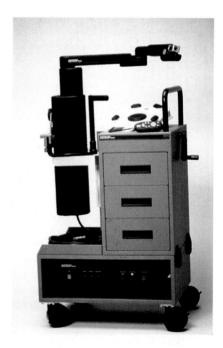

Fig. 9-77 Robotics can be used to hold and maneuver an endoscope. (Courtesy Computer Motion, Goleta, Calif.)

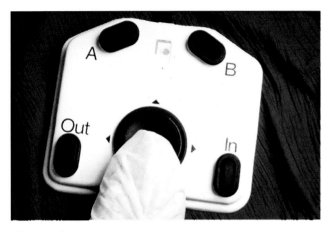

Fig. 9-78   Robotic foot control pad. (Courtesy Computer Motion, Goleta, Calif.)

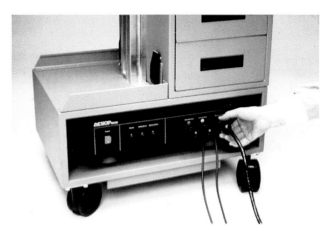

Fig. 9-80   The robotic chassis or controller houses the computer that translates the physician's commands into robotic arm movements. (Courtesy Computer Motion, Goleta, Calif.)

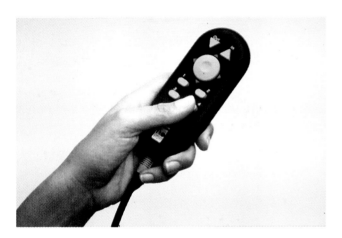

Fig. 9-79   Robotic hand control unit. (Courtesy Computer Motion, Goleta, Calif.)

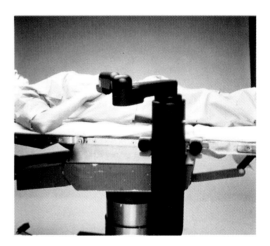

Fig. 9-81   The robotic positioning arm attaches to the surgical table rail. (Courtesy Computer Motion, Goleta, Calif.)

positioner includes the electromechanical device that attaches to the surgical table rail (Fig. 9-81) and connects to the laparoscope with a magnetic coupling device (Fig. 9-82). The control system allows the operator to move the arm for exact laparoscope positioning (Fig. 9-83) and can move the laparoscope quickly or slowly in any direction. A memory feature stores different position coordinates and can quickly restore the laparoscope to a desired preset location. AESOP keeps the laparoscope oriented correctly, which has been a problem with manual holding. For example, if an assistant accidentally turns the scope around, then the anatomy appears upside down.

The fatigue that accrues during long periods of holding and maneuvering the scope has been a concern of surgical team members over the years. Many nurses, physicians, and technologists have been thankful to be relieved of the task of holding the scope. By allowing the

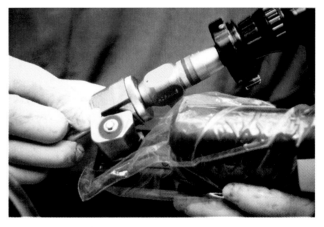

Fig. 9-82   The laparoscope is attached to the robotic positioning arm with a magnetic coupling device, known as a *collar*. (Courtesy Computer Motion, Goleta, Calif.)

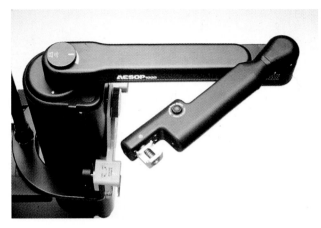

Fig. 9-83   The robotic arm is designed to move the laparoscope in different directions. (Courtesy Computer Motion, Goleta, Calif.)

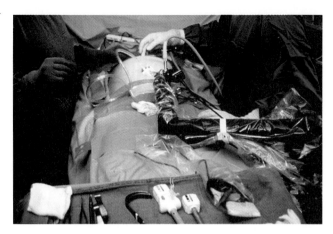

Fig. 9-85   The robotic arm ensures consistent endoscope movement and positioning. (Courtesy Computer Motion, Goleta, Calif.)

physician to remotely control scope movement, the physician can visualize the exact area he or she wants to see (Fig. 9-84). This also has the advantage of preventing miscommunication and arguments among surgical team members.

The following list describes some of the advantages to using a robotic device for endoscope positioning:

- Eliminates the fatigue associated with endoscope holding.
- Minimizes miscommunication between the surgeon and the assistant and frustration on the part of both.
- Returns control of the scope to the surgeon.
- Remembers key locations for immediate scope position changes.
- May shorten the procedure time by eliminating the need to spend extra time on scope positioning.

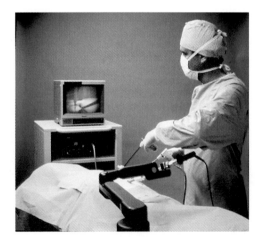

Fig. 9-84   By being able to command the movement of the robotic arm, the surgeon has complete control over laparoscope positioning. (Courtesy Computer Motion, Goleta, Calif.)

- Minimizes the need to remove the scope from the body to clean the lens because inadvertent tissue contact is prevented.
- Enhances the video quality, because unsteady image and video drift is eliminated. This is extremely important if videoconferencing is being done because the image is then being transmitted to another site.
- Provides consistent scope positioning and movement during all hours of the day (Fig. 9-85).
- Ensures the same level of care for every patient.
- Decreases the likelihood of converting the laparoscopic procedure to an open procedure, necessitated by the inexperience or lack of skill of the assistant assigned to hold the scope.
- Frees the physician's hands to perform a more efficient procedure.
- Encourages physicians to attempt more complicated endoscopic procedures.
- Improves staffing efficiency and controls costs.
- Enhances the surgery suite's image as offering the latest in health care technology.

REFERENCES

Ball KA: *Lasers: the perioperative challenge*, ed 2, St. Louis, 1995, Mosby.

Clin Laser Monthly: Use smoke evacuators during electrosurgery, laser procedures, March 1993, p 36.

Frantzides CT: *Laparoscopic and thoracoscopic surgery*, St. Louis, 1995, Mosby, p 3.

Gruendemann BJ, Fernsebner B: *Comprehensive perioperative nursing*, vol 2, practice, Boston, 1995, Jones and Bartlett.

The hazards of surgical smoke (video), Riverside, Calif., 1992, Stackhouse.

Laparosc Surg Update: Insufflation causes fatal gas embolism, 1(10):118,1993.

Laparosc Surg Update: Argon gas used for distention with less postoperative pain, 2(2):21, 1994a.

Laparosc Surg Update: It's true: laparoscopy ORs are more cluttered than others, 3(4):44, 1994b.

Laparosc Surg Update: Solving insufflator problems, 2(9):100, 1994c.

Laparosc Surg Update: Smoke in pneumoperitoneum may be more dangerous than you think, 2(10):118, 1994d.

Laparosc Surg Update: Ultrasonic scalpel safe with nitrous oxide insufflation, 2(10):116, 1994e.

Laparosc Surg Update: Does insufflation spread colon cancer cells? 3(8):94, 1995a.

Laparosc Surg Update: End of ban on nitrous oxide insufflation advocated, 3(8):91, 1995b.

McCracken JE: Endoscopy reveals debris, fluid, and damage in patient-ready GI endoscopes, *Infect Control Steril Technol* 1(6):32, 1995.

Meeker MH, Rothrock JC: *Alexander's care of the patient in surgery*, ed 10, St. Louis, 1995, Mosby.

Mihashi S, et al: Some problems about condensates induced by CO_2 laser irradiation, Department of Otolaryngology and Public Health, Karume University, Karume, Japan, 1975.

Minimally Invasive Surg Nurs: Robotic arm returns direct scope control to surgeon, 8(3):87, 1994.

Molloy D: The diagnostic accuracy of a microlaparoscope, *Assoc Gynecol Laparoscopists* 2(2):203, 1995.

Nezhat CR, Nezhat FR, Luciano AA, et al: *Operative gynecologic laparoscopy principles and techniques*, New York, 1995, McGraw-Hill.

Ott D: Contamination via gynecological endoscopy insufflation. *Gynecol Surg*, 5:2, 1991.

Soderstrom RM: Laparoscopic sterilization: equipment and procedures. In Zatuchni GI, Daly JJ, Sciarra JJ (eds): *Gynecology and obstetrics*, vol 6, Philadelphia, 1986 Harper & Row.

Spellman JR: Laparoscopic equipment troubleshooting, *Today's OR Nurse*, 17(1):19, 1995.

Stengel JM, Dirado R: Laparoscopic Nissen fundoplication to treat gastroesophageal reflux, *AORN J* 61(3):483, 1995.

White RA, Klein SR: *Endoscopic surgery*, St. Louis, 1991, Mosby.

Video Technology

By coupling video technology with endoscopy equipment, it is now possible for an image of what is happening at the end of the endoscope to be displayed on a monitor for the entire surgical team to see. A video system takes light signals of the target, converts them into electricity, and converts them back into light energy to generate a picture on the monitor. A video system basically consists of a camera, monitor, and ancillary components.

VIDEO CAMERA

Evolution of Cameras

Before cameras were used during endoscopy, assistants used eyepiece extensions to obtain a view similar to the surgeon's. This extension was connected to the head of the endoscope and the image went through a beam splitter, which unfortunately reduced the image quality. Often the endoscope images were also not identical as the result of lighting and optical lens problems, thus causing frustration for the surgeon and assistant.

Tube-style cameras were introduced in the 1960s and provided an image that the entire surgical team could observe on a monitor screen (Fig. 10-1), but these tubes were bulky and heavy and were soon replaced with lightweight small-chip cameras. With these advents, video-guided endoscopy suddenly became very popular because it allowed direct visualization, enhanced participation by assistants, and afforded greater surgical accuracy.

Camera Technology

The video camera is the most important component of an endoscopic video system. It is attached to the flexible or rigid endoscope and captures the endoscopic image that is displayed on the monitor screen (Fig. 10-2).

Video camera technology was drastically changed in 1975 when the charged coupled device (CCD) was first introduced. A CCD consists of an arrangement of metal oxides or light-sensitive pieces of silicone called *pixels*, meaning "picture elements." Light is transmitted from the end of the endoscope to the pixels and then the pixels generate electrical impulses or charges proportional to the amount of light that hits the surface of the chip (Fig. 10-3).

The pixels become conductive in the presence of light, and they remain nonconductive in the absence of light. When they are conductive, the charge is transferred into electronic wells cut into the surface of the chip, where they are stored. The CCD then changes the stored charge into an analog signal that is sent to the camera control unit (CCU). The CCU decodes the information and prepares it for output to a video monitor, printer, tape recorder, or other devices. A picture is then generated that is actually a matrix of conductive and nonconductive pixels.

Today's cameras have from one to three chips. A chip is the small silicone wafer on which electronic components are deposited to fabricate circuits.

Single-chip cameras are smaller and lighter, cost less, and are usually more sensitive to light. Using a special filter, they break down the image into red, green, and blue. There is also a stripe filter on the surface of the single chip that allows specific light spectrum colors, such as yellow, cyan, green, and magenta, to pass through. As light enters through the camera, the stripe filter allows

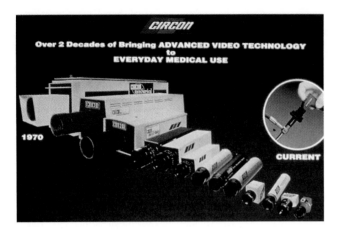

Fig. 10-1 The evolution of medical video cameras. (Courtesy of Circon Corp., Santa Barbara, Calif.)

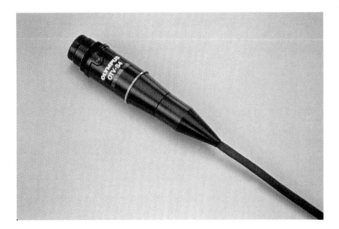

Fig. 10-2 Video camera head designed for both rigid scopes and fiberscopes. (Courtesy Olympus America, Inc., Melville, N.Y.)

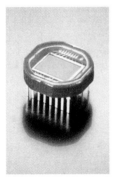

Fig. 10-3 A charged coupled device, which is an arrangement of metal oxides or light-sensitive pieces of silicone called *pixels* that generate electrical impulses to transmit the light signals. (Courtesy Olympus America, Inc., Melville, N.Y.)

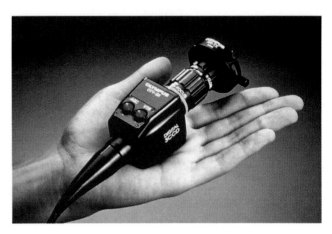

Fig. 10-4 Three-chip camera. (Courtesy Olympus America, Inc., Melville, N.Y.)

only the specified light spectrum colors to activate the pixels. The camera can create shades of color by combining information from the pixels into one image. Advancements in the single-chip camera, such as miniaturizing the pixels and perfecting the types of materials used to produce the CCD, have led to improvements in the image quality.

Newer single-chip cameras are being developed that have digital processors which boost resolution by incorporating three-chip quality into a single chip. The resulting image can be manipulated and enhanced through a processor, thus providing freeze-frame and electronic zoom capabilities.

Three-chip cameras are larger than the one-chip kind but produce better-quality image with enhanced color (Fig. 10-4). Each chip in the three-chip camera is dedicated to one of the primary colors, red, green, or blue. As the light moves into the camera, it passes through a prism block and is evenly distributed among each of the three chips. The electronic information is then passed into the CCU and onto the monitors or printers via the RGB (red, green, blue) system. Colors are created uniformly because the three signals are kept separate throughout the routing inside the camera (Fig. 10-5). Three-chip cameras and CCUs are becoming more compact but provide the same professional video image quality and performance (Fig. 10-6).

Lines of resolution are often used to judge the quality of the image captured by a camera or displayed on a monitor. Resolution is the ability of a video system to make one object distinguishable from another or its ability to produce fine details. Resolution is a measurement in two different axes across the image being viewed by the camera or on the monitor.

The vertical resolution, or the number of horizontal lines, is controlled by a predetermined scanning rate that is regulated and standardized by the National Television Standard Committee (NTSC). A scanning rate of

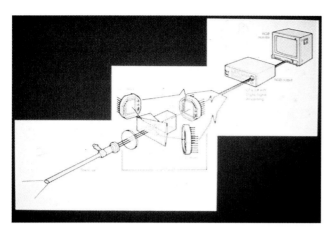

Fig. 10-5 A three-chip camera uses a prism to break down the light coming from the target into three primary colors—red, green, and blue. These colors are picked up separately by the three charged coupled device chips for transmission to the camera control unit and the monitor. (Courtesy Olympus America, Inc., Melville, N.Y.)

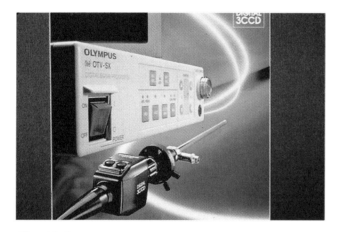

Fig. 10-6 A three-chip camera attached to a rigid endoscope. Also shown is the camera control unit. (Courtesy Olympus America, Inc., Melville, N.Y.)

525 lines is used as the standard video format in the United States, Canada, Japan, and parts of Asia and Central and South America for purposes of video production and broadcasting (Meeker and Rothrock, 1995).

Other standards are used in different countries. Phase alternating line (PAL) is the standard in Great Britain, Australia, and New Zealand and most countries in Europe, Asia, and Africa. Sequential coleur à memoire (SECAM) is losing popularity but is still being used in France and a few other European countries.

The horizontal resolution, or the number of vertical lines, is used as a standard of comparison for video cameras and monitors. Cameras and monitors capture or display a specific number of vertical lines that can be counted visually using a resolution chart of calculated during the manufacturing process. If the horizontal res-

olution is increased, then the device is able to create images that are more defined and clear. A single video chip provides about 450 lines of resolution; three chips provide up to 800 lines of resolution (Frantzides, 1995).

If a camera capable of lower resolution, such as 300 lines of resolution, is connected to a monitor capable of higher resolution, such as 600 lines, the video system will only be able to produce the lower, or 300 lines of resolution. That is, the image clarity can be no greater than that produced by the component of the system with the lowest resolution.

The format is the manner in which the camera's electronic signal information regarding color and brightness is carried to the accessory devices for display or reproduction. A camera can offer any of the different signal transmission options, but the accompanying equipment, such as the monitor, must be compatible with the camera's specific format. The most common video formats are the composite, Y/C, and RGB formats.

All standard systems are capable of handling a composite format. Even systems with RGB or Y/C formats can provide the composite format for video compatibility. Because the composite format has a limited bandwidth, however, it can carry only a small amount of information. Both color and brightness is transmitted on the same signal (Fig. 10-7). An encoding function is required to combine these signals into one video production signal. Because both are carried together, cross-talk and interference can occur, resulting in more video noise or disturbance.

The Y/C format is another common signal transmission method in which the Y (brightness) and the C (color) are carried on two different signals (Fig. 10-8). This is also referred to as *super VHS* or *S-VHS*. Y/C is the next most common format available in the United States. The advantages of this format are that video noise is minimized because two signals are used and that sharper images are produced. A disadvantage is that, because these two signals are carried for long distances at different speeds, extra electronic circuitry may be required to synchronize the two. From the standpoint of its use for medical

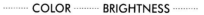

········ **COLOR** ········ **BRIGHTNESS** ········

Fig. 10-7 Standard composite format. (From Meeker MH, Rothrock JC: *Alexander's care of the patient in surgery*, ed 10, St. Louis, 1995, Mosby.)

········ **COLOR** ········

········ **BRIGHTNESS** ········

Fig. 10-8 Y/C or S-VHS format. (From Meeker MH, Rothrock JC: *Alexander's care of the patient in surgery*, ed 10, St. Louis, 1995, Mosby.)

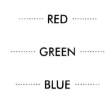

Fig. 10-9 RGB format. (From Meeker MH, Rothrock JC: *Alexander's care of the patient in surgery*, ed 10, St. Louis, 1995, Mosby.)

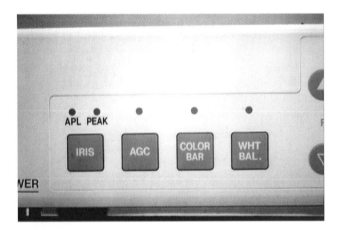

Fig. 10-10 The white-balance control switch is activated when white balancing the camera so that true color detection is provided. (Courtesy Olympus America, Inc., Melville, N.Y.)

purposes, the Y/C format has the advantage of offering higher-resolution recording for video tapes and color prints and clear, bright images for endoscopic viewing.

The RGB format separates the video information into red, green, and blue signals that are each carried separately (Fig. 10-9). A special cable is used to conduct all of these signals at the same time between the camera and monitor. Brightness is then generated as a percentage of each color (30% red, 59% green, 11% blue) (Meeker and Rothrock, 1995). The RGB format generates a sharper picture because of the separate color distinction and the lessened noise interference involved. A disadvantage of this format is that hue and tint color adjustments cannot be made on the monitor. The RGB components may also be more expensive, because the three signals must be synchronized. The RGB format is often used for computer interfacing, which is becoming more popular.

White balancing must be done so that the camera detects different colors relative to pure white. Once the camera is white balanced or white set, the electronic controls within the camera system are then commanded to detect and transmit true colors (Fig. 10-10). Because white is the presence of all colors in proper balance and black

is the absence of natural color, the camera must be shown what white looks like in the context of the lighting system being used. After white balancing is performed, then the colors appearing on the monitor are more accurate.

White balancing can be done in the following way:

- Connect the endoscope to the camera and light source.
- Adjust the light source to obtain adequate imaging on the monitor.
- Position the scope end so that it is perpendicular to the surface of some white material, such as a white lap sponge or towel.
- Focus the scope to obtain a clear picture.
- Depress the white balance switch on the CCU.
- Allow the camera to complete the entire sequence of white balancing before removing the white material from in front of the end of the scope. The camera system is now white balanced and will transmit true colors.

Other features are now available that can enhance camera technology. For example, many camera head controls have now been designed to allow the scrub team to easily white balance the camera, boost the light when extra light is needed (e.g., when small-lumen endoscopes are being used), take hard copy prints, and remotely start and stop the VCR (Fig. 10-11). Many camera units come with remote control pads that can be draped within a sterile sheath and operated by the surgical team at the table.

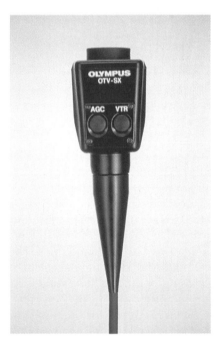

Fig. 10-11 This camera head features a built-in remote control for automatic gain control to reduce glare and to turn the VCR on and off. (Courtesy Olympus America, Inc., Melville, N.Y.)

Most cameras now have an automatic shutter or iris that measures the amount of light sensed and then adjusts itself accordingly. The image quality is improved because the glare from shiny instruments and viscera is reduced.

Camera Cables

A cable is used to connect the camera on the flexible or rigid endoscope to the CCU (Fig. 10-12), but it must be long enough to reach from the surgical field to the CCU. Usually when malfunctions occur, it is the cable that needs to be replaced and not the camera. Therefore, cables that can be disconnected from the camera are the most desirable kind.

Camera cables should be handled gently. They should not be twisted or kinked, because this could break the fiberoptics or wires in the cable. An extra cable should be available in the event replacement of a defective cable is immediately needed, thus eliminating downtime for repairs.

Camera Adapters

A camera adapter or coupler is required to connect the camera to the endoscope. There are a variety of camera adapters available today for rigid or flexible endoscopes (Figs. 10-13 to 10-16). Couplers come in varying focal lengths and optical magnifications. The image size can be controlled by the magnification power of the coupler. There are also different types of couplers. For example, a beam-splitter coupler is used if a physician wants to look directly through the endoscope while the surgical team views the image on the monitor. A direct-link coupler is required if the viewing is to be done only on the monitor.

The degree to which the image on the monitor is magnified is determined by the coupler and the endoscope

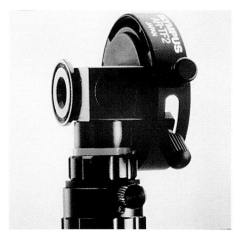

Fig. 10-13 This camera adapter with a beam splitter allows the physician to look through the eyepiece while others view the procedure on the monitor. (Courtesy Olympus America, Inc., Melville, N.Y.)

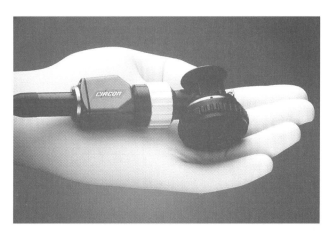

Fig. 10-14 A beam splitter can be very compact. Courtesy Circon Corp., Santa Barabara, Calif.)

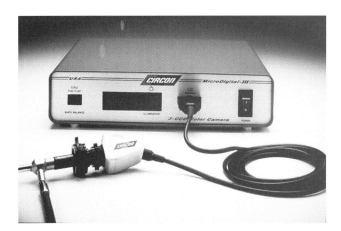

Fig. 10-12 A cable connecting the camera that is attached to the rigid or flexible endoscope to the control unit. (Courtesy Olympus America, Inc., Melville, N.Y.)

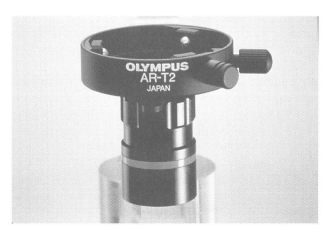

Fig. 10-15 This camera adapter provides a direct link from the camera to the monitor when eyepiece viewing is not desired. (Courtesy Olympus America, Inc., Melville, N.Y.)

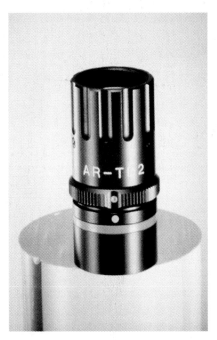

Fig. 10-16 This ultra-slim camera adapter connects directly to an endoscope. (Courtesy Olympus America, Inc., Melville, N.Y.)

lens system. A coupler that produces a larger image on the screen will also cause the brightness of the image to be diminished. Therefore, the picture brightness and quality are usually better if magnification is less. Some physicians prefer using a smaller monitor to obtain a higher-quality image.

An endoscopic camera can be focused at the camera-coupler interface. Some cameras even have a zoom capability that can be used to get a closer look at a structure or abnormality (Fig. 10-17).

There are now videoscopes in which the camera is attached directly to the endoscope without the need for a coupler or in which the camera is incorporated into the endoscope. Because a coupler is not then needed, condensation buildup and fogging are no longer a problem, so the image is usually more clear. The scope and the camera are purchased as one unit, however, so interchangeability is not possible. In addition, the camera cannot then be draped separately. Further, because the camera may be built directly into the endoscope, if there is a problem with the endoscope or the camera, the entire unit must then be returned for repair.

Camera Control Unit

The CCU is connected to the camera with a cable (Fig. 10-18). It provides adjustment capabilities, such as white balancing. The most important feature of a CCU is the automatic shutter that automatically adjusts each pixel's exposure time up to $\frac{1}{15,000}$ of a second. This feature provides a much faster response time to light changes

than the light source. In fact, it reacts as quickly as the human eye to changing light conditions.

Evolving Camera Technology

New technology, called "chip-on-a-stick," has been introduced in which the camera chip has been taken out of the camera head and placed at the distal end of the scope. This eliminates the need for the traditional optical lenses required for cameras located at the head of endoscopes. Chip-on-a-stick cameras also require less illumination than standard cameras because there are no optical lenses or a light cord to cause a loss of transmission (Nezhat, et al, 1995).

The next generation of cameras will use computerized digital information. Instead of providing a continuous waveform of analog information, they will translate the image into thousands of tiny digitized bits of information. Digital signals take up less bandwidth than

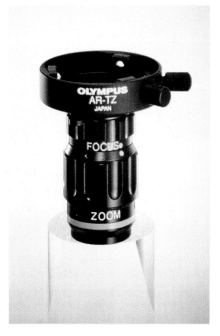

Fig. 10-17 This camera adapter provides a built-in zoom capability that allows the image to be enlarged or reduced so that the ideal image size can be maintained on the monitor. (Courtesy Olympus America, Inc., Melville, N.Y.)

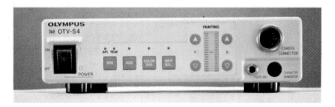

Fig. 10-18 Camera control unit. (Courtesy Olympus America, Inc., Melville, N.Y.)

analog information currently does. Digitized images can also be manipulated so that dual images, freeze frames, and a split screen are possible. In addition, digital information can be stored for later retrieval and even sent to distant places via telephone lines. Digital camera technology is the precursor to the virtual reality simulators and remote telepresence surgery being developed.

Care of the Camera

The camera should be removed from the endoscope so that each component can be cleaned separately during reprocessing (Fig. 10-19). Most cameras today can be immersed in liquid chemicals for disinfection or sterilization (Fig. 10-20). Camera leakage testers are available to identify potential leaks in the camera head that could allow damage to occur during reprocessing. Leakage testing should therefore be done before the camera is immersed in the disinfecting solution (Fig. 10-21).

The camera, coupler, and endoscope are often reconnected before being disinfected or sterilized. This is not ideal, however, because the chemical cannot then reach the surfaces of the sealed-off areas. If possible the endoscope, coupler, and camera should not be reconnected until reprocessing is completed.

Inside the camera coupler is an **O**-ring, or gasket, that provides a moisture-proof seal which is compressed once the camera is connected to the endoscope (Fig. 10-22). This gasket must be inspected during reprocessing to make sure it is intact. Sometimes the gasket becomes worn or damaged during constant use, and this allows moisture to penetrate between the camera head and the coupler, thus affecting the endoscopic image. During an endoscopic procedure, the camera and coupler may need to be disassembled to allow any condensation that

has accumulated to dry. The formation of condensation may indicate failure of the seal within the coupler (Spellman, 1995).

Because a cool endoscope is placed inside a warm body, fogging can occur on the cooler endoscope or camera lenses. If this happens, a sterile antifogging agent can be applied to the lens surfaces to clear the fogging. If the antifogging agent does not work, then the endoscope and the moisture-proof seals in the camera need to be inspected.

Some of the newer cameras can be steam autoclaved. Tight seals are incorporated into the design of these cameras to keep water or steam from penetrating into their interior workings.

To decrease the need to process a camera, and thereby the wear and tear on the camera, cameras are often draped as an alternative to reprocessing (Fig. 10-23).

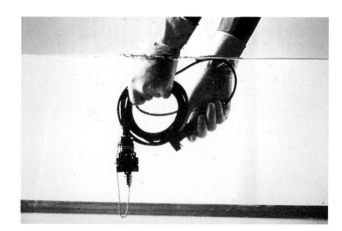

Fig. 10-20 Camera heads and cables that can be immersed in liquid chemical disinfecting solutions. (Courtesy Olympus America, Inc., Melville, N.Y.)

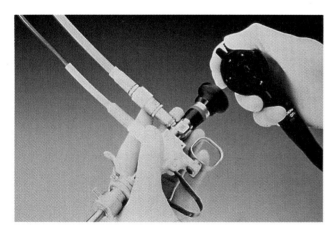

Fig. 10-19 The camera must be removed from the end of the endoscope before reprocessing. (Courtesy Olympus America, Inc., Melville, N.Y.)

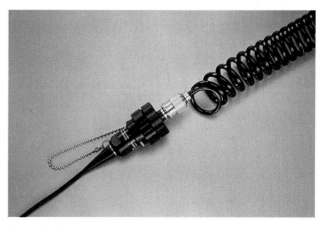

Fig. 10-21 A leakage tester, which can identify a potential leakage problem in the camera head before damage occurs. (Courtesy Olympus America, Inc., Melville, N.Y.)

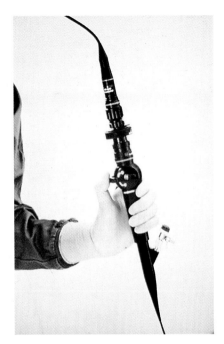

Fig. 10-22 An O-ring or gasket within the coupler that connects the endoscope to the camera. This provides a seal to prevent moisture leakage that could affect the endoscopic image. (Courtesy Olympus America, Inc., Melville, N.Y.)

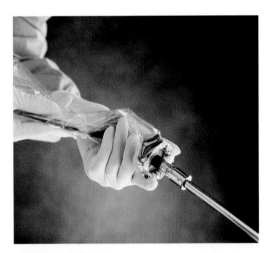

Fig. 10-23 A sterile drape can be placed on the camera to avoid the need to reprocess the camera. (Courtesy Microtek Medical, Inc., Columbus, Miss.)

This can decrease the problems with camera seals leaking, which can lead to camera fogging during an endoscopic procedure. The camera drape is fitted over the camera and light cord, and this prevents the nonsterile camera from contaminating the sterile field. The life expectancy of the camera and coupler is then usually longer because they are not subjected to disinfectant solutions or sterilization processes.

The camera and coupler are draped in the following manner:

- The circulating nurse inserts the camera into the sterile drape, which is held by the scrub nurse (Fig. 10-24).
- The scrub nurse holds the camera with the sterile drape while the circulating nurse assists with telescopically unfolding the length of the drape to cover the light cord (Fig. 10-25).
- The scrub nurse centers the drape lens over the coupler lens that is connected to the camera, taking care not to stretch the drape tightly over the coupler.
- The scope is inserted into the draped coupler, making sure that the alignment is correct (Fig. 10-26).
- The scope and draped camera are ready for use.

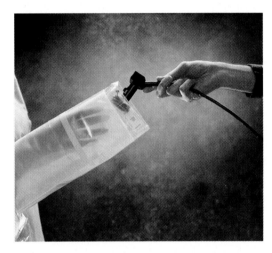

Fig. 10-24 Camera being placed into the sterile drape. (Courtesy Microtek Medical, Inc., Columbus, Miss.)

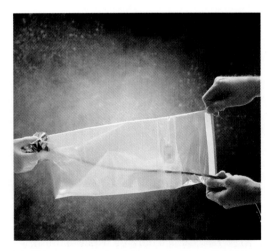

Fig. 10-25 Drape being telescopically unfolded to cover the cord. (Courtesy Microtek Medical, Inc., Columbus, Miss.)

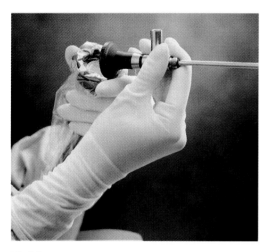

Fig. 10-26   Endoscope head being inserted into the draped camera coupler. (Courtesy Microtek Medical, Inc., Columbus, Miss.)

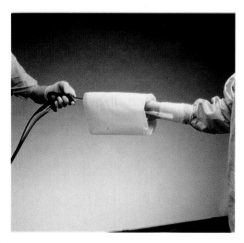

Fig. 10-27   Laparoscope being placed into the rigid plastic sheath and secured as the scope and camera are draped. (Courtesy Medical Dynamics, Inc., Englewood, Colo.)

A single-use sheath and sleeving drape for sterile enclosure of the laparoscope and the camera are now available. This eliminates the need to disinfect or sterilize the laparoscope and camera between procedures, thus possibly increasing the life expectancy of the optical and video equipment. Surgical instruments then must be introduced through other ports, because the laparoscope is fully enclosed (Figs. 10-27 and 10-28).

Three-dimensional Imaging

Most endoscopic procedures are currently performed with the surgical team viewing the image in two dimensions on a monitor, but this causes depth perception to be lost, thus increasing the risk for patient injury, especially if a physician is learning the art of endoscopy or new endoscopic techniques.

Three-dimensional (3D), or stereo vision, imaging helps to restore depth perception by simulating what human eyes do at close distances. Each eye sees the image from a different view, but the brain processes the two pictures into one image that has depth. 3D technology mimics natural vision by making use of right and left cameras to view the surgical site. The images are captured and converted into one image (Fig. 10-29), and team members wear special glasses to see the image in three dimensions (Fig. 10-30). Because 3D images have the depth two-dimensional images do not have, they are clearer and sharper.

The 3D image can be captured using any of the following setups (*Adv Technol Surg Care*, 1995).

1. Two cameras attached to two optical scopes, one set up for the left and one for the right. This dual-lens

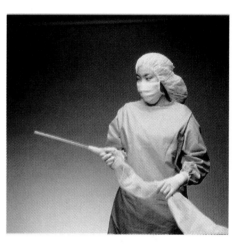

Fig. 10-28   A single-use sheath and sleeve. These provide a sterile enclosure for the entire laparoscope and video system. (Courtesy Medical Dynamics, Inc., Englewood, Colo.)

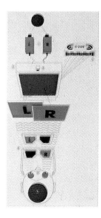

Fig. 10-29   One example of how three-dimensional imaging works. Two cameras mounted side by side collect left and right images. The monitor alternates the images 120 times a second. Shutter glasses are synchronized to the alternating images and the three-dimensional image is perceived. (Courtesy Carl Zeiss Inc., Thornwood, N.Y.)

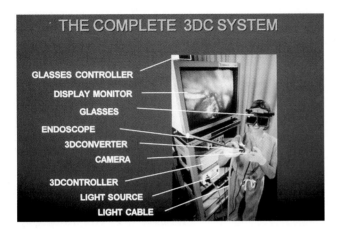

Fig. 10-30   A three-dimensional system. (Courtesy International Telepresence Corp., Vancouver, B.C., Canada.)

system often cannot produce enough light, however, because the channels are each usually only 5 mm in diameter.
2. Two cameras through one optical channel. The image is transmitted to two cameras at the proximal end of the scope. The single image is split by prismlike optics into separate right and left images that are viewed by the two different cameras. Sometimes the prismlike optics may distort the image, however.
3. Two cameras located at the tip of one scope without optical channels or lenses. The laparoscope involved usually needs to be a large 12-mm scope to accommodate the cameras.
4. One camera and one lens with a special device that creates the 3D image. This system can be attached to an existing endoscope and splits the image to create the right and left images and the 3D effect. This system is still being refined for use.

After the image is captured, then it must be perceived by the surgeon. The brain can combine the two images seen by the eyes at a rate of 45 images per second. A typical 2D image system transmits the image at a rate of 60 images per second, so flickering is not noticed. In 3D technology, the camera captures the images at a rate of 60 images per second, and these images are then sent to a conversion unit to alternate them right and left. The special monitor then displays the right and left images at a rate of 120 images per second, resulting in a blur on the screen. The next step is to separate this stereo image so that the eye can perceive the picture. There are two different types of 3D glasses that can do this:
1. Active glasses—these glasses are battery-powered to open and close independent shutters for each eye. They are synchronized with a signal emitted from a device located on the top of the TV monitor to open the right eye shutter to allow the wearer to see the righthand view, and vice versa. The speed at which

each image is seen is $1/120$th of a second, which is twice as fast as the speed of $1/60$th of a second that the eye is used to seeing. Therefore, image flickering is not detected.
2. Passive glasses—The shuttering action is done on the monitor, not on the glasses. A polarized shutter is attached to the front of the monitor and controlled by a camera-signal processing unit. The images are rotated to different directions. The left image is polarized the same as the left lens in the glasses and the right image is polarized the same as the right lens. These glasses are lighter in weight but the lenses may be darker than those of the active glasses.

There are also special rigid endoscopes that provide 3D imaging. In these endoscopes, images from two separate angles are relayed along the length of the endoscope to two cameras, which receive the image from each angle to provide the 3D imagery. Endoscopes are available that provide both straight and oblique angle viewing (Fig. 10-31). Rotatable telescope optics are also available for true image orientation (Fig. 10-32). This is especially important if oblique viewing endoscopes are being used.

Following are some of the advantages of 3D imaging:
- Procedures can be performed more quickly because a more true to life environment is offered.
- Depth perception is provided, which is extremely important if surgery is being performed near complex and vital structures such as the spine.
- Instruments can be manipulated faster and more easily.
- The location of structures and their relationships can be more accurately interpreted.

A study was conducted to compare the viewing capabilities afforded by 2D and 3D video systems by comparing the speed with which certain tasks could be performed through an endoscope. The study did not show any

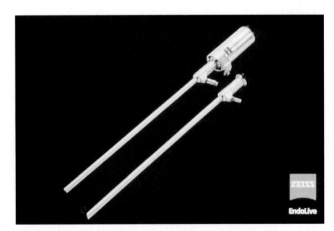

Fig. 10-31   Three-dimensional rigid endoscopes that provide both straight and oblique angle viewing. (Courtesy Carl Zeiss Inc., Thornwood, N.Y.)

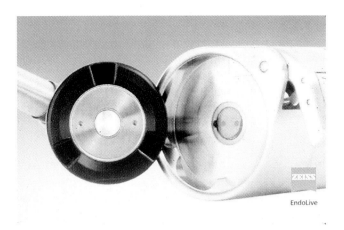

Fig. 10-32 Camera placed on a special rigid endoscope with rotatable telescope optics to provide a three-dimensional imaging system. (Courtesy Carl Zeiss, Inc., Thornwood, N.Y.)

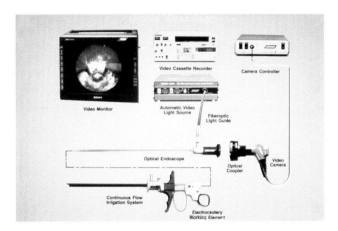

Fig. 10-33 The optical video chain terminates in the monitor. (Courtesy Circon Corp., Santa Barbara, Calif.)

that can occur during cleaning, and decreasing the cost to purchase and maintain the 3D system.

MONITORS

The monitor represents the termination point of the video signal where the image is transmitted for observation (Fig. 10-33). Monitors can receive broadcast signals or input from cables. Many monitors used for endoscopic procedures only receive input from direct cable connections, so they cannot receive broadcast signals and cannot be used as televisions.

The monitor's resolution capabilities must closely match those of the camera. Most monitors have higher resolution capabilities, so the camera used in the video system must also produce high-resolution images.

Often the quality of the image shown on the monitor can be judged by evaluating it next to other models. Monitors used for home viewing tend to show softer colors and less image sharpness; monitors used in surgery need to show more distinct colors, contrast, and definition.

To ensure adequate visualization during endoscopic procedures, the monitor screens should be at least 13 inches (33 cm) diagonally (Fig. 10-34). In some surgical setups the smaller 13-inch monitor is used as the "slave" or second monitor. The 19- or 20-inch (48.3- to 50.8-cm) monitor is usually the main monitor. However, because surgical team members often complain about

significant difference in overall task performance, but some specific outcomes were noted (Birkett, et al, 1994):
- In two thirds of all the tasks performed, the task was accomplished faster at the first attempt using the 3D system.
- The suture and knot tying task was performed 12% faster using the 3D imaging system.
- More complicated tasks were performed 25% faster using the 3D system, but basic tasks were performed at the same rate.

3D video technology continues to pose several problems that are currently being addressed, including the lack of image brightness, the limited visual field, and the need to wear special 3D glasses. Other areas in which solutions are being sought in an effort to help advance this technology include preventing user eye strain and headaches, minimizing the misalignment by the system

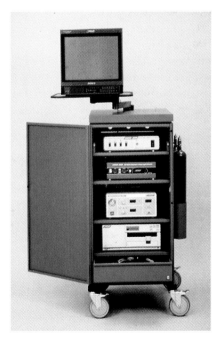

Fig. 10-34 Monitors should have a screen that measures at least 13 inches (33 cm) diagonally to ensure adequate visualization. (Courtesy Circon Corp., Santa Barbara, Calif.)

the difficulty adjusting when having to look from one size monitor to another, some hospitals now provide only the larger-size monitor.

Monitors have numerous adjustment control knobs that can be used to help define the image. Many video monitors also have a reset button that returns the monitor to factory-preset specifications and adjustments. Some monitors have a contrast-adjustment capability that can be used to improve image clarity. The greater the difference between the intensity of the image and that of the background, the greater the contrast.

Because the life expectancy of a monitor is lengthy, a high-end system with at least 600 to 750 lines of resolution should be purchased. As the number of dots per tube increases, the lines of curvature become more sharp and the resolution of the margins of the image become greater. (See earlier discussion of camera resolution for more details.)

Ideally a monitor should accept all three video formats—composite, Y/C, and RGB. However, the most-defined images and best-quality pictures are produced by a monitor and camera with RGB capabilities. As already described in detail, this format separates the red, green, and blue colors, yielding a higher-quality transmission.

High-definition television (HDTV) has been introduced in which the scanning rate has been increased from the traditional 525 lines of resolution to 1100 or 1200 lines per frame, thus more than doubling the quality of the imaging (Nezhat, et al, 1995). HDTV can also receive the digitized signals (instead of the traditional analog signals) now possible with new technological advances. HDTV is already available in Japan and is quickly gaining popularity in the United States.

Although most endoscopic procedures are performed with the surgical team only observing the monitor, often a surgical team member will point to a structure on the monitor screen during an endoscopic procedure. This can result in bacterial contamination, however, because as the gloved hand comes close to the monitor, the probability of bacterial transfer from the screen to the gloved hand increases. A research study has documented that the static electricity generated near the screen of the monitor transfers bacteria to a gloved hand that is near the screen. In fact, transfer occurs more frequently in this way than if the team member were actually to touch the screen (*Laparosc Surg Update*, 1995).

DOCUMENTATION DEVICES

Many different documentation devices are available today that can provide a permanent visual image of the endoscopic procedure. Such visual documentation can be used for provider education, patient education, surgical board approvals, information sharing for consultations, third-party requisitions, and litigation cases.

Video Cassette Recorder

A video cassette recorder (VCR) is needed if a videotaped documentation of the endoscopic procedure is desired. There is a foot switch available that can be used to control the VCR (Fig. 10-35). There are currently different VCR formats that are available with the most versatile being the ½-inch (1.27-cm) tape recorder. The physician or patient can then play these videotapes on home recorders. A ¾-inch (1.9-cm) videotape would have to be converted before it could be used for home viewing, and this would cause some of the quality of the recorded image to be lost. Because the ½-inch systems are the most popular and these units can be used in home environments, theft has become a concern in surgery suites. The use of locking cabinetry helps to prevent this problem.

The professional-grade VCR with ½-inch S-VHS format (with Y/C inputs and outputs) has become popular in surgical settings and produces a high-quality picture. It costs more but cannot be connected to household televisions, thus discouraging theft. The S-VHS recorders can record in the standard VHS format and also in the S format. If recording is done in the S format, however, the videotapes can only be played back on a VCR that is S-compatible (Meeker and Rothrock, 1995). In the future, 8-mm recorders that use ¼-inch tapes will probably become more popular. Because of the compact size of the tape, the tapes take up less storage space.

A character generator can be used to categorize and manage video recordings. The generator can be connected to the CCU for on-screen display and for recording comments, names, dates, times, and other necessary data on a VCR tape (Figs. 10-36 and 10-37).

Following are guidelines for troubleshooting a malfunctioning VCR:
- Make sure a tape is inside the VCR.
- Make sure the tape is rewound.

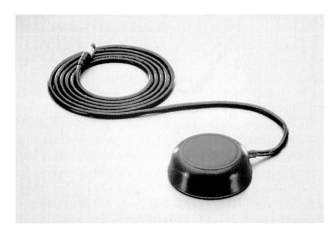

Fig. 10-35 A foot switch may be used to control the VCR. (Courtesy Olympus America, Inc., Melville, N.Y.)

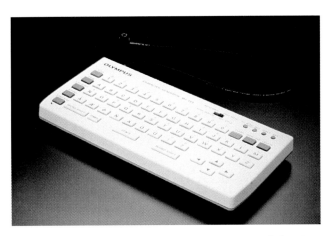

Fig. 10-36 A character generator can be used for data entry on the screen and on the VCR recording. (Courtesy Olympus America, Inc., Melville, N.Y.)

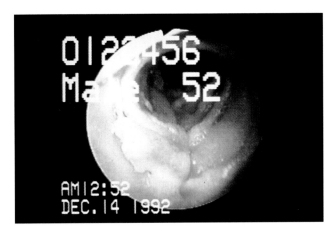

Fig. 10-37 Data are entered on the endoscopic image. (Courtesy Olympus America, Inc., Melville, N.Y.)

- Make sure the VCR is plugged in and turned on.
- Make sure the appropriate settings are indicated on the VCR display panel.
- Follow the manufacturer's instructions regarding the maintenance of the system. For example, if the picture appears fuzzy, a manufacturer may suggest that the tape head be cleaned.

Video Printer

The video printer, sometimes called the *Mavigraph*, is used to record still images during an endoscopic procedure (Fig. 10-38). The system works by freezing the signal from the video system and converting it into a digital image or an instant picture that is printed on special paper using thermal ink-printing techniques. Printing speeds have been decreased from 1 to 2 minutes to approximately 30 to 45 seconds, and systems can record from one to even 25 still pictures on one page. Some video printers can superimpose the patient's name and other information on the side of the print. These prints

are used for patient education and documentation on the patient's chart and may even be given to the patient.

Video Disk Recorder

The video disk recorder is becoming more popular as the means of recording and documenting endoscopic procedures. The recorded disks take less storage space than VCR tapes.

Still-imaging 35-mm Camera

A 35-mm camera with a special adapter can be placed on an endoscope to take pictures for photographs and slides. Attaching the 35-mm camera directly to the endoscope continues to be the best way to produce a photograph, but this requires disconnecting the video camera from the endoscope, which poses a problem in terms of sterility maintenance and asepsis. There are 35-mm cameras that can be gas sterilized, but because gas sterilization takes so long, the camera is then only available for one procedure per day. Camera drapes have also been used to cover the camera to maintain the sterile setup, but this is difficult to do.

A higher-speed film of 400 ASA from a recognized manufacturer is recommended for use. Proper light exposure is needed to produce high-quality slides. To provide such additional lighting or side lights, another light source can be directed through an accessory port. This will intensify images because outlines will be more defined.

Slide-making System

A 35-mm slide-making system is designed to work in tandem with a video printer, which can make 35-mm slides from any standard video signal. Usually the system has 500 lines of resolution, so high-quality images can be produced. A slide-making device produces 35-mm slides much more quickly than the traditional method involving the use of a 35-mm camera attached to the end of the endoscope.

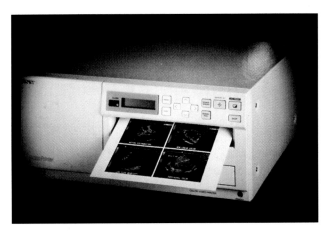

Fig. 10-38 A video printer producing a picture of the endoscopic image. (Courtesy Olympus America, Inc., Melville, N.Y.)

Digital Imaging

Digital imaging allows the camera signal to be processed by a computer. In this process the image information is digitized and then transferred to a disk system on a computer. Software programs can be used to modify or store the image, import it into presentations, or transport it to other clinical sites for review. However, optical memory drives and disk storage systems need to be refined to advance this technology.

VIDEO CABINETRY

Special cabinets have been designed for the placement and storage of video equipment and other endoscopic devices (Fig. 10-39). These cabinets usually are mobile, so the video system can be moved from room to room. The wheels need to be large enough to allow for easy mobility and need to lock to stabilize the cabinet after positioning.

The video system components should be strategically arranged in the cabinet and connected according to the manufacturer's suggestions. The ends of the cords can be color coded or identified so that reconnection is simplified should a piece of equipment have to be removed. A schematic drawing of the connection layout should be available to assist surgical team members with reconnection.

The video cabinet usually has a lock to secure the equipment and prevent theft. After a video system has been installed and is operational, the back of the cabinet also may be locked so that connections and settings cannot be changed. The key must be stored in a secure place so that it is accessible to the experienced video technician or nurse.

An electrical power bar can be used to supply electricity to each piece of equipment in the cabinet. Only

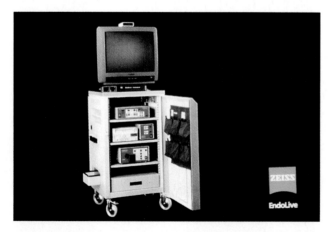

Fig. 10-39 All video components can be stored easily and securely in a video cabinet. (Courtesy Carl Zeiss Inc., Thornwood, N.Y.)

the power bar then has to be connected to the electrical outlet, but the power bar needs to be on for electricity to flow to the component pieces. A power bar makes it easier to set up the video system because all of the components are already plugged into it.

TROUBLESHOOTING VIDEO EQUIPMENT

Surgical team members should become very familiar with the many different pieces of equipment in a video system and should work closely with the video technician to learn how to operate the system and how to solve minor problems that may arise. The manufacturers' operating and service manuals should also be readily accessible so that they can referred to for help dealing with video technology challenges.

If problems with video transmission are noted, then the components, equipment, and connections should be checked in an organized manner. One way to do this is to start at the top of the stack of video equipment and work down through the devices, checking all connections and settings on the front before moving to the back panels. Sometimes the problem may be as minor as a switch not being completely turned on. Checklists can also be used to help organize this troubleshooting process.

Sometimes there may not be enough time to investigate the source of a video problem during an endoscopic procedure, so a replacement system must be brought in. For this reason, such systems must be readily available. If the patient's condition is stable and time is not too critical, the nurse may take the time during the procedure to investigate the situation using an organized approach to identify and solve the problem.

Troubleshooting a video system should progress from the most simple or basic solution to the most complex. For example, a monitor may not be producing a video image simply because the monitor is unplugged or the multiplug power strip is not switched on.

Listed in the box are some common problems that are encountered and the questions to be asked when troubleshooting video equipment (*Laparosc Surg Update*, 1994).

VIDEOCONFERENCING

Videoconferencing has gained much popularity over the past few years as the potential applications of this technology in health care environments have been appreciated. The necessary equipment is being purchased for and connectivity is being established in a variety of patient care settings, including surgery and endoscopy suites. Because videoconferencing holds great promise from the standpoint of enhancing communication, education,

---

Box 10-1 *Troubleshooting video equipment*

PROBLEM: There is no picture on the monitor.
- Is the power switch on?
- Are any fuses blown or circuit breakers tripped?
- Do all the pieces in the system have to be on for one component to work?
- Are the camera cables connected to the correct ports?
- Are the cable connections secure? (Moving equipment around the surgery suite may loosen some connections. Try wiggling the cable at the camera end and then at the camera control unit end. If wiggling the camera cord corrects the problem or affects the image, then cable is usually the problem.)
- Is the monitor on the correct channel?
- Is the problem with only one piece of equipment? (Try switching each component until the problem is identified.)
- Can the problem be solved by bypassing the peripheral equipment?
- Has the peripheral equipment been correctly programmed?

PROBLEM: The picture is not clear.
- Has the camera been white balanced?
- Does the color control need to be adjusted?
- Does the color control on the video printer need to be adjusted? (Sometimes this may affect the monitor.)
- Are all of the cables connected securely? (Sometimes the video image is sent to the monitor over several cables. If one is not connected well, then the monitor image is affected.)

PROBLEM: The picture is cloudy or not in focus.
- Does manipulating the focus control on the camera before inserting the endoscope into the patient correct the problem?
- Is the endoscope lens fogged?
- Is there debris or condensation on the end of the endoscope?
- Has an antifog solution or other defogging methods been tried?
- Is the lens fogging because the endoscope was too cold when it was inserted into the warm body cavity?
- Has moisture accumulated between the endoscope and the camera?

PROBLEM: There is no light from the light source.
- Are there broken fibers in the fiberoptics? (Extensive fiber breaks will prevent the light from getting to the surgery site.)
- Is there a problem with the light bulb? (A light bulb

that may be ready to burn out usually does not produce adequate amounts of light.)
- Are the camera and light cable connections correct?

PROBLEM: The image is dark.
- Is there any moisture on the optics?
- Have the connections been made correctly?
- Is the light source set to automatic?
- Has the integrity of the fiberoptics been examined?
- Can the image be brightened by adjusting the camera control unit's automatic gain control?

PROBLEM: The image on the monitor flickers.
- Is the auto iris in the "on" position on the camera or light source? (Sometimes if they are both on, they will compete with each other over the light settings. One of the auto iris settings needs to be deactivated.)
- Has the camera cable been inspected for pin holes, cuts, or other damage?

PROBLEM: The image on the monitor is excessively bright.
- Is the camera properly connected to the light source? (If the connection is not secure, then the light source will assume the camera needs more light and will increase to the maximum power.)
- Is the camera or light source on "auto iris"? (One device should have this setting in the "on" position to ensure the correct amount of light is provided from the light source to the camera.)

PROBLEM: There is static interference.
- Is the cable that extends between the monitors damaged?
- Are the camera cable and electrosurgical cable tangled?
- Is the electrosurgical cable damaged?
- Are the electrosurgery unit and the camera control unit plugs attached to separate three-prong hospital grade outlets?

PROBLEM: There is too much glare on the image.
- Is the light source set to automatic?
- Can the automatic light intensity be adjusted?
- Are the light source cables securely connected?

PROBLEM: The color is not accurate.
- Are the camera control unit adjustment knobs properly positioned?
- Has the camera been white balanced?
- Have all color settings been returned to the initial factory settings?
- Can the color intensity and tint be adjusted?
- Have the color adjustments on the printer been checked?

---

and accessibility, its use may be very critical to ensuring the expanding acceptance and continued development of endoscopic procedures. Videoconferencing can provide a communication avenue to enhance training of the endoscopy team, assess dysfunctioning equipment, provide quick responses to new endoscopic product development, and even evaluate patients postoperatively.

Videoconferencing involves telecommunications, which is the art and science of taking services and technology and applying them to the development of the means to communicate audio, video, graphics, and other information over distances (Trowt-Bayard, 1994) and thereby enhance communication. Health care environments have discovered it can be applied in various ways to benefit the patient and health care team, provide education, minimize decision-making time, and provide cost efficiency.

Videoconferencing Technology

Videoconferencing requires basic telecommunications equipment and a way to connect different sites. However, planning must be done in advance to identify the applications of videoconferencing technology pertinent to endoscopy so that appropriate equipment is procured. Cost comparisons must also be done to identify the type of connectivity that would be most beneficial and cost-effective.

Equipment

To participate in videoconferencing for endoscopy, each site must have certain basic equipment, including a monitor, camera, codec, and other various devices.

The high-resolution color monitors used for viewing endoscopic procedures can be used for videoconferencing (Fig. 10-40). These monitors should have composite and Y/C formats (Ball, et al, 1995). Sometimes two monitors are used for videoconferencing, one to receive the image from the distant site and one to display the view being sent from the near site (Fig. 10-41). One monitor can be used instead of two if a picture-in-picture feature is available. The distant site image would constitute the main picture on the monitor and the near site image would be in a small window at the bottom of the screen (Fig. 10-42), which could be turned off if the near site

participants do not need to see their own transmission. If videoconferencing is done during an endoscopic procedure, the monitor should be placed where the endoscopic team can easily see it.

A panoramic camera is needed at each site so participants can see each other (Fig. 10-43). This camera can be mounted on top of the monitor or on a tripod stand; its position is usually controlled by the video conferencing system's keypad (Fig. 10-44). The video room camera should have remote pan, tilt, and zoom controls. The existing endoscopic camera can be used to provide the endoscopic image. Both cameras are connected to the videoconferencing system so that either site can switch between the endoscopic and room camera views.

A codec (compressor/decompressor or coder/decoder) is a critical component of the videoconferencing system (Fig. 10-45). It changes the analog (waveform) signal to a digital signal and then compresses it for transmission to the distant site (Preston, 1992). At the distant site, the

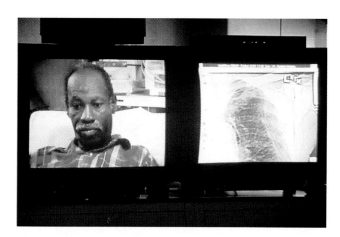

Fig. 10-41   Two-monitor setup for videoconferencing. (Courtesy United Medical Network, Dublin, Ohio.)

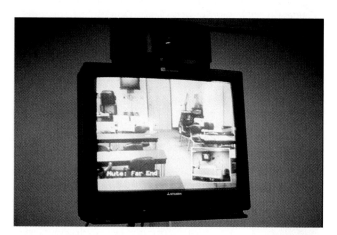

Fig. 10-42   A picture-in-picture feature, seen on the lower righthand part of this screen, provides a view of the near end while the view of the far end is displayed on the rest of the screen.

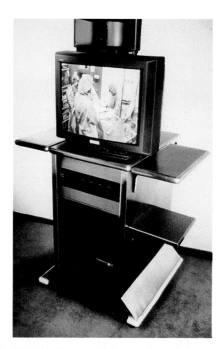

Fig. 10-40   The high-resolution color monitor used for endoscopic procedures can be used for videoconferencing. (Courtesy United Medical Network, Dublin, Ohio.)

codec decompresses the information and transforms the digital signal into an analog signal, so it can be viewed on the monitor. There are codecs offering different transmission speeds and bandwidth options so that the image

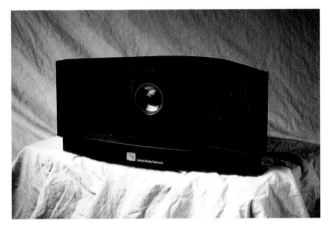

Fig. 10-43 A panoramic camera, which can provide a view of the entire room. (Courtesy United Medical Network, Dublin, Ohio.)

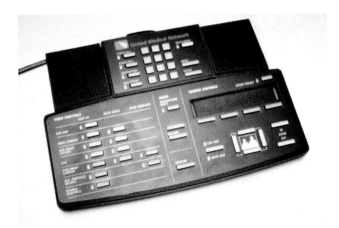

Fig. 10-44 The keypad controls the camera movement. (Courtesy United Medical Network, Dublin, Ohio.)

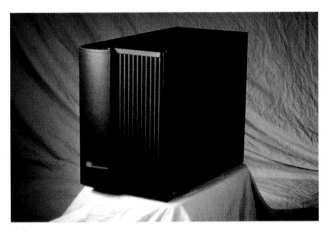

Fig. 10-45 A codec compresses and decompresses the video signal. (Courtesy United Medical Network, Dublin, Ohio.)

quality can be controlled. If the codecs are similar, then the control keypad can control video camera movement at both the distant and near sites.

Until recently, dissimilar codecs could not interact with each other at different sites unless the message was first transmitted through a digital video bridge, which can be very expensive. Today manufacturers are offering codecs that can communicate with each other because an industry standard must now be met that ensures internetwork compatibility (Preston, 1992).

Other devices may be needed for videoconferencing, depending on the applications. A remote microphone can be placed on the outside of the physician's mask if the spoken commentary regarding an endoscopic procedure is to be transmitted. The microphone should not be placed inside the mask, because then the audio transmission will be muffled. The proper placement of microphones in a classroom or auditorium is also critical when a presentation or the proceedings of a conference are being transmitted (Fig. 10-46). Questions from the distant site need to be heard at the near site for interactive communication to take place.

Often a video slate annotation pad is used to draw, illustrate, and point out details on freeze-frame images for transmission to the other end (Fig. 10-47). The annotated image can be viewed at each site so that areas of interest can be discussed.

Other equipment that may be needed, depending on the intended application, include a document camera (Fig. 10-48), VCR, laser printer, FAX machine, and remote assessment tools (e.g., stethoscope, otoscope) (Fig. 10-49). As this technology becomes more widely used, new devices will be developed to enhance its capabilities.

Connectivity

Information is transmitted to one or more sites during videoconferencing. There are many different modes of transmission or connectivity.

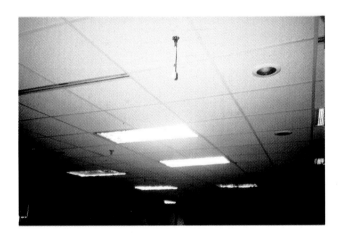

Fig. 10-46 Microphones are suspending from the ceiling so that questions from the audience can be heard.

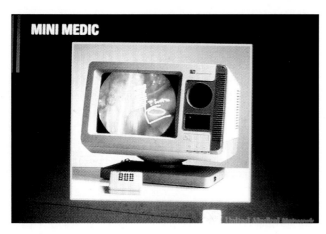

Fig. 10-47 An annotated image as it appears on the monitor at the far end. An annotation pad was used at the near end to draw, illustrate, and point out details on a freeze-frame image that was transmitted. (Courtesy United Medical Network, Dublin, Ohio.)

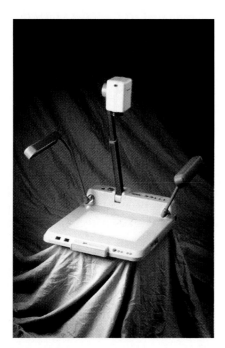

Fig. 10-48 A document camera that can capture the image of a photograph, x-ray study, or other pictures. (Courtesy United Medical Network, Dublin, Ohio.)

Satellite transmission provides a full-motion broadcast-quality picture but requires an uplink to a satellite and a downlink to a specific location. Satellite transmission can be carried on KU-band or C-band. A KU-band satellite dish is relatively small and portable, while a C-band satellite dish is much larger. If the satellite transmission is digital, then each site must have a device that can translate the analog signal to a digital signal (Preston, 1992).

Because satellite time for the transmission must be purchased, satellite transmission can become very ex-

pensive. In one report it was noted that satellite transmission is approximately eight times more expensive than transmission over telephone lines (Preston, 1992).

Satellite connectivity is useful for transmission to and from remote areas where terrestrial transmission is impossible. Very small aperture satellite dishes that can be placed on mobile units are being developed for these purposes. The dish can then be easily transported and set up at the remote area for videoconferencing transmissions.

Telephone lines can be used for terrestrial videoconferencing transmission to sites linked by the appropriate lines. This has gained much popularity in the health care community because prescheduling is not needed and the costs are considerably less. Videoconferencing transmission usually requires a bandwidth or carrying capacity of 90 million bits per second (Mbps). In comparison, a normal telephone call requires only 64 thousand bits per second (Kbps). With current technology, the fastest speed that can be provided is 1.54 Mbps, or the bandwidth of a T-1 line. A T-1 line consists of 24 voice channels or lines of 64 Kbps each (Preston, 1992). Connectivity with T-1 technology is available in many places throughout the world (Fig. 10-50). Because a higher bandwidth is needed, more lines within the T-1 can be combined. Generally a higher bandwidth yields better image quality and transmission. When lower bandwidths or fewer lines are used, visual anomalies occur, such as motion artifact and less clear images.

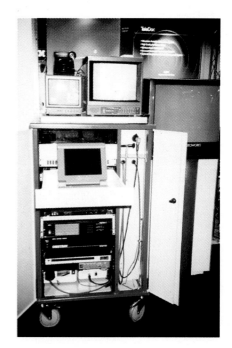

Fig. 10-49 Remote assessment tools are contained within a cabinet.

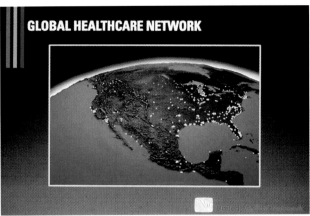

Fig. 10-50 Connectivity is being established throughout the world. (Courtesy United Medical Network, Dublin, Ohio.)

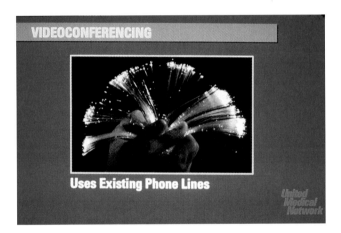

Fig. 10-51 T-1 telephone lines can be used to transmit the information for videoconferencing. (Courtesy United Medical Network, Dublin, Ohio.)

For videoconferencing in the health care environment to be effective, at least six lines or channels of the T-1 (¼ T) should be used, representing a 384-Kbps transmission. Two lines, or a 112-Kbps bandwidth, can be used to achieve a "talking head" type of transmission, but the clarity will be diminished. Some facilities prefer to use the entire T-1 for the transmission, which provides the clearest image and quickest transmission. With the appropriate equipment, multiple videoconferencing calls using six lines each can be transmitted concurrently over the same T-1 (Fig. 10-51).

If multiple channels are used, an inverse multiplexer (I-Mux) is needed to make sure that the channels are sent or recombined into a cohesive single transmission. The I-Mux is used at each site to connect to the T-1 network and interface with the codec.

Microwaves can also be used to transport the signal, but microwaves are sent from one tower to another and a disadvantage of this system is that the towers must be

in sight of each other. This transmission method is also susceptible to atmospheric disturbances.

Fiberoptic lines are also being used to provide connectivity. These lines consist of strands of thin glass fibers that use light to transmit the telecommunication signals.

Videoconferencing Applications

Videoconferencing has been shown to be effective for many health care applications. As usage increases, new applications are being discovered that provide greater patient access, control costs, and ensure the delivery of quality services.

Education

Continuing education is vital to the maintenance of a concentrated knowledge base and multidisciplined skill level in today's changing health care environment. State boards mandate that continuing education is needed to maintain licensure and certification. Providers, such as nurses and physicians, are constantly challenged to understand new devices and advanced endoscopic techniques. With the evolution of videoconferencing technology, a new and exciting means of providing education has come available.

Videoconferencing technology can be used to transmit inservices, presentations, grand rounds, conferences, and college classes, and to provide preceptorships. The exchange of information for the purposes of learning about endoscopic procedures has been shown to be greatly enhanced by videoconferencing (Ball, et al, 1995).

Lectures and educational panel discussions, such as grand rounds, are being transmitted to distant sites thereby eliminating the need to physically transport the speaker or panelists to that area (Fig. 10-52). Because the transmission is a two-way exchange, questions can be asked at

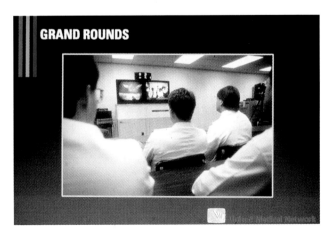

Fig. 10-52 Grand rounds are being transmitted to professionals at other sites using videoconferencing technology. (Courtesy United Medical Network, Dublin, Ohio.)

the distant site and everyone at each end is able to see each other. This technology has helped to control the cost of education for providers and has helped to minimize the feeling of isolation among practitioners located in remote or rural areas.

Often nurses do not have the time or financial resources to attend a professional conference. Videoconferencing has helped bring conferences to distant sites (Fig. 10-53). For example, in 1994 a session on unlicensed assistive personnel delivered at the Association of Operating Room Nurses Congress in New Orleans was transmitted to nurses in Denver, Colorado, and Cincinnati, Ohio (Ball, 1994). The nurses at the distant sites could be seen by those at the actual session and those at the actual session could be seen by those at the distant sites. Questions and answers were exchanged throughout the presentation. Those nurses in Denver and Cincinnati who could not physically attend the AORN Congress were able to electronically attend and actively participate in it, and were even awarded contact hours for their attendance.

College classes are also being offered to students at distant areas to minimize the travel needed to attend these sessions. Through the medium of videoconferencing, course offerings are no longer confined to one site, with the result that there are now greater educational opportunities and pursuing an advanced degree is more attainable.

Distant preceptorships are another videoconferencing application. To receive or maintain practice privileges for endoscopic procedures, a physician or nurse may have to be observed by an experienced practitioner. Sometimes a preceptor may not be readily available for this. Videoconferencing technology allows an expert at one site to precept another professional at a different site, thus making available more preceptors.

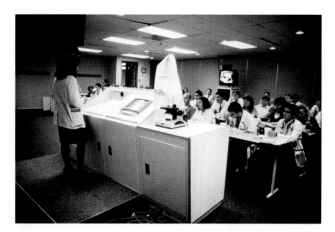

Fig. 10-53 Videoconferencing can allow people to remotely attend conferences. (Courtesy United Medical Network, Dublin, Ohio.)

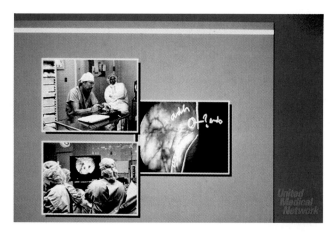

Fig. 10-54 The first remote preceptorship took place at Doctors Hospital in Columbus, Ohio. (Courtesy United Medical Network, Dublin, Ohio.)

The first interactive surgical preceptorship was conducted at Doctors Hospital in Columbus, Ohio, in 1992. A surgeon in a classroom at one site was able to observe and interact with a surgeon performing a laparoscopic procedure at another site (Fig. 10-54). The precepting surgeon used an annotation board to draw, illustrate, and point to areas on still images captured during the operation as single-freeze frames. Both surgeons were able to discuss the procedure in "real" time. This remote preceptorship provided an effective means to evaluate another surgeon's ability to perform a laparoscopic procedure (Ball, et al, 1995).

The educational applications of videoconferencing continue to grow. Education is usually the primary driving force behind the purchase or procurement of videoconferencing equipment. Other applications will evolve as usage increases.

Remote consultations

Long-distance consultations are being effectively conducted using videoconferencing technology. A provider at one end can assess a patient at another end while communicating the requisite plan of care to the patient and the other provider. This type of remote assessment using videoconferencing is called *telemedicine* (Fig. 10-55), and it eliminates the need for travel distances to be assessed by the consultant. This interactive technology can save a lot of money and time for patients and providers.

For example, a patient may have to travel from a rural clinic to a metropolitan hospital for a preoperative assessment to be done and then again for an endoscopic procedure to be performed. The preoperative assessment can be conducted using videoconferencing technology, that links the hospital with the rural clinic. A nurse may be with the patient at the rural clinic while the anesthesiologist at the hospital remotely examines the

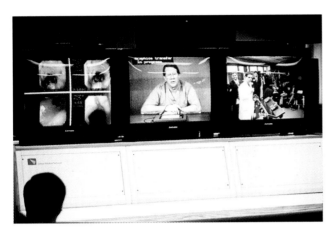

Fig. 10-55 During a remote consultation, the physician is able to assess the patient's condition and discuss possible treatment options. (Courtesy United Medical Network, Dublin, Ohio.)

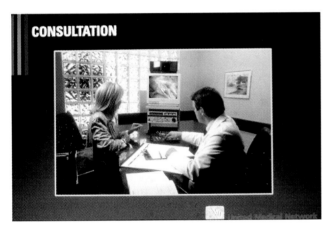

Fig. 10-56 Remote consultation can link providers with providers. (Courtesy United Medical Network, Dublin, Ohio.)

patient and discusses the anesthesia choice. The patient does not then have to make an extra trip to the hospital for the preoperative assessment.

Remote consultations are also being performed where access to patients is difficult (rural areas), where the transport of patients can be a problem (nursing homes), and where continual security measures must be employed (prisons). Remote consultation or telemedicine is being widely used today to link patients with providers and providers with providers (Fig. 10-56).

Other medical videoconferencing applications are teleradiology and telepathology. In these applications, the expert physician can remain at his or her facility, where radiographic images or pathology smears and other information are transmitted for his or her evaluation. A diagnosis can be made and a treatment plan suggested without the practitioner needing to travel to the distant site. Professional organizations are setting standards for transmission to ensure that a clear image is received and an accurate diagnosis rendered. For example, the American Radiology Association has developed transmission standards that must be followed by radiologists participating in teleradiology.

Administrative meetings

Videoconferencing can also be used for administrative and other meetings (Fig. 10-57). Because many hospitals today are merging to form health systems, communication among the facilities is of paramount importance. The exchange of information afforded by videoconferencing is instant, so decisions can be made more quickly and open communication fostered. This type of communication is also very cost-effective because the expense of travel and the time away from work are eliminated. Sometimes in places where a videoconferencing program has been developed, however, it has become difficult to arrange time to transmit educational programs because of the telecommunicated administrative meetings that quickly fill up the schedule.

Product development

Health care and surgical manufacturing and sales companies are quickly discovering the advantages of videoconferencing. Many industries are linking their offices, classrooms, manufacturing sites, and research laboratories with their key customers in an effort to facilitate endoscopic product evaluation and development. By directly and immediately assessing the needs and concerns of their customers, manufacturers can develop more practical and beneficial endoscopic products. Educational sessions and marketing presentations that promote a new technique or instrument can also be transmitted among sites. This technology not only allows health care providers to actually see how a new

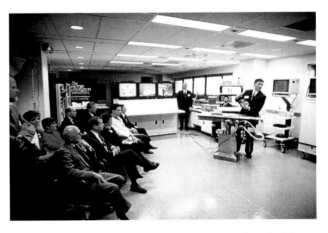

Fig. 10-57 Videoconferencing can be used for administrative meetings.

instrument is used during an endoscopic procedure, but it also allows two-way communication between the observers and the surgeon performing the procedure.

Future applications

Videoconferencing has been the inspiration behind remote telepresence surgery. With the advent of robotics and videoconferencing equipment and connectivity, a physician can now perform surgery on a patient at a distant site. The physician merely places his or her hands into special gloves that control instrument movement and views the patient via a telecommunications linkup to the far site. The actual movements made by the physician are transmitted to the far site, where the surgery is actually being performed. In the future, the perioperative nurse may be the only licensed professional at the sterile field. This technology has advanced quickly from its original purpose of providing remote telepresence surgery on the battlefield and in space.

Videoconferencing Issues

There are numerous issues that surround the use of videoconferencing. Once these concerns are addressed and potential solutions offered, videoconferencing can become an even more acceptable and popular tool.

Standardization

The need to be able to communicate using different brands of equipment has made it necessary to develop standards for the industry. Governmental mandates now require manufacturers to meet the agreed upon criteria so that interactivity can be accomplished. However, transmission is best when all the equipment used has been purchased from the same manufacturer, because this allows full advantage to be taken of the different equipment features. For example, if a different codec is used at each site, it will usually not be possible to remotely control the camera. The cameras can be controlled remotely if two similar codecs are used.

Confidentiality

Confidentiality is a vital and fundamental component of patient care. The patient must always be assured that privacy is maintained by anyone involved with his or her care. Videoconferencing is now challenging this patient right because of the patient information, assessment data, and treatment results being shared with providers at remote sites. Therefore, the health care team utilizing videoconferencing must constantly strive to ensure confidentiality.

Today many non–health care companies are getting involved in the sale of videoconferencing equipment and connectivity, but some of these companies are not versed in the protocols, expectations, and ethics surrounding patient care. Therefore, they are not concerned about methods or procedures that guarantee patient privacy. As an example of one situation that could happen, suppose an insurance salesman is thinking he is calling a colleague for a videoconferencing meeting but accidentally dials a surgical suite where a female patient is being prepped for a laparoscopy. When the call is connected, the patient's privacy is invaded because the salesman is then actually entering the surgical suite remotely.

Every health care provider, hospital, clinic, or other setting that is purchasing videoconferencing equipment and establishing connectivity must be cognizant of this major problem. Providers can ensure patient confidentiality only by using a private network for health care services. Therefore, before procuring equipment and determining the appropriate network for connectivity, users must find out from the vendor or person integrating the system who can directly call into the network.

Practicing across state lines

State boards of medicine and state boards of nursing control the practices of medicine and nursing, respectively. This means that to practice within a certain state, one must hold a license awarded by that state. By allowing providers to interactively communicate to provide care for a patient across state boundaries, videoconferencing threatens to violate this arrangement. For example, a family practice physician in West Virginia may seek a remote consultation for a patient from a urologist in Ohio. Does this then mean that the urologist is actually being telephonically transmitted to West Virginia to treat the patient? If this is the case, then the urologist would need a license to practice in West Virginia. Or is the patient being telephonically transported to Ohio for treatment? If the latter is the case, a problem would not exist because the urologist is licensed to practice in Ohio.

This problem becomes even more of an issue if it is a nurse who is at one end of the transmission. That is, a nurse assessing a patient in West Virginia cannot carry out an order from a consulting physician in Ohio because both practitioners must be licensed within the same state.

At first glance one would think there is an easy solution to this problem. For example, health care providers who use videoconferencing could be granted a national license that would allow them to care for and treat patients across state lines. Such a licensing arrangement would be similar to the one pertaining to military nurses and physicians that allows them to practice in the different states they are sent to. However, one major question that must still be resolved is where does jurisdiction reside if national licensure is granted—in the state where the patient has been treated or in the state where the remote consultation originated?

These are problems that are currently being addressed in the health care field as videoconferencing evolves. The American Telemedicine Association is serving as a valuable resource to the American Medical Association and the Federation of the State Medical Boards in their effort to resolve this quandary. The National Council of State Boards of Nursing and the American Nurses Association are also exploring solutions to this problem that apply to the nursing community.

Reimbursement

The provision of a remote consultation by an expert requires reimbursement for services rendered, but currently there are no guidelines for determining the amount of such reimbursement or whether reimbursement should even be granted. The Health Care Financing Administration (HCFA) is reviewing this predicament and has designated some pilot project sites where reimbursement for remote consultations is to be studied. As the results from this study are published, other third-party carriers will be able to address the issue of reimbursement.

Capitation will have a direct effect on the popularity of videoconferencing. Because income is already determined in a capitated environment, reimbursement is not a concern. Capitated health care delivery is focused on keeping costs down while still providing quality services. The use of videoconferencing to obtain remote consultations with experts may facilitate the delivery of more immediate care that maintains the patient's optimal health, whereas sending a patient to a distant site for assessment and treatment will only increase expenditures, especially if the patient's condition is compromised as a result of the need to be transported and the delay in treatment.

Return on investment

The return on investment needs to be determined to justify the cost of videoconferencing equipment and connectivity for use in an endoscopic program. To this end, a business plan should be developed in a consistent and organized fashion that validates the need to get involved with videoconferencing in the delivery of health care. The following outline can be used as a model for creating a business plan for a videoconferencing program.

  I. External assessment of videoconferencing technology
    A. Evolution of videoconferencing
    B. External environment assessment
      1. Local competition
        a. Videoconferencing applications
        b. Administrative support
        c. Equipment and connectivity
        d. Promotion of program
        e. Physician use and interest
      2. Community needs (rural sites, clinics)
      3. Regulatory issues
        a. State licensure
        b. Reimbursement
        c. Standardization
  II. Internal assessment of videoconferencing potential
    A. Administrative support
    B. Financial resources and needs
    C. Proposed applications
      1. Equipment needed
      2. Connectivity capabilities
      3. Anticipated usage
      4. Capital and operating budget needs
    D. Technical support within facility
    E. Education required to foster support of program
    F. Internal marketing capabilities
    G. Benefits for the patient, provider, hospital
  III. SWOT analysis of facility concerning videoconferencing
    A. Strengths
    B. Weaknesses
    C. Opportunities
    D. Threats
  IV. Proposed goals of the videoconferencing program
    A. Short-term goals (less than 1 year)
      1. Financial performance
      2. Program development, maintenance, and expansion
      3. Applications
      4. Equipment maintenance and service
      5. Staffing
      6. Marketing
    B. Intermediate goals (1 to 3 years)
    C. Long-term goals (over 3 years)
  V. Proposed evaluation methods
    A. Satisfaction surveys
      1. Physicians
      2. Nurses
      3. Other health care professionals
      4. Patients
    B. Written annual report
      1. Overview of videoconferencing program
      2. Trends in videoconferencing program
      3. Highlights during the year
      4. Return on investment
        a. Resources used
        b. Cost savings
      5. Achievement of set goals
      6. Proposed future goals

Increased use of videoconferencing in health care environments will justify the cost of the equipment and connectivity, provide increased accessiblity to patients and experts, enhance the quality of patient care services, validate improved patient outcomes, promote cost-efficiency, and advance communications and networking technology in health care.

REFERENCES

Adv Technol Surg Care: 3D technology may be next surgical standard, 13(6):74, 1995.

Ball KA: Riding the superhighway of education with video teleconferencing, *Minimally Invasive Surg Nurs* 8(3):114, 1994.

Ball KA, Perez J, Theslof G: Video conferencing in surgery: an evolving tool for education and preceptorships, *Telemed J* 1(4):297, 1995.

Birkett DG, Josephs LG, Este-McDonald J: A new 3-D laparoscope in gastrointestinal surgery, *Surg Endosc* 8(1):1448, 1994.

Frantzides CT: *Laparoscopic and thoracoscopic surgery*, St. Louis, 1995, Mosby.

Laparosc Surg Update: Video troubleshooting tips, 2(10):114, 1994.

Laparosc Surg Update: Close encounter with the video screen may contaminate gloves, should be avoided, 3(4):43, 1995.

Meeker MH, Rothrock JC: *Alexander's care of the patient in surgery*, ed 10, St. Louis, 1995, Mosby.

Nezhat CR, Nezhat FR, Luciano AA, et al: *Operative gynecologic laparoscopy principles and techniques*, New York, 1995, McGraw-Hill.

Preston J: *The telemedicine handbook*, Austin, Tex., 1992, Telemedicine Interactive Consultive Services.

Spellman JR: Laparoscopic equipment troubleshooting, *Today's OR Nurse* 17(1):13, 1995.

Trowt-Bayard T: *Videoconferencing, the whole picture*, New York, 1994, Flatiron Publishing.

11

Endoscopic Energies and Diagnostic Tools

Different types of energies are now available that can be used through flexible or rigid endoscopes for therapeutic and diagnostic purposes. This chapter reviews the critical details about these various energies, as well as the details about various diagnostic tools that can be used endoscopically, so that nurses and others will have a thorough understanding of how to use this technology safely and appropriately in health care setting.

LASER

History of Laser Technology

In 1917 Albert Einstein formulated the theory of stimulated emission that became the basis for laser technology (Einstein, 1917). This theory basically states that the ability of molecules to absorb radiation depends on the number of molecules present and whether the molecules are in their upper- or lower-energy states. Molecules in the upper state are more stimulated to emit rather than absorb radiation.

In 1958 A. L. Schawlow and C. H. Townes explored this concept and developed the principle of LASER, which is an acronym for light amplification by the stimulated emission of radiation. They thought that mirrors could be used to amplify this stimulated emission (Schawlow and Townes, 1958).

Guided by these earlier concepts, Dr. Theodore H. Maiman built the first true laser in 1960 (Fig. 11-1). A ruby crystal was used as the lasing material, and mirrors were used to amplify the lasing action. This was the first of many lasers to be developed for medical use (Ball, 1995).

Since then, laser technology has expanded tremendously, and, as new wavelengths and delivery devices have been introduced, it has continued to grow in popularity. During this time, laser systems have become less complex, extremely mobile, and very user friendly. Today lasers are used as the standard tool for many ophthalmologic and dermatologic procedures. The versatility and effectiveness of the laser as a cutting and coagulating tool has also made it a popular instrument for many endoscopic procedures. However, with the health care reform issues and cost containment concerns of the 1990s, the cost-efficiency of laser technology has been challenged. In addition, many laser systems purchased in the late 1980s and early 1990s have fallen into disuse because of inappropriate patient charges for the system, which deterred their use. However, for those physicians who have mastered the art of controlling the laser beam and helped to establish realistic patient charges for use of the technology, lasers remain the preferred means of cutting, coagulating, ablating, and vaporizing tissue (Fig. 11-2).

Laser Physics

The acronym LASER describes the process by which a form of energy is converted into light energy. This term is also used to refer to the device that produces the light, and to the light itself.

Light is measured in wavelengths. A wavelength is the distance between the peaks of two successive waves, usually measured in microns or nanometers. The wavelength determines the color of the light (Fig. 11-3). Wavelengths can be graphed along a continuum, known

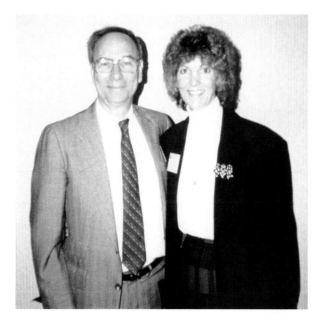

Fig. 11-1 Dr. Theodore Maiman and author, Kay Ball. (From Ball KA: *Lasers: the perioperative challenge*, ed 2, St. Louis, 1995, Mosby.)

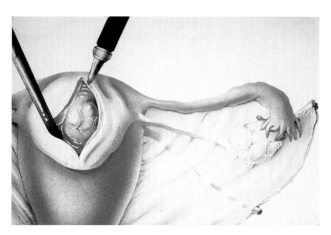

Fig. 11-2 The Nd:YAG laser energy delivered through a contact tip is used to precisely excise a uterine lesion during laparoscopy. (Courtesy Surgical Laser Technologies, Inc., Oaks, Penn.)

sists of negatively charged electrons rotating around a positively charged nucleus. The electrons orbit at discrete energy levels at various distances from the nucleus. These electrons are able to move from one orbital path to another, and in the process produce energy.

Laser energy is generated in the following way. When a negatively charged electron rotates close to the nucleus, the atom is in its ground state, or resting phase. When the atom is excited by an outside energy source, the energy is absorbed and the electron jumps into a higher orbital shell and becomes unstable. Almost immediately the electron returns to its normal resting state, but as it does so, a tiny bundle of surplus energy, called a *photon*, is spontaneously emitted. While it is excited this photon can interact with a neighboring atom, causing it to emit a photon. Stimulated emission has thus occurred because two photons have been emitted that travel together in perfect harmony (Fig. 11-6). The excitation process continues until there are more atoms in the excited state

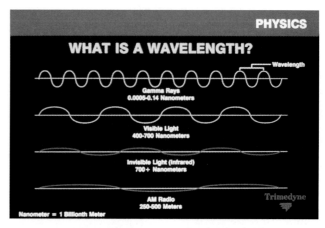

Fig. 11-3 Wavelength is the distance between the peaks of two successive waves. The wavelength can be very long to very short. (Courtesy Trimedyne, Inc., Irvine, Calif.)

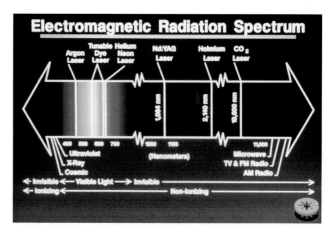

Fig. 11-4 The electromagnetic spectrum. (Courtesy Coherent, Inc., Palo Alto, Calif.)

as the *electromagnetic spectrum* (Fig. 11-4). They can range from very long, in the infrared region, to very short, in the ultraviolet area (Fig. 11-5). Wavelengths in the infrared area are 750 nm 1 mm long. Examples of light with long wavelengths are radio waves, television waves, and microwaves. The carbon dioxide laser has a wavelength of 10,600 nm. Visible light exists in the midregion of 400 to 750 nm. The blue-green light emitted by the argon laser exists in this range. Ultraviolet wavelengths, or short waves, are in the 100- to 400-nm region. The light emitted by excimer lasers exists in this range. X rays and cosmic rays have much shorter wavelengths.

An understanding of basic atomic activity is needed to comprehend how laser energy is formed. An atom con-

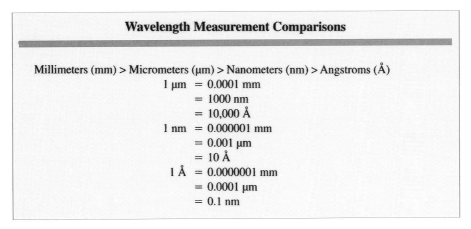

Fig. 11-5   The range of wavelengths in the electromagnetic spectrum. (From Ball KA: *Lasers: the perioperative challenge*, ed 2, St. Louis, 1995, Mosby.)

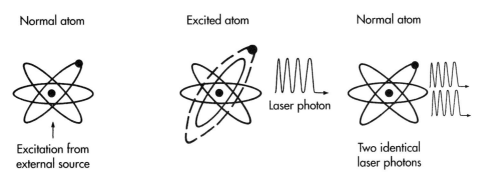

Fig. 11-6   Photon generation. An external energy source excites the atom to spontaneously emit a photon. This photon can stimulate the emission of two identical photons. (From Ball KA: *Lasers: the perioperative challenge*, ed 2, St. Louis, 1995, Mosby.)

than in the resting state, a condition known as *population inversion of the laser medium*. At this point, laser energy can be emitted from the system.

Laser Light Characteristics

Laser light differs from ordinary light in three ways: It is monochromatic, collimated, and coherent.

Monochromatic means one color or one wavelength. Laser light produces photons that are all the same color or wavelength. Red laser light is usually 630 nm and is a pure red. In contrast, white light coming from a light bulb consists of array of different colors or wavelengths.

Laser light is considered collimated because the light waves are parallel to each other as they travel in space, unlike the uncollimated light from a flashlight, for example, which diverges and spreads out as it travels away from its source (Fig. 11-7).

Laser light waves are also considered coherent because they travel in phase and in the same direction. All of the peaks and troughs of the waves are synchronized with each other. On the other hand, ordinary light waves from a light bulb travel in random directions, making them incoherent (Fig. 11-8).

Power Density

The power of the laser beam is measured in watts. Wattage is equal to the amount of laser energy, measured in joules, divided by the duration of exposure, measured in seconds:

$$\text{Watts} = \frac{\text{Joules}}{\text{Seconds}}$$

Power density refers to the amount of laser power that is concentrated within a spot. It is determined by dividing the power (watts) by the diameter of the spot size, measured in centimeters squared:

$$\text{Power density} = \frac{\text{Watts}}{\text{Spot size (cm}^2\text{)}}$$

Power density therefore is the amount of power that is distributed within the area of the beam diameter. The smaller the spot size, the more concentrated the power; thus, the greater the power density, the more intense the beam. With increased power density, the depth of penetration into the tissue is greater. If the laser energy

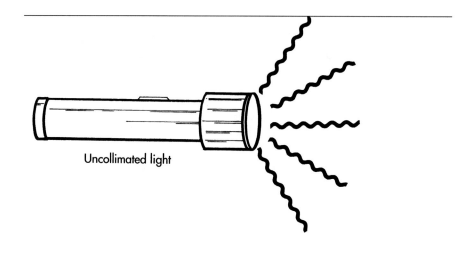

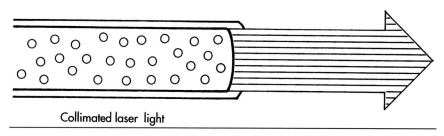

Fig. 11-7 Collimated laser beam compared with the noncollimated beam from a flashlight. (From Ball KA: *Lasers: the perioperative challenge*, ed 2, St. Louis, 1995, Mosby.)

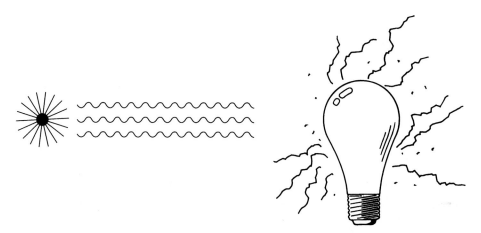

Fig. 11-8 Coherent laser beam compared with the incoherent waves from a light bulb. (From Ball, KA: *Lasers: the perioperative challenge*, ed 2, St. Louis, 1995, Mosby.)

is spread out over a larger spot size, then the same wattage is disseminated over a larger area, thus decreasing the power density and depth of penetration.

Tissue Effects

When laser energy strikes tissue, reflection, scattering, transmission, or absorption occurs, depending on the laser wavelength, the energy delivered, and the type of tissue.

Reflection occurs if the laser beam hits an obstacle and is reflected off of it (Fig. 11-9). If a shiny instrument is in the path of the laser beam, then direct reflection occurs, causing potential injury at another site. For example, a CO_2 laser beam can be reflected off the surface of the laparoscope, causing an accidental burn to other tissue. Instruments that could be in the path of the laser beam can be ebonized or anodized to minimize direct reflection.

Some of the laser beams, especially the noncontact neodymium:yttrium-aluminum-garnet (Nd:YAG) laser beam, can scatter as the energy is distributed in many different paths after hitting the surface (Fig. 11-10). Backscattering could occur during endoscopy if the laser beam scatters backward up through the endoscope. This could damage the operator's eye or the optics of the telescope. Backscattering can also cause damage to the distal end of the scope.

Some of the laser energies cause little or no thermal energy to be produced when transmitted through tissue (Fig. 11-11). For example, the argon laser beam can be transmitted through clear structures and solutions of the eye (cornea, aqueous, lens, and vitreous) to coagulate a bleeding vessel on the retina, but because the energy is not absorbed by the clear structures and solutions, no tissue effect is observed in these nontargeted areas.

Thermal effects and a tissue response occur when the laser energy is absorbed (Fig. 11-12). Most laser light causes a thermal response when it strikes tissues, thus causing the laser beam to be absorbed by the cells. As the laser energy strikes the tissue, the cells are heated to the point of boiling (100°C). Vaporization and carbonization occur as the pressure within the cell rises and the membrane ruptures, spewing the cellular contents into the air. Adjacent cells are affected as the target cells continue to be heated (Fig. 11-13). The degree of thermal damage depends on the temperature to which the cells are heated. If only coagulation is desired, then the cells should only be heated to 60° to 65°C, the point at which the tissue begins to blanch. If less heat is produced, there is less adjacent conductive thermal spread and less tissue damage. The length of exposure of the laser energy to the tissue is important in determining the amount of thermal spread (Table 11-1).

Laser Systems

There are a variety of laser systems that are currently being used for medical purposes. Following are the characteristics of each type of laser used for such purposes, going

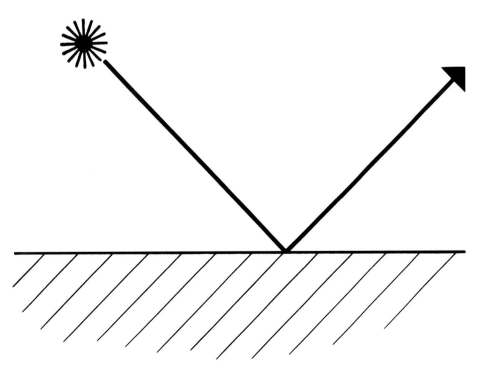

Fig. 11-9   Reflection. (From Ball KA: *Lasers: the perioperative challenge*, ed 2, St. Louis, 1995, Mosby.)

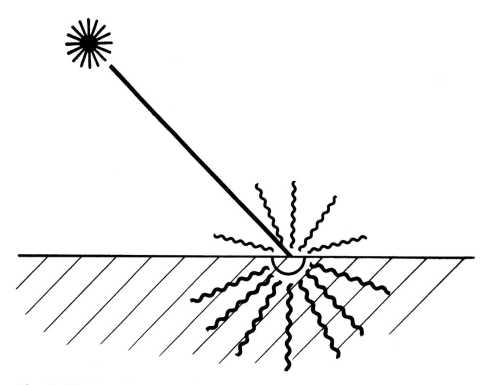

Fig. 11-10 Scattering. (From Ball, KA: *Lasers: the perioperative challenge*, ed 2, St. Louis, 1995, Mosby.)

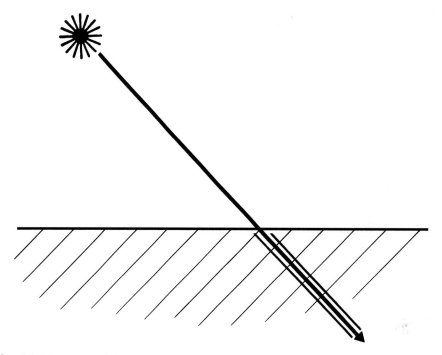

Fig. 11-11 Transmission. (From Ball KA: *Lasers: the perioperative challenge*, ed 2, St. Louis, 1995, Mosby.)

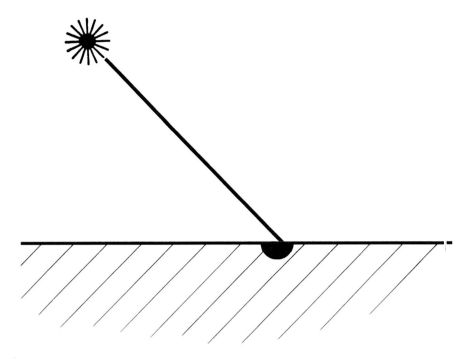

Fig. 11-12 Absorption. (From Ball KA: *Lasers: the perioperative challenge*, ed 2, St. Louis, 1995, Mosby.)

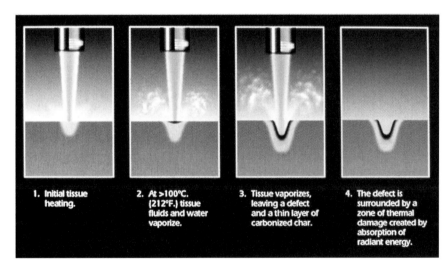

1. Initial tissue heating.

2. At >100°C. (212°F.) tissue fluids and water vaporize.

3. Tissue vaporizes, leaving a defect and a thin layer of carbonized char.

4. The defect is surrounded by a zone of thermal damage created by absorption of radiant energy.

Fig. 11-13 Absorption of laser energy in tissue. (Courtesy Surgical Laser Technologies, Inc., Oaks, Penn.)

from those that emit longer-wavelength light to those that emit shorter-wavelength light.

Carbon dioxide laser
- 10,600-nm wavelength
- Complex delivery system within an articulated arm with mirrors or a waveguide system
- Continuous or pulsed modes
- Transmitted through air
- Shallow depth of penetration (0.1 to 0.2 mm)

Table 1 ▪ *Tissue changes with temperature increases*

Temperature	Visual change	Biologic change
37°–60°C	No visual change	Warming, welding
60°–65°C	Blanching	Coagulation
65°–90°C	White/gray	Protein denaturization
90°–100°C	Puckering	Drying
100°C	Smoke plume	Vaporization, carbonization

- Highly absorbed by water
- Not color selective
- Used with rigid endoscopes

Erbium:YAG laser
- 2900-nm wavelength
- Fiber delivery system
- Pulsed mode
- Highly absorbed by water
- Shallow depth of penetration
- Being explored for use with endoscopes

Holmium:YAG laser
- 2100-nm wavelength
- Fiber delivery system
- Pulsed mode
- Produces a vapor bubble to transmit the beam to the tissue in fluid environments
- Shallow depth of penetration (0.4 to 0.6 mm)
- Used with rigid or flexible endoscopes

Neodymium:YAG laser
- 1064-nm wavelength
- Fiber delivery system (noncontact or contact)
- Continuous or pulsed modes
- Transmitted through clear solutions
- Great depth of penetration with noncontact (2 to 6 mm)
- Shallow depth of penetration with contact (0.1 to 0.5 mm)
- Used with flexible or rigid endoscopes

Frequency-doubled YAG laser
- 1064-nm wavelength
- 532-nm wavelength when potassium titanyl phosphate (KTP) crystal is placed in front of the 1064-nm wavelength laser beam
- Fiber delivery system
- Continuous or pulsed modes
- Depth of penetration dependent on wavelength
- 532-nm wavelength very selective to pigmented tissue
- Used with flexible or rigid endoscopes

Argon laser
- Blue-green color at 488- and 515-nm wavelengths
- Fiber delivery system
- Continuous or pulsed modes
- Transmitted through clear structures and solutions
- Moderate depth of penetration (0.5 to 2 mm)
- Highly selective to pigmented tissue (hemoglobin and melanin)
- Used with flexible or rigid endoscopes

Tunable dye laser
- 400 to 1000-nm wavelengths variable with dyes
- Red dye laser (approximately 630 nm)

- Yellow dye laser (approximately 577 to 585 nm). This wavelength is highly selective to pigmented tissue (hemoglobin)
- Fiber delivery system
- Depth of penetration dependent on laser wavelength
- Used with flexible or rigid endoscopes

Excimer laser
- 100- to 360-nm wavelengths variable with laser media
- Complex delivery systems
- Excellent cutting capabilities
- Laser media may be carcinogenic
- Currently not being used for endoscopy

Laser Safety

To use laser technology the surgical team members must attend special training classes that educate them about laser biophysics, safety, and applications. This helps ensure that the laser is used safely and appropriately during surgery. However, even though there are many safety factors that should be understood, the three most important ones pertaining to laser endoscopy are eye protection, smoke evacuation, and fire safety.

Eye protection

Laser energy can damage unprotected eyes during surgery. Because there are numerous different wavelengths that can be used during endoscopy, there is a variety of eyewear that can be worn. The eye protection must block the specific wavelength of the laser beam being used. According to the American National Standards Institute Z136.3 guidelines, the wavelength that the lens is protecting against and the optical density or filtering capacity of the lens material must be inscribed on the eyewear (Fig. 11-14). The eyewear should also have side shields to protect the wearer's eyes when his or her head is turned (Fig. 11-15).

Different laser beams have different effects on the eye (Fig. 11-16). The CO_2, holmium:YAG, and excimer lasers can cause corneal damage because these beams are highly absorbed by the cells of the cornea. The noncontact Nd:YAG and argon lasers can damage the retina because these wavelengths are transmitted through the clear anterior structures and solutions of the eye.

Eyewear should be worn whenever a laser system is in use during endoscopy, even though the beam may appear to be confined within an enclosed area. This is because problems can easily occur that would allow the beam to be emitted outside the enclosed endoscopic site, thus creating a hazardous situation. For example, the fiber may accidentally become dislodged from the endoscope during activation, allowing the laser beam to be emitted outside the confined endoscopic area. Or the laser fiber could be broken somewhere along its length, allowing the laser energy to exit at the site of the break.

Eye protection should also be worn whenever the CO_2 laser is used during laparoscopic procedures. This is necessary, because, for example, the articulated arm could become disconnected, thus allowing the laser energy to exit, or the CO_2 laparoscope could be removed from the cannula, also allowing the CO_2 beam to cause harm if it should be inadvertently activated.

The patient's eyes must also be protected during endoscopic procedures. If general anesthesia is being used, the anesthesia provider usually makes sure of this (Fig.

11-17). If the patient is awake during the endoscopic procedure, then he or she should be instructed as to the rationale for wearing eye protection and should wear the appropriate eye glasses or goggles.

Smoke evacuation

One of the major safety concerns associated with laser technology is the hazards posed by the surgical plume or smoke that is emitted as tissue is vaporized. The laser is not the only thermal surgical tool that causes a plume to be generated, however. The electrosurgical unit can also produce surgical smoke that must be evacuated.

Whenever a thermal tool impacts tissue, cellular destruction occurs as the cellular contents heat to the point of boiling, thus causing the cell membrane to rupture and a plume to be emitted. Surgical smoke consists of water, carbonized particles, possibly viruses and bacteria, and an offensive odor. The odor is caused by the toxins in the smoke, such as acrolein, benzene, formaldehyde, polycyclic aromatic hydrocarbons, and toluene.

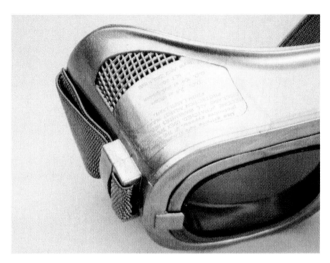

Fig. 11-14 The wavelength and optical density should be inscribed on the lens or elsewhere on the protective eyewear. (From Ball KA: *Lasers: the perioperative challenge*, ed 2, St. Louis, 1995, Mosby.)

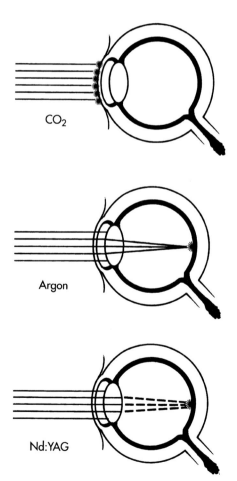

Fig. 11-16 The CO_2 laser can cause corneal damage; the argon and Nd:YAG lasers can cause retinal damage. (From Ball KA: *Lasers: the perioperative challenge*, ed 2, St. Loius, 1995, Mosby.)

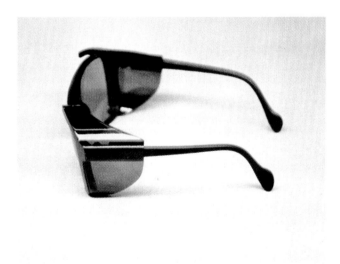

Fig. 11-15 Side shields prevent the laser beam from striking the eye from the side. (From Ball KA: *Lasers: the perioperative challenge*, ed 2, St. Louis, 1995, Mosby.)

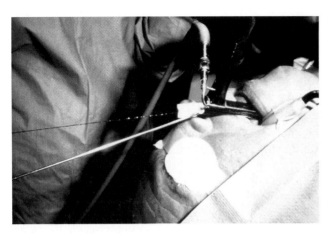

Fig. 11-17   The patient's eyes are protected with moistened gauze pads during laser microlaryngoscopy. (From Ball KA: *Lasers: the perioperative challenge*, ed 2, St. Louis, 1995, Mosby.)

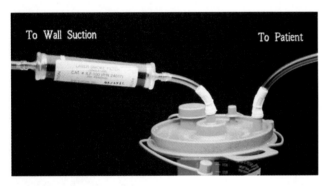

Fig. 11-18   An inline filter is placed between the suction canister and the wall outlet and is used to evacuate small amounts of plume. (Courtesy Stackhouse, Inc., Palm Springs, Calif.)

The two chief concerns pertaining to surgical smoke are the size of the particulate matter and the viability of the cells within the plume. Research has conclusively shown that 77% of the particulate matter in the plume is 1.1 μm in diameter or smaller (Mihashi et al, 1975). This extremely small particulate matter can easily be inhaled into the alveoli of the surgical team members' lungs if not evacuated adequately. This can lead to chronic irritation or infection and possibly bronchitis or emphysema-like conditions.

Surgical masks are not adequate protection, however, because they usually only filter particulate matter that is 5 μm in diameter or larger. High-filtration surgical masks can filter particulate matter that is 0.1 μm, but these masks should not be used as the first line of protection. The plume needs to be evacuated at the point of origin.

The viability of the cells contained in the plume continues to be researched. Garden et al (1988) conducted research that proved intact DNA from bovine papilloma virus can be extracted from laser smoke. In a continuation of this study, the DNA was then reinoculated into cows, with the result that the same papilloma virus grew in these animals (*Clin Laser Monthly*, 1993). Because the route of entry was through inoculation and not through the respiratory tract, further studies are needed to conclusively prove whether viable cells can be transmitted in surgical smoke.

A smoke evacuation system should be used whenever a surgical plume is generated. An inline suction filter can be used to evacuate small amounts of plume without its contaminating the suction line system (Fig. 11-18). Larger plumes can be adequately evacuated using an individual smoke evacuator (Fig. 11-19). Most units on the market today have an ultra low penetration air (ULPA) filter that filters particulate matter down to 0.1 μm in diameter. The ULPA filter needs to be changed periodically, however, to maintain this filtering capability. A charcoal filter usually is included in the smoke evacuator filtration system to absorb the offensive odor.

The plume released during laparoscopy is difficult to evacuate without removing the insufflation gas, too. A low-pressure suction valve can be placed on the suction line to minimize the amount of gas removed. By depressing the plunger, the resulting gentle suction will cause the plume to dissipate without destroying the pneumoperitoneum (Fig. 11-20). A high-flow insufflator is also needed, however, to provide a continual flow of insufflation gas.

Ott et al conducted research to determine the effects of surgical smoke that is left inside the abdomen during laparoscopy (*Laparosc Surg Update*, 1994). It was found that the smoke can cause an increase in the carboxyhemoglobin level, thus decreasing the patient's perfusion intraoperatively. If the plume is evacuated during the procedure, the patients experience less postoperative symptoms, such as nausea.

Fire safety

Any tool, such as a laser, that produces heat energy is capable of starting a fire during surgery. Ignition can

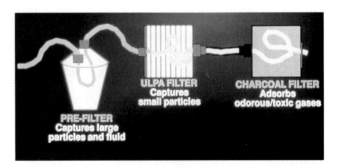

Fig. 11-19   Smoke evacuation may involve the use of multiple filtering systems. (Courtesy Stackhouse, Inc., Palm Springs, Calif.)

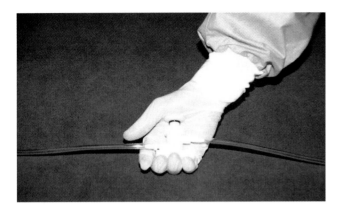

Fig. 11-20   Gentle suctioning of the plume generated during laparoscopic procedures can be achieved by depressing a special low-pressure suction valve. (From Ball KA: *Lasers: the perioperative challenge*, ed 2, St. Louis, 1995, Mosby.)

occur if a reflected laser beam or a direct laser beam comes in contact with a dry, combustible item. Therefore, whenever a laser is used during endoscopy, the delivery system, such as the fiber, must never be placed on drapes, sponges, or plastic instruments that are combustible. The laser must be put in the standby mode whenever it is not being used.

If the surgical drapes or something near the surgical site catches fire, the flames need to be smothered immediately. Sterile water or saline is usually readily available to help douse the fire. If the laser unit is on fire, then a fire extinguisher should be used. A halon (hydrogenated halocarbons) fire extinguisher may be recommended, depending on state regulations. Because halon disrupts the ozone layer of the atmosphere, halon fire extinguishers are considered an environmental concern.

Other fire extinguishers can also be used, but only with caution, because each can cause damage to the laser unit. A carbon dioxide fire extinguisher freezes the target site with its pressurized contents but can damage the internal components of the laser. A dry chemical (ABC) fire extinguisher emits a very fine dust, but this can damage the optics or circuitry of the laser. Pressurized water should not be sprayed on a laser system, however, because the high-voltage current can be conducted by water and cause electrocution.

Instrument safety

A laser delivery device must be compatible with the instrumentation or endoscope to prevent damage to the fiber and to the endoscope or instrument. For example, a laser fiber must be small enough to fit easily into the endoscopic instrument or endoscope (Fig. 11-21).

Because the tip of a bare fiber can tear the inside lumen of the operating port of a flexible endoscope

upon insertion, a length of medical grade tubing (approximately 3 feet [1 meter] long) can be used to protect the end of the fiber during insertion. To do this the fiber is placed inside the tubing with the end of the fiber recessed within the tubing. The fiber and tubing are then inserted into the operating channel of the flexible endoscope. When the tubing and fiber tip can be seen through the endoscope, then the tubing is withdrawn to expose the fiber tip. This protects the inside lumen of the channel.

If the fiber is too close to the scope end, the energy emitted from the fiber tip and the backscatter from the laser beam can cause thermal damage, resulting in lens pitting, operating port trauma, and other related problems (Fig. 11-22). To prevent this the distal end of the fiber must extend at least 1 cm past the tip of the endoscope before the laser is activated (Fig. 11-23). Both the end of the fiber and the position of the

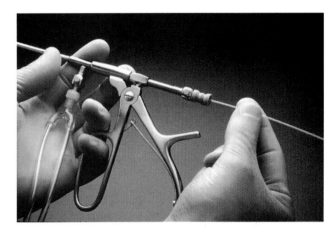

Fig. 11-21   To prevent damage to a laser fiber, it must fit easily into an endoscopic instrument.

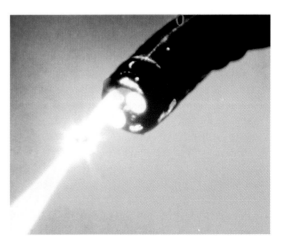

Fig. 11-22   The tip of the laser fiber must extend past the end of the endoscope to protect the lens and the end of the scope from thermal damage.

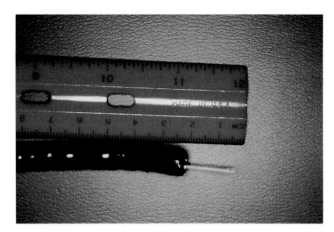

Fig. 11-23 Before the laser is activated the operator should make sure the laser fiber extends past the end of the endoscope.

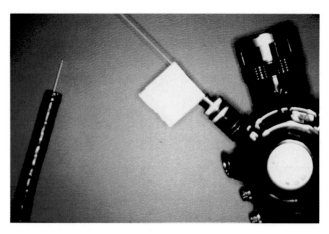

Fig. 11-24 By flagging the fiber, the team can determine whether the fiber tip is extending past the end of the endoscope.

aiming beam on the target site should be observed. If the endoscopic procedure is being viewed by the endoscopic team, then the laser operator can also note the position of the fiber before placing the laser in the ready mode.

To ensure that the laser fiber extends adequately beyond the tip of the endoscope, it can be marked before the procedure to determine the appropriate positioning. To do this the fiber is first passed through the endoscope to position the tip past the end of the endoscope. A piece of tape is then placed on the fiber at the level of the operating channel entry port (Fig. 11-24). The fiber is then withdrawn with the tape in place. As the fiber is inserted through the endoscope during the procedure, the physician and endoscopic team members can observe the location of the tape to determine whether the fiber is far enough beyond the end of the endoscope before they activate the laser.

Benefits of Laser Technology

There are many benefits to using laser technology in endoscopic procedures. These include (Ball, 1995):

- The sealing of smaller blood vessels (less bleeding)
- The sealing of lymphatics (decreases postoperative edema and the spread of malignant cells)
- The sealing of nerve endings (in selective tissues, decreases postoperative pain)
- The sterilization of tissue (resulting from thermal response)
- A decrease in the extent of postoperative stenosis (resulting from decreased scarring)
- Quicker recovery time and return to normal activities (for many procedures)
- Shorter surgery time (for many procedures)
- A shift to outpatient and local anesthesia (for many procedures)

ELECTROSURGICAL UNIT

For many years, electrosurgery has been a popular energy used for endoscopic procedures. However, many endoscopic team members have never attended a formal training class in this technology. Education is vital to ensuring the safe use of electrosurgery, and some of the important points are covered here.

History of Electrosurgery

The use of electrosurgery became popular around 1926 when Dr. Harvey Cushing, a neurosurgeon, and Dr. William T. Bovie, a biophysical engineer, worked together to develop the technology for use in neurosurgical procedures (Fig. 11-25). They were very impressed with its coagulative capabilities and concluded that it was a vital instrument in providing the hemostasis needed during vascular procedures, such as neurosurgical procedures.

The first commercially electrosurgery unit (ESU) was available in the early 1930s (Fig. 11-26). It stood chest high and weighed about 300 pounds (136 kg). The entire cabinet was crafted out of wood.

As an interesting aside, Dr. Bovie tried to sell the patent for his invention to Harvard University, but they were not interested. He ultimately sold the patent for $1.00 to the Liebel Flarshiem Company, who manufactured it. Dr. Bovie died destitute in Maine.

Electrosurgery Physics

The basic physics of electricity must be understood to comprehend how electrosurgery is accomplished. As mentioned earlier, atoms have electrons that orbit the nucleus of each atom. As electrons flow from one atom to the orbit of an adjacent atom, an electrical current is generated. The properties of electricity—current, voltage,

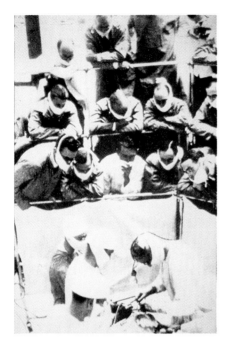

Fig. 11-25 Dr. Harvey Cushing and Dr. William Bovie working collaboratively to develop electrosurgery. (Courtesy Valleylab, Inc., Boulder, Colo.)

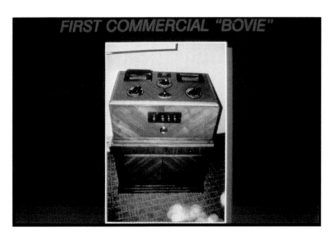

Fig. 11-26 The first commercially available electrosurgery unit weighed about 300 pounds (136 kg). (Courtesy Valleylab, Inc., Boulder, Colo.)

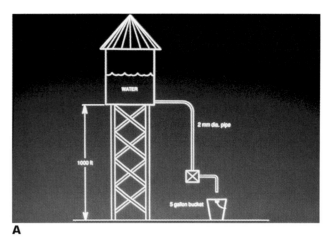

A

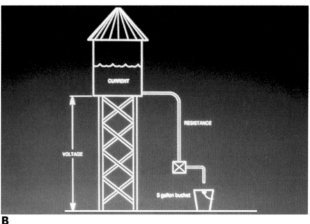

B

Fig. 11-27 **A** and **B**, The properties of electricity can be compared to the behavior of water in a water tower. (Courtesy Valleylab, Inc., Boulder, Colo.)

Resistance: The impedance that is present to obstruct the flow of electrons. It is measured in ohms. Resistance can be compared to the diameter of the water pipe through which the water flows from the water tower. A smaller-diameter pipe will restrict the flow, and a larger-diameter pipe will facilitate the flow of water. Resistance is produced by the various body tissues during electrosurgery. As electrons encounter resistance, heat is produced and a tissue effect is noted.

A completed circuit or an intact pathway must be present so the electrons can flow. That is, if an electrical current originates from earth, then the electricity must be returned to the ground to complete the circuit.

Two forms of electrical energy are used today: direct current (DC) and alternating current (AC). In DC the electrons flow only in one direction; in AC the electrons flow back and forth as the polarity changes, depending on the frequency of the device being operated (Fig. 11-28). During electrosurgery, AC actually enters the patient's body and the patient becomes part of the circuit.

and resistance—can be compared to the behavior of water in a water tower, as follows (Fig. 11-27):

Current: The flow of electrons measured in amperes. It can be compared to the water that flows from a water tower.

Voltage: The force or push that allows the electrons to travel or flow from one atom to another. Voltage is measured in volts. Voltage can be compared to the height of the water tower that determines the force with which the water flows.

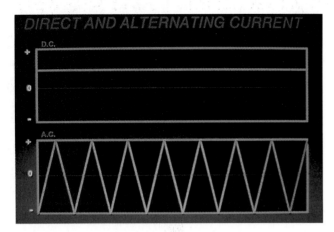

Fig. 11-28   Direct current versus alternating current. (Courtesy Valleylab, Inc., Boulder, Colo.)

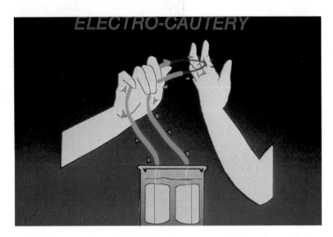

Fig. 11-29   During electrocautery, direct current is used to heat a wire but the electrical current does not enter the patient's body. (Courtesy Valleylab, Inc., Boulder, Colo.)

The term *electrocautery* is often misused in reference to electrosurgery. Electrocautery devices make use of DC as the electrons flow in one direction into a wire element. Because the wire produces a high impedance to the electrical flow, heat is produced. The wire is then held in contact with tissue to provide coagulative effects (Fig. 11-29), but no electrical current actually passes into the patient's tissue. Electrocautery energy can be created in battery-operated units, such as the small disposable electrocautery devices used to coagulate blood vessels during cataract extraction.

Frequency is the number of waves passing through a given point. It is measured in hertz units. The electrical current in a normal household wall outlet alternates at 60 cycles per second (Hz) at approximately 110 volts. If a person were to stick his or her finger into a wall outlet, then nerve and muscle tissues would be electrostimulated. Prolonged exposure could result in electrocution.

Neuromuscular stimulation ceases when the frequency of the electrical current is increased to more than 100,000 Hz (100 kHz). Electrosurgical systems operate at frequencies well over 100 kHz so that nerve and muscle stimulation does not occur. Therefore, electrocution is not a problem (Fig. 11-30).

Electrosurgical Modes

Monopolar electrosurgery is the mode commonly used today. In a monopolar system, the electrical current is delivered to the tissue through an active electrode, or pencil. The energy then flows through the patient's body to a dispersive or return electrode pad positioned somewhere else on the patient's body (Fig. 11-31). The purpose of the dispersive pad is to safely remove the current from the patient. The energy is then taken back to the ESU generator as the circuit is completed (Fig.

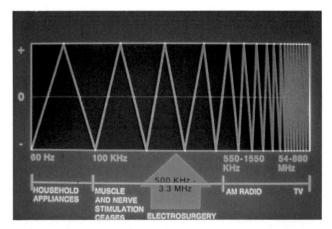

Fig. 11-30   The electrical current used in electrosurgery is well over 100 kHz. (Courtesy Valleylab, Inc., Boulder, Colo.)

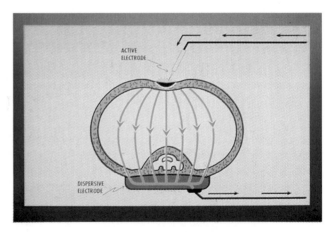

Fig. 11-31   In monopolar electrosurgery systems, the active electrode delivers the electrical energy to the target and the dispersive electrode collects the energy. (Courtesy Ethicon Endo-Surgery Inc., Cincinnati, Ohio.)

11-32). The only difference between the active electrode and the dispersive electrode is size. The active electrode concentrates the electrical energy into a small area to produce a tissue effect; the dispersive electrode collects the electrical energy over a larger area and the skin temperature under the dispersive pad only increases a couple of degrees as the electron flow is gathered, thus minimizing the risk of a burn.

Bipolar electrosurgery has become very popular in recent years. In a bipolar system, there is no need for a dispersive pad because the electrical energy flows from one tine of the bipolar instrument and is received by the other, which returns the current back to the generator. The two tines of the bipolar instrument serve as the active and dispersive electrodes, thus eliminating the flow of current through the patient's body. The path of the electrical energy is confined to the tissue touching the bipolar instrument tines (Fig. 11-33).

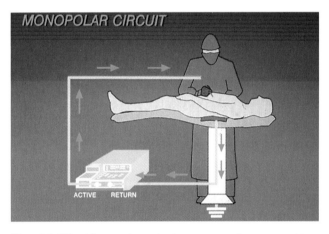

Fig. 11-32 Monopolar electrosurgery. (Courtesy Ethicon Endo-Surgery Inc., Cincinnati, Ohio.)

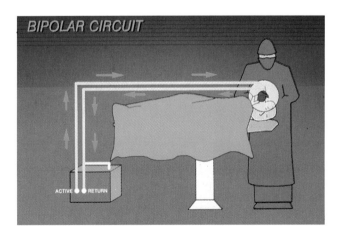

Fig. 11-33 Bipolar electrosurgery. (Courtesy Ethicon Endo-Surgery, Inc., Cincinnati, Ohio.)

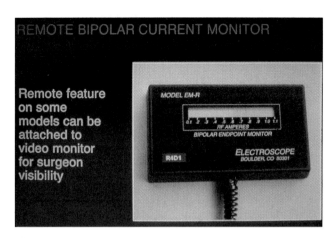

Fig. 11-34 Bipolar impedance monitor. (Courtesy Valleylab, Inc., Boulder, Colo.)

During bipolar electrosurgery, the flow of the electrical energy is stopped if a certain impedance level is reached. Usually this level is 100 ohms. Even though the electrosurgical generator appears to still be activated because an audible sound is heard while the pedal is pressed, the current is actually stopped from flowing when the specified resistance is met. There are meters available today that measure the impedance between the tines of the bipolar instrument; they are useful for letting the surgeon know tissue desiccation is occurring or that complete desiccation has been achieved. The surgeon can then decide whether further tissue interaction is needed in adjacent areas. Usually the bipolar meter can be mounted on the video monitor so that the surgical team can observe the status of the bipolar current (Fig. 11-34).

Tissue Effects

Different tissue effects can be achieved as the variables change; these include:
- Waveform
- Power setting
- Length of exposure
- Active electrode size
- Type of tissue
- Eschar presence

Waveforms

As the waveforms change from a pure cut to a pure coagulation action, so do the tissue effects change (Fig. 11-35). The endoscopic team must therefore be aware of the effects of the various waveforms.

To be in a pure cut mode the generator must be on a 100% duty cycle, meaning that the electrical flow is continually being applied and heat is quickly being generated for cutting and vaporization of the tissue. The frequency is high, but the voltage is low. Because less force,

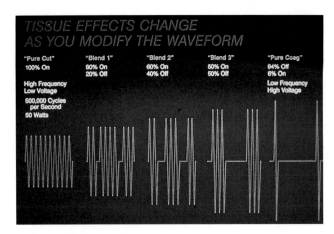

Fig. 11-35 Cut versus coagulation waveforms. (Courtesy Valleylab, Inc., Boulder, Colo.)

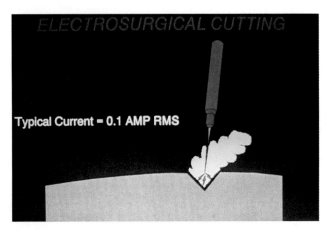

Fig. 11-36 For effective cutting, the active electrode is held slightly above the target tissue. (Courtesy Valleylab, Inc., Boulder, Colo.)

or volts, are used to push the current, the cut mode becomes more safe than the other modes.

When the cut mode is being used, the electrons are constantly bombarding the tissue, causing extensive heat to be produced. As the cellular contents begin to boil, the cell membrane ruptures and the tissue is cut. For cutting to be most effective, the active electrode should be held slightly above the tissue so that the electrons jump through the impedance of the air to the target site (Fig. 11-36). The current concentration is at its maximum when the active electrode is held slightly away from the tissue. The cellular structure also causes resistance, and this in turn causes great heat to be generated, resulting in cellular destruction. Because heat is produced so quickly, most of it dissipates into steam and plume and peripheral heating of the adjacent tissue is minimized.

Desiccation occurs when the active electrode in the cut mode is held in contact with the tissue (Fig. 11-37).

This happens because the current concentration is reduced while the electrode is in contact with the tissue and less heat is produced. Instead of exploding, the cells are gently heated, causing denaturization and cellular dying, and hence tissue desiccation.

In a pure coagulation mode, the frequency is lowered and the voltage is increased. The duty cycle is only on 6% of the time, thus 94% of the time the flow of electrons to the surgical site is stopped. Therefore the voltage must be increased to compensate for this duty cycle.

During coagulation or fulguration, the intermittent delivery of the electrons causes the cells to heat up and then cool, thus producing a coagulative effect. The higher voltage allows a spraying effect of the electrical energy to coagulate a larger area. The tissue effect is very superficial, such that cells only collapse and this produces a coagulum. Because more voltage is required, this mode is less safe, especially if insulation failure occurs.

Most electrosurgical generators also have a blend mode that allows different combinations of the cut and coagulation modes to be used. Different blend modes may be desired, depending on the tissue involved, the tissue effect desired, or the technique used.

Power setting

The power setting of the ESU also determines the tissue effect. Obviously the higher the power setting, the more distinctive the tissue effects. If a higher voltage is used, a coagulative effect is achieved; lower voltages provide precise cutting capabilities.

Length of exposure

The longer the length of exposure, the more distinctive the tissue result, because heat is generated as the active electrode delivers the electrical energy to the target site. Therefore the longer the electrical current is applied,

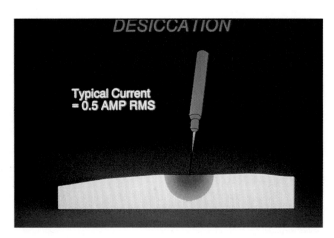

Fig. 11-37 Electrosurgical tissue desiccation. (Courtesy Valleylab, Inc., Boulder, Colo.)

the more thermal spread occurs in adjacent tissue and the more tissue damage occurs.

Active electrode size and configuration

The smaller the active electrode, the more concentrated the electrical current; thus, an increased tissue effect can be achieved. A smaller active electrode requires less power, however, because the current is concentrated within a smaller area.

There are a variety of tips of different geometric configurations available today for monopolar or bipolar electrosurgery (Fig. 11-38). The surgeon has a full complement of instruments to choose from, and the instrument chosen depends on the type of tissue, the tissue response desired, and physician preference (Fig. 11-39).

Type of tissue

The characteristics of the tissue also determine the tissue effect achieved. Tissue varies in density and resistance. For example, tissue that is not well vascularized, such as adipose tissue, is less dense and therefore more resistant. As a result it does not conduct electrical energy well. Higher-power settings are therefore necessary when cutting adipose tissue, unlike those needed when cutting muscle tissue, which is well vascularized and more dense.

Another example of this is the cervix. A postmenopausal woman's cervix is less vascular than that of a premenopausal woman, meaning that it is therefore less dense and more resistant. Therefore, when a cervical procedure is performed on a postmenopausal woman, the power setting may need to be increased.

Eschar presence

The amount of eschar present also determines the amount of electrosurgical energy needed. Because eschar is less

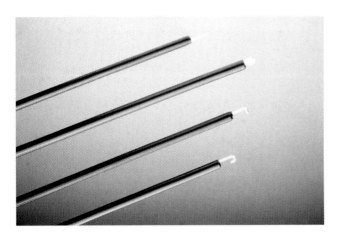

Fig. 11-38 Electrosurgical tips. (Courtesy Aesculap, Inc., South San Francisco, Calif.)

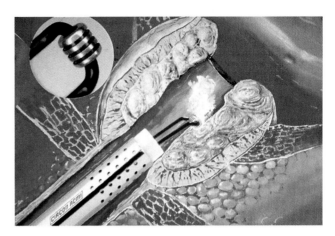

Fig. 11-39 A vaporization electrosurgical probe is used to resect the prostate gland during an endoscopic procedure. (Courtesy Circon Corp., Santa Barbara, Calif.)

dense, it impedes or resists electrical energy; therefore more power is needed to achieve the desired tissue effect in the presence of eschar. The active electrode must also be kept clean and free from debris to maintain lower resistance within the electrosurgical circuit. There are electrosurgical tips with a special coating that can reduce eschar buildup during surgery. The nonstick surface also allows for a more consistent and cleaner cut at lower-power settings.

Electrosurgical Units

There are three main types of ESUs: grounded, isolated, and return-electrode monitoring (REM) systems.

Grounded electrosurgical system

The grounded electrosurgical system, which made its debut in the 1920s, was the first type to be invented and is still available today. In the system the AC energy is taken from the wall outlet and its frequency is increased to more than 300,000 cycles per second. The current travels from the ESU, enters the patient's body, and then is returned back to ground through the patient's return electrode or dispersive pad (Fig. 11-40). However, there are many grounded conductive objects that may be touching the patient during surgery, and electricity can follow any of these alternative paths in seeking to return to ground. Because electricity takes the path of least resistance, such alternative return paths can divert the current from the dispersive pad (Fig. 11-41). For example, the current may seek to return to ground through an electrocardiographic monitoring pad. Because the monitor pad then disperses the electrical energy over a small area, heat is created and a burn is sustained (Fig. 11-42). This type of incident illustrates a drawback of the grounded electrosurgical system.

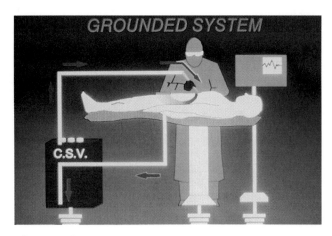

Fig. 11-40   Grounded electrosurgical system. (Courtesy Valleylab, Inc., Boulder, Colo.)

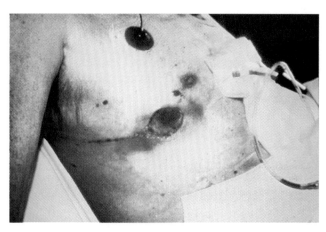

Fig. 11-42   Alternate path burn. (Courtesy Valleylab, Inc., Boulder, Colo.)

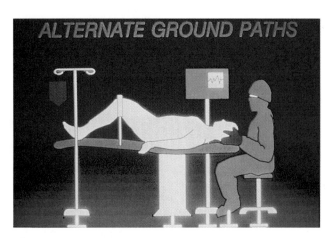

Fig. 11-41   Alternate paths for electrical current. (Courtesy Valleylab, Inc., Boulder, Colo.)

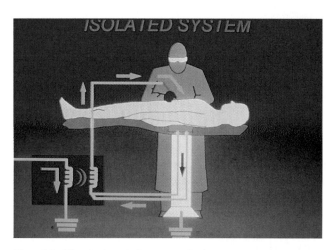

Fig. 11-43   Isolated electrosurgical system. (Courtesy Valleylab, Inc., Boulder, Colo.)

Isolated electrosurgical system

In 1968 isolated generator technology came available that revolutionized electrosurgery technology. In this system the wall current received into the generator is passed through a transformer to create an isolated current that is not ground referenced but is referenced only to itself. Therefore the current that flows into the patient's body cannot flow through an alternative path. It only flows back through the dispersive pad to return to the generator to complete the circuit. If the pad is not on the patient, the electrical current does not flow (Fig. 11-43).

However, although an isolated electrosurgical system prevents patients from being burned at alternative pathway sites, dispersive pad site burns can occur. These burns have been estimated to account for 70% of the injuries incurred during electrosurgery procedures (Valleylab, 1995) (Fig. 11-44). To prevent these burns, the dispersive pad must be properly positioned and adhered so that the electrical current is led back to the generator.

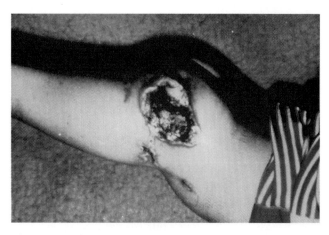

Fig. 11-44   Burn at the dispersive pad site. (Courtesy Valleylab, Inc., Boulder, Colo.)

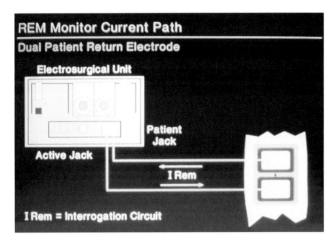

Fig. 11-45 Return-electrode monitoring system. (Courtesy Valleylab, Inc., Boulder, Colo.)

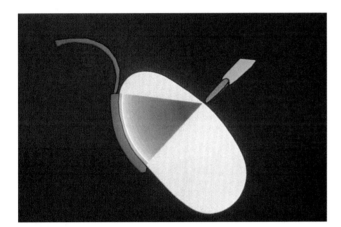

Fig. 11-46 The electrical energy is collected over the large area of the dispersive pad. (Courtesy Valleylab, Inc., Boulder, Colo.)

Return-electrode monitoring system

REM was introduced in the early 1980s as a means to protect patients from dispersive pad site burns. This system continually monitors the impedance or heat buildup underneath the dispersive pad as it communicates with the patient's skin (Fig. 11-45). The temperature of the resting epidermis is approximately 22°C, and irreversible skin damage or a burn can occur at 44°C. The system deactivates the current flow if a high impedance level is detected at the patient-pad interface, thus preventing a burn.

Dispersive Pad Placement

Proper placement of the dispersive pad is of vital importance so that the electrical energy is sufficiently dispersed over a large area and burns are prevented (Fig. 11-46). To ensure this the pad should be placed over an area that is well vascularized, such as a muscle mass. It should not be placed over sites where there is excessive hair,

bony prominences, excessive adipose (fat) tissue, or exceedingly dry skin because of the impedance that can occur. Irregular body contours should also be avoided. If the patient is repositioned during a procedure, the pad should be checked for proper adherence, because if there is reduced contact, the current flow would then be concentrated into a smaller area and a burn could occur (Fig. 11-47).

In summary, surface area impedance or resistance to the flow of electrical current can occur in the presence of:

- Adipose tissue
- Excessive hair
- Fluid invasion
- Bony prominences
- Scar tissue
- Adhesive failure

Depending on the position of the patient during the endoscopic procedure, the pad is placed as near to the surgical site as possible. If it is likely that the patient will be repositioned during the procedure, then the pad should be placed in an area where proper contact is ensured throughout the procedure (Fig. 11-48).

Minimally Invasive Electrosurgery Safety

Certain problems are unique when electrosurgery is used during endoscopic procedures. These include insulation failure, direct coupling, and capacitive coupling.

Insulation failure

Insulation is used on endoscopic electrosurgical instruments to ensure that the electrical energy stays within the instrument until it reaches the exit area. Sometimes, however, this insulation fails. This can occur in reusable instruments as the result of repeated processing, but some disposable instruments can also be affected if only a thin layer of insulation is used to coat them. In either

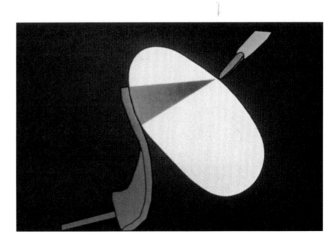

Fig. 11-47 If the dispersive pad becomes detached from the skin, then the electrosurgical energy becomes concentrated within a smaller area and a burn can occur. (Courtesy Valleylab, Inc., Boulder, Colo.)

event, electrosurgical energy is allowed to escape, causing a burn to a nontargeted structure that may be out of the operator's endoscopic field of vision (Figs. 11-49 and 11-50).

This is of particular concern during use of the coagulation mode because of the high-voltage current involved. This energy can push through compromised insulation and possibly blow a hole in weakened insulation. If the current exiting is concentrated, then significant injuries can occur. As noted earlier, less volts are needed to push the current in the cut mode, therefore the cut mode is much safer for use during endoscopy. It can also be used as a safer means of achieving coagulation. When the active electrode in the cut mode is held in contact with the tissue, it can no longer cut because the current and heat are dissipated, hence coagulation occurs rather than cutting.

Direct coupling

Direct coupling occurs if the electrosurgical energy is flowing while the active electrode is near or touching metal instruments or objects (clips). The current can energize the uninsulated metal, potentially causing patient injury (Fig. 11-51). The electrosurgery unit should therefore not be activated whenever the active electrode is near or touching a metal object.

Capacitive coupling

A capacitor is created when two conductors are separated by a nonconductor or insulator. Electrical energy can then flow from one conductor to another. This can be shown by positioning two conductive wires near each other. The electrical current flowing through the first wire can cross the high impedance of air, causing the current to flow into the second wire. The insulator in this example is the air.

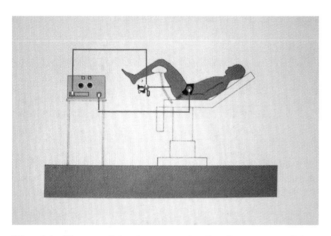

Fig. 11-48 Possible placement for the dispersive pad during laparoscopy. (Courtesy Karl Storz, Culver City, Calif.)

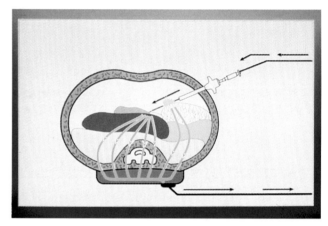

Fig. 11-50 Insulation failure during laparoscopy. (Courtesy Ethicon Endo-Surgery Inc., Cincinnati, Ohio.)

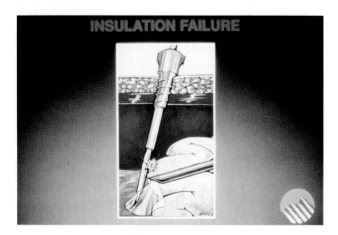

Fig. 11-49 Insulation failure during laparoscopy. (Courtesy Everest Medical Corp., Minneapolis, Minn.)

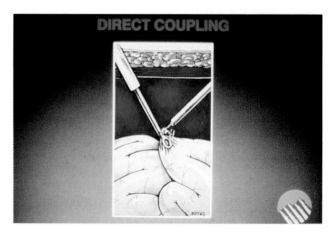

Fig. 11-51 Direct coupling during laparoscopy. (Courtesy Everest Medical Corp., Minneapolis, Minn.)

During endoscopic procedures a capacitor is formed because the active electrode, which is conductive and surrounded by insulation, is passed through the metal laparoscope or trocar sheath, which then serves as the other conductor (Fig. 11-52). The current from the active electrode can then flow to the metal laparoscope or trocar sheath.

The amount of capacitance that may be created on the second metal sheath depends on many variables. It may be increased if either instruments with thin insulation or instruments that are long and narrow are employed (Fig. 11-53). The higher voltage produced by the active electrode in the coagulative mode also can cause capacitance to be increased. If the electrosurgery energy is delivered using an open-circuit method while the active electrode is not in contact with the tissue, then the chance of capacitive coupling also increases.

The electrical charge will then remain in the second instrument until it can find a path to the patient dispersive pad and complete the circuit. Ordinarily this energy can be safely dissipated through contact with the large surface area of the abdominal wall (Fig. 11-54). However, if there is a plastic collar, such as a stabilizing anchor, on the metal trocar sheath then the energy cannot be discharged on the surface of the abdominal wall but will be concentrated in the charged metal instrument. If the metal surface of the charged trocar sheath or laparoscope then touches other tissue, the electrical current will be emitted and cause a thermal tissue response or burn (Figs. 11-55 and 11-56). This injury may go undetected by the surgical team and may not

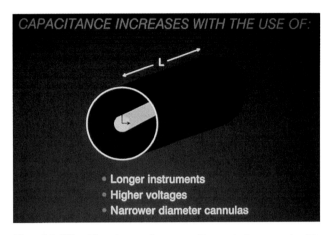

Fig. 11-53 The chance for capacitance is increased with longer, more narrow instruments. (Courtesy Valleylab, Inc., Boulder, Colo.)

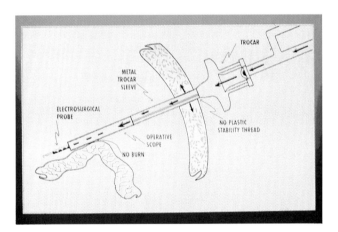

Fig. 11-54 Electrical energy can be safely discharged over the larger surface area of the abdominal wall during laparoscopy. (Courtesy Ethicon Endo-Surgery, Inc., Cincinnati, Ohio.)

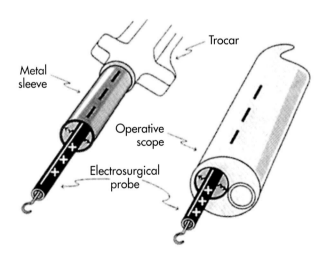

Fig. 11-52 Capacitive coupling occurs when electrical energy flowing from an instrument charges a nearby metal trocar sheath or laparoscope. (Courtesy Ethicon Endo-Surgery, Inc., Cincinnati, Ohio.)

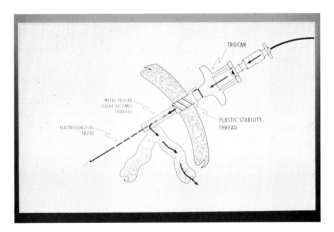

Fig. 11-55 Capacitive coupling to the metal trocar sheath and the resulting bowel injury. (Courtesy Ethicon Endo-Surgery, Inc., Cincinnati, Ohio.)

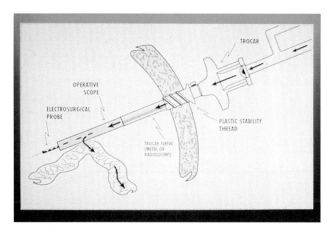

Fig. 11-56   Capacitive coupling to the metal laparoscope and the resulting bowel injury. (Courtesy Ethicon Endo-Surgery, Inc., Cincinnati, Ohio.)

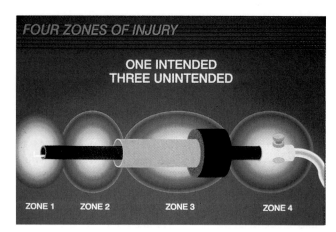

Fig. 11-58   Four zones of potential injury during endoscopy. (Courtesy Valleylab, Inc., Boulder, Colo.)

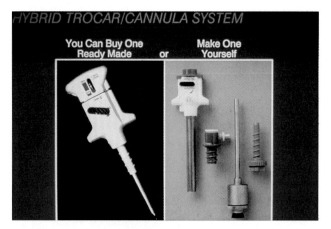

Fig. 11-57   Hybrid mixtures of nonconductive and conductive instruments during laparoscopy can lead to problems with capacitive coupling. (Courtesy Valleylab, Inc., Boulder, Colo.)

the operator. Zone two and three are the areas where accidental injury, which often goes undetected, occurs as a result of insulation failure, direct coupling, or capacitive coupling. Zone four is the area on the endoscope where the surgical team can sustain a burn as the result of problems with the electrosurgical instrumentation. Advancements in instrument design and energy monitoring are helping to reduce the risks of these injuries to patients and surgical team members.

Monitoring systems

Monitoring systems are now available that detect electrical energy leakage and faults in insulation and then deactivate the electrosurgical device if the electrical leakage exceeds the predetermined setting. These protective systems provide a return path so that electricity does not have to flow through the patient to the dispersive pad. The active electrode used in this system is surrounded by a protective shield that collects any stray electrical energy and safely returns it to the generator, thus preventing patient injury (Fig. 11-59). There are protective shields that can be applied to existing instruments or individual active protective electrodes (Fig. 11-60). This monitoring system should not, however, be relied on in lieu of the regular inspection of the surgical instruments used for electrosurgery.

Minimizing ESU hazards during laparoscopy

The surgical team must thoroughly understand the art and science of electrosurgery, especially as it applies to the performance of minimally invasive procedures. Following are some important tips to remember.

- Never use metal cannulas with plastic anchors, because the plastic anchors will prevent energy from being dispersed to the abdominal wall. Do not use cannula systems that mix plastic with metal.

be identified until the patient exhibits complications during the postoperative phase.

The use of hybrid mixtures of instruments made of nonconductive and conductive materials must therefore be avoided to minimize the problem of capacitive coupling (Fig. 11-57). For example, a plastic anchor should not be used with a metal trocar sheath because the sheath could become electrically charged and this energy would not be safely discharged through the large surface of the abdominal wall. On the other hand, if an all plastic nonconductive system is used, then the elements needed to create capacitve coupling are entirely eliminated.

Zones of injury

There are four zones where injury can occur during an endoscopic procedure (Fig. 11-58). Zone one is the area of the intended tissue reaction that can be visualized by

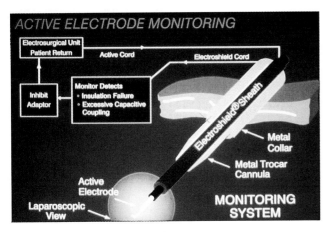

Fig. 11-59 An active-electrode monitoring system provides a protective shield that collects any stray electrical energy and safely returns it to the generator, thus preventing patient injury. (Courtesy Valleylab, Inc., Boulder, Colo.)

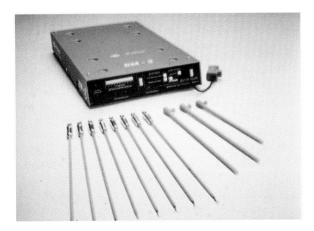

Fig. 11-60 Protective shields or individual active electrodes are available to prevent patient injury resulting from stray electrical current. (Courtesy Valleylab, Inc., Boulder, Colo.)

- Desiccated or thermal injury to the abdominal wall can also prevent dispersion of the electrical energy.
- Improper cleaning and reprocessing can damage the insulation on instruments. Inspect all reusable instruments. If damage is noticed, document the problem and remove the instrument from service for repair. If an insulation break or damage is noted after the surgery, then closely observe the patient for any postoperative complications.
- Keep the active electrode tip clean and free from debris to prevent overheating resulting from the accumulation of charred tissue.
- Use intermittent activations instead of prolonged activation.
- Carefully insert and remove instruments through the cannula so they are not damaged.

- Use active electrode monitoring to help eliminate concerns about insulation failure and capacitance.
- Use low-voltage current (cutting mode) and the lowest power setting whenever possible.
- If more operating space is needed inside the abdomen, then a nasogastric tube can be inserted to decompress the stomach or an indwelling catheter can be used to empty the bladder. Evacuation of the bowel during the preoperative preparation can also create more operative space.
- Do not activate the electrode in open space; only activate it when near or in direct contact with the target tissue.
- To keep the surgical team from being burned by the ESU, place the active electrode in a safety holster whenever it is not in use. If an open laparoscopy is being performed and a long hemostat is used for coagulation through the direct coupling effect, then the hemostat should be held firmly so that any electrical energy transfer is dispersed over a larger area. If the hemostat is held lightly, the electrical energy may concentrate at the point of contact and possibly cause a burn. The surgical team member should also not lean on the patient or table while activating the ESU, because this could place him or her within the electrical circuit.
- Retain all instruments that may have malfunctioned and injured the patient.
- Always check the return or dispersive electrode to ensure proper placement.
- Do not activate the ESU when it is near or in direct contact with another instrument.
- Minimize the chance of direct coupling, capacitive coupling, or insulation failure by using active electrode monitoring devices.
- Use bipolar electrosurgery whenever possible.

ARGON-ENHANCED ELECTROSURGERY

An argon-enhanced electrosurgery device incorporates argon gas with electrosurgical energy, thus improving the effectiveness of the electrosurgical current (Fig. 11-61). Argon gas, which is inert and noncombustible, can be used safely with electrosurgical energy. It is heavier than air and, as a result, creates an efficient pathway for the electrosurgical energy between the electrode and the target tissue, such that the electrical current forms an ionized arc (Fig. 11-62).

The flow of the argon gas also helps to increase visibility because it clears the surgical site of fluids and plume so that coagulation can be achieved and carbonization reduced.

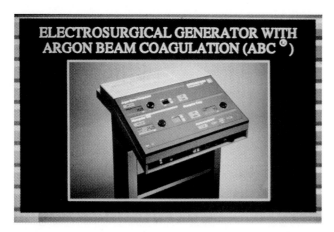

Fig. 11-61 Argon-enhanced electrosurgical device. (Courtesy Valleylab, Inc., Boulder, Colo.)

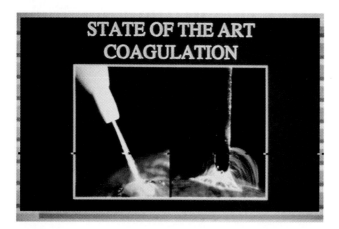

Fig. 11-62 Argon gas (*left*) is used to more effectively deliver the electrical energy to the target tissue than is possible with electrosurgery devices not employing argon gas (*right*). (Courtesy Valleylab, Inc., Boulder, Colo.)

There are also other benefits to the use of argon-enhanced electrosurgery technology, including:
- More rapid coagulation with reduced blood loss
- No need to be in contact with the tissue for coagulation
- Reduced risk of rebleeding
- Less tissue adherence to the electrode when in contact with tissue
- Less depth of penetration of the energy, thus less adjacent tissue damage
- Less surgical plume

The argon-enhanced electrosurgical device should be used with caution during laparoscopic procedures, however, because intraabdominal overpressurization resulting from the steady flow of argon gas can cause the formation of a gas embolism. Since argon gas is less soluble in the blood than CO_2, such an embolism may last long enough to reach the heart. Therefore another

port should be left open during activation to allow any excess gas to escape and thus minimize overpressurization. Insufflators that have an audible overpressurization alarm should also be used. In addition, the patient should be closely monitored so that any early symptoms of an embolism can be quickly detected and treated.

ULTRASONIC DEVICES

Vibrating energy devices that produce ultrasonic energy were developed as a safe alternative to devices using laser or electrosurgical energy (Fig. 11-63). In these ultrasonic devices, high-frequency sound waves are propagated to a blade tip to produce energy.

An "infrasonic" longitudinal wave has a frequency of less than 20 cycles per second, or 20 Hz. The rumblings of an earthquake produce infrasonic waves. "Audible" sound waves have a frequency of 20 to 20,000 Hz. These sounds cause the brain to be stimulated and sound to be heard. "Ultrasonic" waves have a frequency of over 20,000 Hz and, like a dog whistle, cannot be sensed by the human ear.

There are two devices popular today that make use of ultrasonic energy; one is the cavitational ultrasonic aspirator (CUSA) and the other is the harmonic ultrasonic scalpel.

The production of ultrasonic energy begins with an electrical current. A generator sends an electrical signal through a coaxial cable to the transducer in the handpiece. The transducer then converts the electrical energy to mechanical motion through the contraction and expansion of ceramic elements (Fig. 11-64). This mechanical motion then provides a longitudinal vibratory response that moves the tip at the end of the handpiece from 23,000 (CUSA) to more than 55,000 (harmonic scalpel) cycles per second (Fig. 11-65). As the power level on the generator is increased, the longitudinal excursion of the

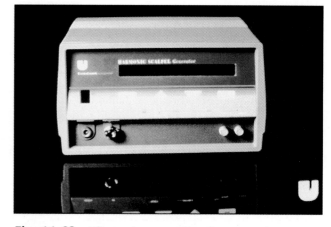

Fig. 11-63 Ultrasonic generator. (Courtesy Ethicon Endo-Surgery, Inc., Cincinnati, Ohio)

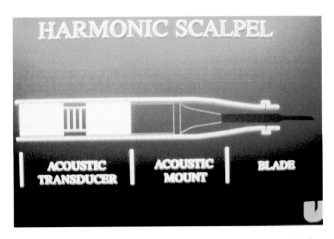

Fig. 11-64 A transducer within the ultrasonic device handpiece converts electrical energy into mechanical motion. (Courtesy Ethicon Endo-Surgery, Inc., Cincinnati, Ohio)

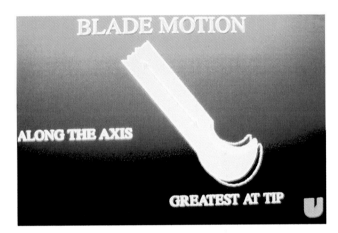

Fig. 11-65 An ultrasonic blade may move longitudinally more than 55,500 times per second. (Courtesy Ethicon Endo-Surgery, Inc., Cincinnati, Ohio)

50 to 150 μm. In comparison, noncontact laser energy may cause damage to a depth of 2 to 4 mm.

Different tip configurations are available for different applications (Fig. 11-66). Tips come in various shapes, such as a blade, ball, or hook. It is important to apply countertraction to obtain the desired tissue response while the energy is most acute at the end of the

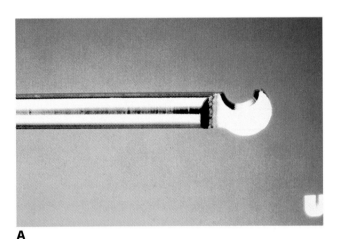

A

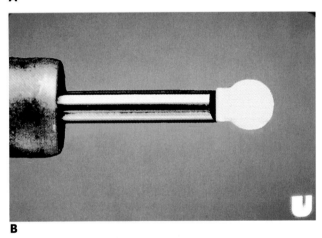

B

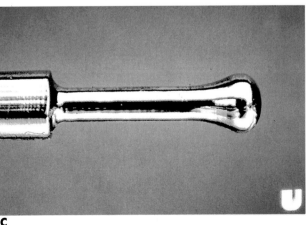

C

Fig. 11-66 A, B, and C, Different ultrasonic tip configurations. (Courtesy Ethicon Endo-Surgery, Inc., Cincinnati, Ohio)

tip becomes longer but the frequency remains the same. Some vibratory systems have a safety mechanism that continually adjusts the tip motion to offset the resistance. If too much impedance is encountered, the system's alarm sounds and the system may shut down.

When the tip is in contact with tissue, its mechanical motion causes denaturing of the tissue protein. The hydrogen bonds, which give the tissue structure, are then broken, causing protein molecules to become disorganized. A sticky coagulum forms that welds and coagulates smaller bleeding vessels. No tissue plume is generated as the result of cellular destruction, and only a small amount of water vapor is produced but dissipates quickly.

Because such a small amount of thermal energy is generated from the mechanical energy, the adjacent tissue damage is minimal, usually limited to a depth of tip or in the middle of the hook (Fig. 11-67). A shear-grasper that eliminates the need for countertraction may also be used. Tissue is placed between the blade and the tissue pad to stabilize the target (Fig. 11-68), and the ultrasonic energy is then delivered to cut or coagulate the tissue.

The ultrasonic device can be used for cavitational cutting, especially of low-protein-density tissues, such as the liver parenchyma and fat. Because the ultrasonic energy causes fluids between the tissue planes to vaporize and expand at low temperatures, the tissue planes are easily visualized and separated (Fig. 11-69). The minimal amount of thermal energy generated also promotes this, because the tissue layers then tend to disconnect instead of melting together.

A study was conducted comparing the results of laparoscopic Nissen fundoplications in which the short gastric vessels were dissected either with the ultrasonic device or a multifire clip applier. When the clip applier was used, the average surgery time was 37.4 minutes, an average of 20 ml blood was lost, and the average cost of the procedure was $849. When the ultrasonic device was used, the average surgery time was 24.2 minutes, an average of 14 ml of blood was lost, and the average cost was $545 (*Laparosc Surg Update*, 1995).

There are many advantages to using the ultrasonic device for cutting and coagulation during endoscopy. Including some already mentioned, these are:

- No surgical plume or odor is produced.
- Less adjacent tissue is damaged than that damaged using the laser or an ESU.
- It provides tactile feedback for the surgeon.
- Precision and control are possible during cutting or coagulation.
- No nerve or muscle is stimulated because electrical current is not conducted to the tissue.
- No stray electrical or laser energy is produced.
- Visibility is enhanced because no tissue smoke is generated.

CRYOSURGICAL UNITS

For years, cryosurgery has been used to destroy small quantities of diseased or unwanted tissue. Now cryosurgical systems have been perfected that can ablate large quantities of targeted tissue. For cryosurgery to be effective, however, the cryosurgery system must generate an iceball capable of producing a temperature that is sufficient to induce cellular death. Cells are usually destroyed at approximately $-50°C$ or colder. The farther away the cryoprobe tip is from the target tissue, the greater the potential for cells to remain viable because the temperature is not then sufficiently lowered.

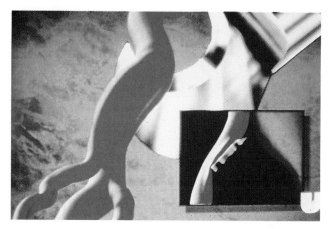

Fig. 11-67 Ultrasonic hook is used to coagulate a blood vessel. (Courtesy Ethicon Endo-Surgery, Inc., Cincinnati, Ohio)

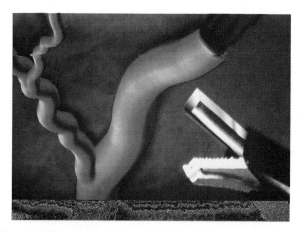

Fig. 11-68 Ultrasonic shears-grasper can cut and coagulate tissue without the need for countertraction. (Courtesy Courtesy Ethicon Endo-Surgery, Inc., Cincinnati, Ohio)

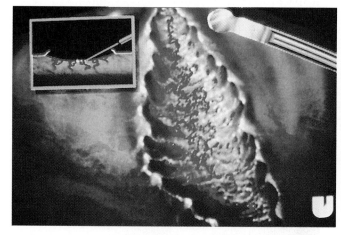

Fig. 11-69 Ultrasonic cavitational cutting. (Courtesy Ethicon Endo-Surgery, Inc., Cincinnati, Ohio)

The cryosurgery devices available today come in the form of gaseous nitrogen systems or super-cooled liquid nitrogen systems. However, the super-cooled liquid nitrogen system tends to be more efficient in extracting heat. In this system the liquid nitrogen is delivered to the probe to form the iceball. Some of the single-use cryoprobes transfer and then return the super-cooled liquid nitrogen for recycling. The cryoprobe has an insulated shaft that confines the freezing zone to the distal tip (Fig. 11-70). Smaller cryoprobes (e.g., 3 mm in diameter) have been perfected that can be inserted through smaller trocar sites. Recent improvements in this technology have allowed cryoprobes to be placed under ultrasonic imaging guidance for more controlled tissue destruction.

Cryosurgery is currently being used to treat malignant tumors, such as prostatic cancer and hepatic neoplasms. More research is needed, however, to validate the effectiveness of cryosurgery technology in the destruction of other diseased tissue.

HYDRODISSECTION SYSTEMS

In hydrodissection, pulsed-flow or continual-flow irrigation solutions are used to separate and delineate tissue planes (Fig. 11-71). This technology offers precise dissection and increased removal of char and debris, thus enhancing visualization so that anatomic structures can be more readily identified. Either a continuous pressure of more than 500 mm Hg or a variable pressure of up to 2500 mm Hg is needed to achieve hydrodissection. A trumpet valve is used to deliver the irrigant and also provide suction (Fig. 11-72).

Hydrodissection has been used for tissue dissection during laparoscopic-assisted vaginal hysterectomies and laparoscopic cholecystectomies. It has also been used to break up clots. The use of this technology for endoscopic procedures continues to be explored.

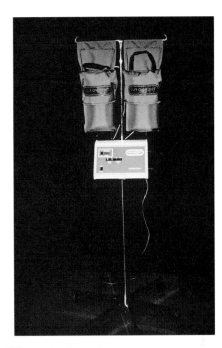

Fig. 11-71   Hydrodissection system. (Courtesy Sanese Medical Corp., Columbus, Ohio.)

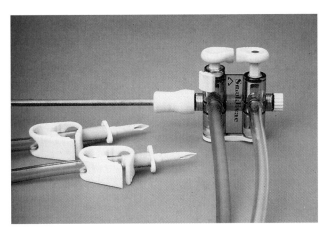

Fig. 11-72   A trumpet valve controls the flow of irrigant and suction. (Courtesy Davol, Inc., Cranston, R.I.)

DIAGNOSTIC TOOLS

Ultrasound Devices

Ultrasonographic imaging is being developed for use during laparoscopy to determine the presence of stones and to visualize the common bile duct, though it cannot yet replace cholangiography (Fig. 11-73). It involves the insertion of a special probe (Fig. 11-74). It can also be used during hysteroscopy to detect uterine fibroids and other abnormalities (Fig. 11-75).

Ultrasound devices have also been developed that are used on the abdominal surface to determine the

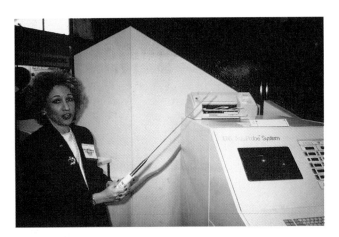

Fig. 11-70   Cryosurgery probe.

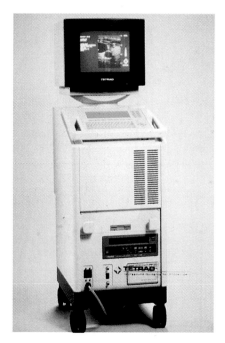

Fig. 11-73 Laparoscopic ultrasonography system. (Courtesy Tetrad Corp., Englewood, Colo.)

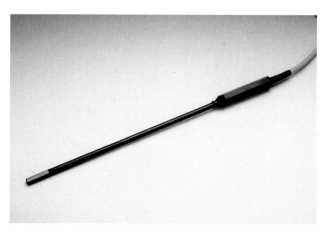

Fig. 11-74 An endoscopic ultrasonography probe. (Courtesy Tetrad Corp., Englewood, Colo.)

presence and location of abdominal wall adhesions before the start of a laparoscopic procedure. The goal is to find an adhesion-free window for the initial trocar placement. Subsequent trocar placements can be guided visually through the laparoscope.

Spectral Analyzer

A biomedical spectral analyzer is currently being developed to serve as an endoscopic fiberoptic device that measures the light-scattering properties of tissue to detect cancer in situ in the colon or bladder (*Adv Technol Surg Care*, 1995). The probe, which is inserted endo-

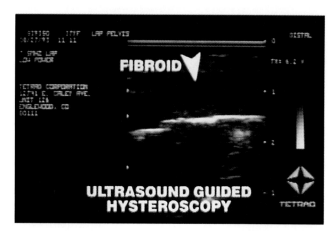

Fig. 11-75 A fibroid is detected with ultrasound imaging during hysteroscopy. (Courtesy Tetrad Corp., Englewood, Colo.)

scopically, contains two fibers, one that delivers the light from a xenon light source to the target being touched and the other that collects the light scatter after it hits the target. This light is conducted to an analyzing spectrometer that compares this information with the light signatures of normal tissue. This method of diagnosis is less expensive than standard biopsy and offers immediate results. The system is continuing to be refined and its effectiveness for other various endoscopic procedures investigated.

Radioimmunoguided Device

The primary goal of the surgical removal of solid tumors is to perform a complete resection, even at the microscopic level. Radioimmunoguided surgery has been developed to help the surgeon identify microscopic tumor cells. For example, most solid adenocarcinomas have a tumor-associated mucin on their surface that can attract a radiolabeled monoclonal antibody. The radiolabeled antibody is introduced into the patient weeks before surgery by means of injection through a peripheral intravenous line. A laparotomy is then performed and a hand-held, gamma-detecting device is used to detect the antibody that has attached to the tumor. In this way the tumor can be excised very accurately (Kim, 1993). Laparoscopic probes utilizing this technology will be developed in the future.

REFERENCES

Adv Technol Surg Care: Fiber-optic light device spots cancerous tissue, 13(9):111, 1995.

Ball KA: *Lasers: the perioperative challenge*, ed 2, St. Louis, 1995, Mosby.

Clin Laser Monthly: New research confirms laser plume can transmit disease, 11(6):81,1993.

Einstein A: On the quantum theory of radiation, *Physio Z* 18:121, 1917.

Garden JM, O'Banion K, Shelnitz L, et al: Papillomavirus in the vapor of carbon dioxide laser–treated verrucae, *JAMA* 8:1199, 1988.

Kim JA, Triozzi PL, Martin EW: Radioimmunoguided surgery for colorectal cancer, *Oncology* 1993.

Laparosc Surg Update: Smoke in pneumoperitoneum may be more dangerous than you think, 2(10):118, 1994.

Laparosc Surg Update: Harmonic scalpel saves time, money dividing short gastrics, 3(9):104, 1995.

Mihashi S, et al: Some problems about condensates induced by CO_2 laser irradiation, Department of Otolaryngology and Public Health, Karume University, 1975.

Schawlow AL, Townes CH: Infrared and optical lasers, *Phys Rev* 112:1940, 1958.

Valleylab, *Principles of electrosurgery*, Boulder, Colo, 1995, Valleylab.

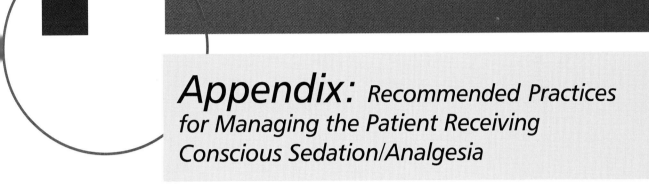

Appendix: Recommended Practices for Managing the Patient Receiving Conscious Sedation/Analgesia

The following recommended practices were developed by the AORN Recommended Practices Committee and have been approved by the AORN Board of Directors. They were published as proposed recommended practices through the AORN fax-on-demand system for comments by members and others. They are effective January 1, 1997.

These recommended practices are intended as achievable recommendations representing what is believed to be an optimal level of practice. Policies and procedures will reflect variations in practice settings and/or clinical situations that determine the degree to which the recommended practices can be implemented.

AORN recognizes the numerous types of settings in which perioperative nurses practice. The recommended practices are intended as guidelines adaptable to various practice settings. These practice settings include traditional ORs, ambulatory surgery units, physicians' offices, cardiac catheterization suites, endoscopy suites, radiology departments, and all other areas where operative and other invasive procedures may be performed.

Purpose

"Sedation and analgesia describes a state which allows patients to tolerate unpleasant procedures while maintaining adequate cardiorespiratory function and the ability to respond purposefully to verbal command and/or tactile stimulation. Patients whose only response is reflex withdrawal from a painful stimulus are sedated to a greater degree than encompassed by sedation/analgesia."

These recommended practices provide guidelines for RNs managing patients receiving conscious sedation/analgesia. Patient selection for conscious sedation/analgesia should be based on established criteria developed through interdisciplinary collaboration of health care professionals. The type of monitoring used with patients who receive conscious sedation/analgesia, the medications selected, and the interventions taken must be within the defined scope of perioperative nursing practice.

Certain patients are not candidates for conscious sedation/analgesia with monitoring by RNs. These patients may require more extensive monitoring and sedation, as provided by anesthesia care providers, and should be identified in consultation with anesthesiologists, surgeons, and other physicians. It is not the intent of these recommended practices to address situations that require the services of anesthesia care providers.

The patient care and monitoring guidelines in these recommended practices may be exceeded at any time. Their intent is to encourage quality patient care; however, implementation of these recommended practices cannot guarantee specific patient outcomes. These recommended practices are subject to revision as warranted by advances in nursing practice and technology.

RECOMMENDED PRACTICE I

Registered nurses should understand the goals and objectives of conscious sedation/analgesia.

195

Interpretive statement 1:

The primary goal of conscious sedation/analgesia is to reduce the patient's anxiety and discomfort so as to facilitate cooperation between the patient and the caregivers. Conscious sedation/analgesia can be used as an adjunct to local anesthesia during the procedure.

Rationale:

Adequate preoperative preparation and verbal reassurances from RNs facilitate the desired effects of conscious sedation/analgesia and may allow for a decrease of the dosages of opioids, benzodiazepines, and sedatives used.

Interpretive statement 2:

Objectives for the patient receiving conscious sedation/analgesia include
- alteration of mood;
- maintenance of consciousness;
- enhanced cooperation;
- elevation of pain threshold;
- minimal variation of vital signs;
- some degree of amnesia; and
- a rapid, safe return to activities of daily living.

Rationale:

Conscious sedation/analgesia produces a condition in which the patient exhibits a depressed level of consciousness but retains the ability to independently respond appropriately to verbal commands or physical stimulation. Misunderstanding the objectives of conscious sedation/analgesia may jeopardize the quality of care.

RECOMMENDED PRACTICE II

The RN monitoring the patient who receives conscious sedation/analgesia should have no other responsibilities that would require the nurse to leave the patient unattended or compromise continuous patient monitoring during the procedure.

Interpretive statement 1:

The RN should provide continuous monitoring of the patient who receives conscious sedation/analgesia. The RN must be able to immediately recognize and respond to adverse physiologic and psychological changes during the procedure.

Rationale:

It is unrealistic to assume that one RN can perform circulating duties and also provide continuous monitoring, physical care, and emotional support for the patient who receives conscious sedation/analgesia.

RECOMMENDED PRACTICE III

The RN monitoring the patient's care should be clinically competent in the function and in the use of resuscitation medications and monitoring equipment and be able to interpret the data obtained from the patient.

Interpretive statement 1:

The RN who is monitoring the patient should understand how to operate monitoring equipment used during conscious sedation/analgesia.

Rationale:

Knowledge of the function and proper use of monitoring equipment is essential for providing safe patient care.

Interpretive statement 2:

The nurse who is monitoring the patient should demonstrate knowledge of
- anatomy and physiology;
- pharmacology of medications used for conscious sedation/analgesia;
- cardiac arrhythmia interpretation;
- possible complications related to the use of conscious sedation/analgesia; and
- respiratory functions (ie, oxygen delivery, transport, uptake).

Rationale:

Medications used for conscious sedation/analgesia may cause rapid, adverse physiologic responses in the patient. Early detection of such responses allows for rapid intervention and treatment.

Interpretive statement 3:

The RN who is monitoring the patient should be competent in the use of oxygen delivery devices and airway management.

Rationale:

Rapid intervention is necessary in the event of complications from the undesired effects of conscious sedation/analgesia.

Discussion:

The airway management skill level of the RN who is monitoring the patient receiving conscious sedation/analgesia should be defined by the health care facility's policies and procedures. Basic cardiac life support, which includes maintenance of the patient's airway by use of the head-tilt or chin-lift maneuver, is considered a basic competency for all RNs. The use of oxygen delivery devices (eg, respirator bag, face mask device) may be included as part of the orientation and continuing education process for RNs who monitor patients receiving conscious sedation/analgesia. Advanced cardiac life support (ACLS) certification may be required in some health care facilities. Health care professionals with ACLS skills (eg, ACLS team members, anesthesia care providers) should be readily available to every location in which conscious sedation/analgesia is being administered.

Interpretive statement 4:

Health care facilities should provide competency-based education programs for all RNs who manage patients undergoing conscious sedation/analgesia. These programs should offer a variety of learning opportunities based on learners' needs.

Rationale:

The facility should have an education/competency validation mechanism in place that includes a process for evaluating and documenting RNs' demonstration of knowledge, skills, and abilities related to the management of patients receiving conscious sedation/analgesia. Evaluation and documentation of competence should occur on a periodic basis according to the health care facility's policies and procedures.

RECOMMENDED PRACTICE IV

Each patient who will receive conscious sedation/analgesia should be assessed physiologically and psychologically before the procedure. The assessment should be documented in the patient's record.

Interpretive statement 1:

A preprocedure patient assessment should include a review of:
- physical examination findings;
- current medications;
- drug allergies/sensitivities;
- current medical problems (eg, hypertension, diabetes, cardiopulmonary disease, liver disease, renal disease);
- tobacco smoking and substance abuse history;
- chief complaint;
- baseline vital signs, including height, weight, and age;
- level of consciousness;
- emotional state;
- communication ability; and
- perceptions regarding the procedure and conscious sedation/analgesia.

Rationale:

A preprocedure assessment provides health care professionals baseline data and identifies the patient's risk factors.

RECOMMENDED PRACTICE V

Each patient who receives conscious sedation/analgesia should be monitored for adverse reactions to medications and for physiologic and psychological changes.

Interpretive statement 1:

The RN who administers medications for conscious sedation/analgesia should be responsible for understanding the medications'
- indications and dosages,
- contraindications,
- adverse reactions and emergency management techniques,
- interactions with other medications,
- onset and duration of action, and
- desired effects.

Rationale:

Patient anxiety and medications used for conscious sedation/analgesia may cause rapid, adverse physiologic and psychological changes in the patient.

Interpretive statement 2:

The RN who monitors the patient receiving conscious sedation/analgesia should be knowledgeable of the desirable and undesirable medication effects of conscious sedation/analgesia.

Rationale:

Observation of the patient for desired therapeutic medication effects, prevention of avoidable medication reactions, early detection and management of unexplained adverse reactions, and accurate documentaion of the patient's response are integral components of the monitoring process.

Discussion:

Desirable effects of conscious sedation/analgesia include
- intact protective reflexes,
- relaxation,
- comfort,
- cooperation,
- diminished verbal communication,
- patent airway with adequate ventilatory exchange, and
- easy arousal from sleep.

Potential complications of conscious sedation/analgesia include

- aspiration
- severely slurred speech,
- unarousable sleep,
- hypotension,
- agitation,
- combativeness,
- hypoventilation,
- respiratory depression,
- airway obstruction, and
- apnea.

Interpretive statement 3:

Before conscious sedation is administered, an oxygen delivery device should be in place or immediately available, an IV access line should be established, and appropriate monitoring devices should be in place.

Rationale:

Sedatives and benzodiazepines used for conscious sedation/analgesia may cause somnolence, confusion, coma, diminished reflexes, and depressed respiratory and cardiovascular functions. Opioids used for conscious sedation/analgesia may cause respiratory depression, hypotension, nausea, and vomiting. Overdosage and adverse reactions may occur at any time during the procedure and may be reversible.

Discussion:

The following equipment should be present and ready for use in the room in which conscious sedation/analgesia is administered:

- oxygen,
- suction apparatus,
- oxygen delivery devices,
- noninvasive blood pressure device,
- electrocardiograph, and
- pulse oximeter.
  Monitoring parameters should include
- respiratory rate,
- oxygen saturation,
- blood pressure,
- cardiac rate and rhythm,
- level of consciousness, and
- skin condition.
  Undesirable changes in patient condition should be reported immediately to the physician.

Interpretive statement 4:

Each patient who receives conscious sedation/analgesia intravenously should have continuous IV access. If medications are not administered intravenously, the need for IV access should be determined on a case-by-

case basis. In all instances, an individual with the skills to establish IV access should be immediately available.

Rationale:

Continuous IV access provides a means for administering medications used for conscious sedation/analgesia and for implementing emergency medications and fluids to counteract adverse medication effects.

Discussion:

Continuous IV access may be obtained using an IV access device or by infusing IV fluids through an access port. The type of continuous IV access chosen will vary depending on health care facilities' policies and procedures and physicians' preferences.

Interpretive statement 5:

An emergency cart with appropriate resuscitative medications, including narcotic and sedative reversal medications, and equipment (eg, defibrillator) should be immediately available to every location in which conscious sedation/analgesia is being administered.

Rationale:

Medication overdoses or adverse reactions may cause respiratory depression, hypotension, or impaired cardiovascular function requiring immediate intervention and/or cardiopulmonary resuscitation (CPR). Equipment for CPR or emergency medication reversals should be available for immediate use because diminished reflexes, depressed respiratory function, and impaired cardiovascular function may occur within seconds or minutes after the administration of medications used for conscious sedation/analgesia.

RECOMMENDED PRACTICE VI

Documentation of patient care during conscious sedation/analgesia should be consistent with the AORN "Recommended practices for documentation of perioperative nursing care" wherever conscious sedation/analgesia is administered.

Interpretive statement 1:

Nursing diagnoses applicable to patients receiving conscious sedation/analgesia may include the potential for

- anxiety related to the unfamiliar environment and procedure,
- ineffective breathing patterns or impaired gas exchange related to altered level of consciousness or airway obstruction,
- knowledge deficit related to poor recall secondary to medication effects,

- cardiac output changes related to medication effects on the myocardium, and
- injury related to altered level of consciousness.

Rationale:

Use of nursing diagnoses for planning the care of patients who receive conscious sedation/analgesia provides for patient care that focuses on patients' responses to the procedures and/or nursing interventions. Nursing interventions are directed toward positive patient outcomes.

Interpretive statement 2:

Documentation should include:
- preprocedure assessment;
- dosage, route, time, and effects of all medications and fluids used;
- type and amount of fluids administered, including blood and blood products, monitoring devices, and equipment used;
- physiologic data from continuous monitoring at 5- to 15-minute intervals and upon significant events;
- level of consciousness;
- nursing interventions taken and the patient's responses; and
- untoward significant patient reactions and their resolution.

Rationale:

Documentation of nursing interventions promotes continuity of patient care and improves communication among health care team members. Documentation also provides a mechanism for comparing actual versus expected patient outcomes.

RECOMMENDED PRACTICE VII

Patients who receive conscious sedation/analgesia should be monitored postprocedure, receive verbal and written discharge instructions, and meet specified criteria before discharge.

Discussion:

Postprocedure patient care, monitoring, and discharge criteria should be consistent for all patients. Patients and their family members or caregivers should receive verbal and written discharge instructions and verbalize an understanding of the instructions to the nurse. Preprocedure and postprocedure instructions, as well as verbalization of understanding, is encouraged because medications used for conscious sedation/analgesia may cause significant patient amnesia that directly affects recall ability.

Discharge guidelines provide specific criteria for assessing and evaluating the patient's readiness for discharge and home care. Discharge criteria should reflect indications that the patient has returned to a safe physiologic level. These indicators should include
- adequate respiratory function;
- stability of vital signs, including temperature;
- preprocedure level of consciousness;
- intact protective reflexes;
- return of motor/sensory control;
- absence of protracted nausea;
- skin color and condition;
- satisfactory surgical site and dressing condition when present; and
- absence of significant pain.

The presence of a responsible adult escort is necessary for discharge. Discharge criteria should be developed by representatives from the medical staff, anesthesia, nursing, and other departments as appropriate.

RECOMMENDED PRACTICE VIII

Policies and procedures for managing patients who receive conscious sedation/analgesia should be written, reviewed periodically, and readily available within the practice setting.

Discussion:

Policies and procedures for managing patients receiving conscious sedation/analgesia should include
- patient selection criteria
- extent of and responsibility for monitoring,
- method of recording patient data,
- data to be documented,
- frequency of the patient's physiologic data documentation,
- medications that may be administered by the RN, and
- discharge criteria.

Policies and procedures are operational guidelines that are used to minimize patient risk factors, standardize practice, assist staff members, and establish guidelines for continuous quality improvement activities by establishing authority, responsibility, and accountability.

GLOSSARY

Benzodiazepines: A pharmacologic family of central nervous system depressants possessing anxiolytic, hypnotic, and skeletal muscle-relaxant properties. These medications are used to allay anxiety and fear and produce varying amnesic effects during conscious sedation/analgesia. Diazepam and midazolam are two benzodiazepines commonly used for conscious sedation/analgesia.

Conscious sedation/analgesia: A minimally depressed level of consciousness that allows a surgical patient to retain the ability to independently and continuously maintain a patent airway and respond appropriately to verbal commands and physical stimulation.

Managing the patient: The use of the nursing process to deliver and direct comprehensive nursing care during a procedure in a practice setting.

Monitoring: Clinical observation that is individualized to patient needs based on data obtained from preprocedure patient assessments. The objective of monitoring patients who receive conscious sedation/analgesia is to improve patient outcomes. Monitoring includes the use of mechanical devices and direct observation.

Opioid: Natural or synthetic pharmacologic agents that produce varying degrees of analgesia and sedation and relieve pain. Fentanyl and meperidine hydrochloride are two opioid analgesic medications that may be used for conscious sedation/analgesia.

Sedatives: Pharmacologic agents that reduce anxiety and may induce some degree of short-term amnesia.

Index